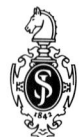

# Contents

| | | |
|---|---|---|
| **A** | **Introduction and Historical Landmarks** | **1** |
| A.1 | Definition of the Photodynamic Action | 1 |
| A.2 | Optimum Photosensitizing Agent for Photodynamic Action | 1 |
| A.2.1 | Hematoporphyrin Derivative (HpD) and Porfimer Sodium (Photofrin) | 1 |
| A.2.2 | Porphines | 2 |
| A.2.3 | Phthalocyanines | 2 |
| A.2.4 | Chlorine Derivatives | 2 |
| A.2.5 | Lutetium texaphyrin (Lu-Tex) | 3 |
| A.2.6 | Porphycenes | 3 |
| A.2.7 | Other Photosensitizers | 3 |
| A.2.8 | Endogenous Porphyrins | 3 |
| A.3 | Definition of Fluorescence Detection with ALA-Induced Porphyrins (FDAP) | 4 |
| A.3.1 | Physical Background of the Fluorescence in FDAP | 6 |
| A.4 | Mechanisms of Action in PDT | 7 |
| | | |
| **B** | **δ-Aminolevulinic Acid (ALA)** | **9** |
| B.1 | Chemistry of ALA and ALA Methylester (ALA) | 9 |
| B.2 | Metabolism of ALA | 10 |
| B.3 | Pharmacodynamics of ALA | 12 |
| B.3.1 | Systemic Administration of ALA | 12 |
| B.3.2 | Topical Application of ALA | 16 |
| | | |
| **C** | **Light Used in FDAP and PDT** | **19** |
| | | |
| **D** | **Unresolved Issues in FDAP and PDT** | **21** |
| | | |
| **E** | **Fluorescence Detection of ALA-induced Porphyrins (FDAP)** | **23** |
| E.1 | FDAP: Evaluation of the ALA-Induced Fluorescence in Skin Diseases | 23 |
| | | |
| **F** | ***Ex vivo* – Investigations on ALA-induced Porphyrins** | **33** |
| F.1 | Porphyrin Accumulation in Cells (*in vitro*) | 33 |
| F.2 | Porphyrin Accumulation in Skin Tumors, Colon and Bronchial Carcinomas after Administration of ALA (*ex vivo*) | 34 |
| | | |
| **G** | ***In vivo* – Investigations on ALA-Induced Porphyrin /FDAP** | **37** |
| G.1 | FDAP: Kinetics of ALA-Induced Porphyrins in Human Cutaneous Tumors, Psoriasis Lesions and Normal Skin | 37 |
| G.2 | FDAP: Kinetics of Porphyrin Accumulation in Solar Keratoses: ALA versus ALA Methylester | 39 |
| G.3 | FDAP: Use of the *in vivo* – Fluorescence for Surgical Planning | 43 |
| G.4 | FDAP: Evaluation of the Optimum Photosensitizing Substance or its Prodrug | 44 |
| G.5 | FDAP: Evaluation of the Optimum Exciting Light Source | 46 |
| G.6 | FDAP: Correlation of *in vivo* – Tumor Fluorescence and Histopathology | 46 |
| G.7 | FDAP: Course of FDAP in Relation to the Number of PDT-Sessions | 50 |

Contents

| | | |
|---|---|---|
| **H** | **The Clinical Use of FDAP**  55 | |
| H.1 | FDAP in Clinically Well-defined Tumors  55 | |
| H.2 | FDAP in Clinically Ill-defined Lesions  56 | |
| H.3 | FDAP in Pretreated or Damaged Skin  59 | |
| H.4 | Limitations of FDAP  61 | |
| H.5 | Usefulness of FDAP in Guiding Tumor Therapies  62 | |

| | | |
|---|---|---|
| **I** | **Photodynamic Therapy in Cutaneous Diseases**  65 | |
| I.1 | PDT: Evaluation of the Efficacy in Solar Keratoses  65 | |
| I.2 | PDT: Evaluation of the Efficacy in Bowen's Disease  71 | |
| I.3 | PDT: Evaluation of the Efficacy in Basal Cell Carcinoma  72 | |
| I.4 | PDT: Evaluation of the Efficacy in Squamous Cell Carcinoma  76 | |
| I.5 | PDT: Evaluation of the Efficacy in Psoriatic Lesions  78 | |
| I.6 | PDT: Evaluation of the Efficacy in Selected Cutaneous Diseases  84 | |
| I.6.1 | PDT in Skin Cancers and Preranceroses Others than Discussed Above  85 | |
| I.6.2 | PDT in Tumors of the Oral Mucosa  86 | |
| I.6.3 | PDT in Non-neoplastic Skin Diseases  86 | |
| I.6.4 | PDT in Non-dermatological Indications  89 | |
| I.7 | PDT: Evaluation of the Optimum Photosensitizing Substance or its Prodrug  89 | |
| I.8 | PDT: Evaluation of the Optimum Exciting Light Source  91 | |

| | | |
|---|---|---|
| **J** | **General Discussion**  97 | |
| J.1 | FDAP: Indications and Limits  97 | |
| J.2 | PDT: Indications and Limits  101 | |
| J.3 | Safety and Tolerability of ALA-PDT  107 | |
| J.4 | Regulatory Affairs Concerning Aminolevulinic Acid  108 | |
| J.5 | Regulatory Affairs Concerning Aminolevulinic Acid Methylester  108 | |

**K  Conclusion  109**

**L  Summary  111**

Acknowledgements  113
Bibliography  115

# Abbreviations

| | |
|---|---|
| ALA | Aminolevulinic acid |
| ALA methylester | Aminolevulinic acid methylester |
| ALA-S | Aminolevulinic acid synthase |
| BCC | Basal cell carcinoma |
| BD | Bowen's disease |
| BPD-MA | Benzoporphyrin derivative-monacid ring A |
| b.w. | Body weight |
| DMSO | Dimethylsulfoxide |
| EDTA | Ethylendiaminetetraacetic acid |
| FDAP | Fluorescence diagnosis with ALA-induced porphyrins |
| HpD | Hematoporphyrin derivative |
| Lu-Tex | Lutetium texaphyrin |
| NPe6 | N-Aspartyl-chlorine e6 |
| NS | Normal skin |
| PBG | Porphobilinogen |
| PC | Phthalocyanine |
| PD | Paget's disease |
| PDL | Pumped dye laser |
| PDT | Photodynamic therapy |
| PP IX | Protoporphyrin IX |
| PS | Photosensitizer |
| SCC | Squamous cell carcinoma |
| SK | Solar keratosis |
| $SnET_2$ | Tin etiopurpurin |
| m-THPC | Meso-tetra(hydroxyphenyl)-chlorine |
| $TPPS_4$ | Tetra-sodium-meso-tetraphenylporphine-sulfonate |

# A  Introduction and Historical Landmarks

## A.1  Definition of the Photodynamic Action

The selective uptake of a photosensitizer into neoplastic tissue and its selective destruction by subsequent irradiation (principle of photodynamic therapy (PDT)) is a fascinating but not a new idea. The ability of several dyes (e.g., acridine) to sensitize microorganisms (e.g., paramecium) for their destruction by a following exposure to light was first mentioned in 1900 (Raab, 1900). At that time, the author and his co-workers also recognized that the described reaction depended on oxygen and therefore they called it "photodynamic action" or "photodynamic effect" (Fig. 1) (von Tappeiner, 1904).

As early as 1903, this photodynamic action was used to treat different skin diseases (i.e., condylomata lata, lupus vulgaris and skin tumors) for the first time (Figs. 2 and 3).

Other indications tested as target of photodynamic action were herpes simplex, molluscum contagiosum, pityriasis versicolor and psoriasis vulgaris (von Tappeiner and Jesionek, 1903; Jesionek and von Tappeiner, 1905). In these early days eosin was applied as photosensitizer and irradiation was performed with white light.

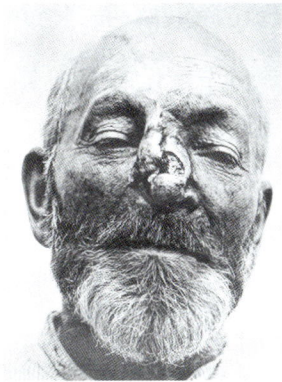
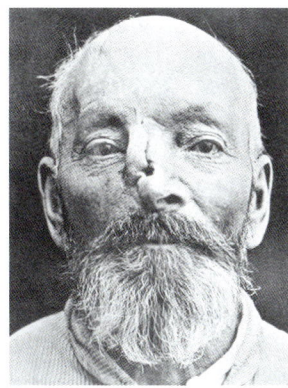

Fig. 2 (left) and Fig. 3 (right). Original photos from the publication of von Tappeiner before and after photodynamic treatment. The ulcerating tumor was treated by eosine and white light

## A.2  Optimum Photosensitizing Agent for Photodynamic Action

For optimization and standardization of PDT, various photosensitizing substances, especially porphyrins, were tried in the following years. The first experiments with the photosensitizer hematoporphyrin were done in 1911. Since then, porphyrins remained the most effective and most frequently examined substances in PDT. Concerning the diagnostic potential of porphyrin compounds, the diagnosis of tumors was performed using hematoporphyrin for the first time in 1924 (Policard, 1924). Hematoporphyrin caused a bright red fluorescence in tumor tissues when illuminated with UV-light. In the 40's further investigations in experimentally induced sarcomas and mammary carcinomas confirmed the affinity of hematoporphyrin to neoplastic tissues measured by the typical red fluorescence (Figge et al, 1948). In the 50's it was also shown that an intravenous application of hematoporphyrin in carcinoma patients led to a preferred accumulation of porphyrins in the tumor tissue. This was again proven by the characteristic red fluorescence during UV-illumination.

### A.2.1  Hematoporphyrin Derivative (HpD) and Porfimer Sodium (Photofrin)

In 1960, Lipson et al presented the hematoporphyrin derivative (HpD) that consists of a mixture of roughly ten porphyrin derivatives – dihemato-

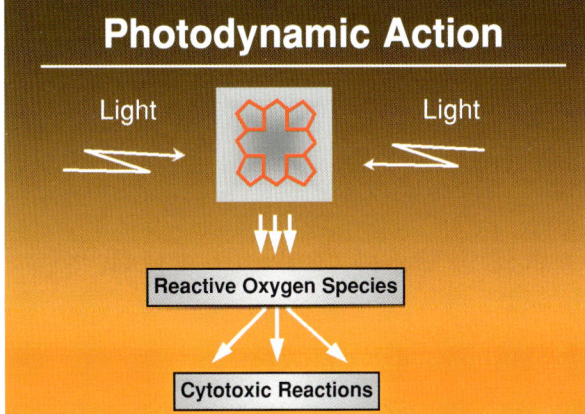

Fig. 1. Photodynamic action involves the activation of a photosensitizer by light. Subsequent energy and electron transfer from the photosensitizing molecules to oxygen induces the formation of reactive oxygen species which themselves are responsible for cytotoxic reactions

porphyrin esters and dihematoporphyrin ethers (Lipson et al, 1961). HpD has been used to aid in identification and localization of human cancers since their red fluorescence can be observed readily upon activation with blue light. Apparent selective HpD uptake has been demonstrated in a wide range of animal and human cancers (Gregorie et al, 1968; Doiron et al, 1979; Kinsey et al, 1978). Until the 80's, HpD remained the most important photosensitizer in PDT.

To date porfimer sodium (Photofrin), the purified compound of HpD, is the only approved photosensitizer for clinical PDT. The first registration was obtained in Canada in 1993 for the treatment of bladder cancer. During the following years, porfimer sodium received approvals for PDT of selected stages of lung, esophageal, gastric, and cervical cancer in several European countries and Japan (Evenson, 1995). In 1995, the US Food and Drug Administration approved Photofrin for the treatment of advanced esophageal tumors, followed by a recent approval for the ablation of early-stage lung cancer (Dougherty et al, 1998; Reynolds, 1997). The intravenous administration of porfimer sodium or HpD at doses of 0.5 to 2.0 and 3.0 to 5.0 mg/kg b.w., respectively, leads to maximal tumor-to-normal cell concentration ratios after 24 to 48 hours (Ochsner, 1997). The cutaneous accumulation of porphyrin-based photosensitizing drugs and their slow clearance from the skin leads to long-lasting cutaneous photosensitivity, requiring photoprotective measures during 4 to 6 weeks after PDT (Ochsner, 1997; Gomer, 1991). An approach to avoid this side effect is the use of topical porphyrin formulations (McCullough et al, 1983; Pres et al, 1989; Steiner et al, 1995; Santoro et al, 1990). However, these reports as well as personal research findings (Table 19) indicate that local photosensitivity is also strong after topical application of porphyrin products. The number of reports is very limited and major studies using PDT with topical porphyrins are lacking.

Chemical purity, specific accumulation in neoplastic tissue, short time interval between the administration of the drug and its maximal accumulation in the tumor, short half life and rapid clearance from normal tissues, activation at wavelengths with optimal tissue penetration, high quantum yields for the generation of singlet oxygen, and lack of toxicity in the absence of light are desirable features of an ideal photosensitizer (Moan, 1990). The time interval between drug administration and sufficient photosensitizer concentration within the malignant lesion determines the time point of light application and varies considerably between different types of cancer and different photosensitizers. Newer drugs are distinguished by drug-to-light intervals in the range of a few hours, keeping the irradiation within practicable time limits.

### A.2.2 Porphines

Porphines are synthetic porphyrins with high potency to photosensitize tumorous and normal tissues (Kreimeier-Birnbaum, 1989). TPPS4 (tetra-sodium-meso-tetraphenylporphine-sulfonate) has been evaluated intensively for topical treatment of skin tumors (Santoro et al, 1990). The hydrophilic compound is activated by light at 630 nm and localizes preferentially in the tumor stroma (Kessel et al, 1987; Evenson, 1985). If administrated systemically, the major limitation of TPPS4 is its neurotoxicity (Winkelmann et al, 1987).

### A.2.3 Phthalocyanines

Since the first description of the photosensitizing property of phthalocyanines (PCs) (Ben Hur and Rosenthal, 1985), PCs have been intensively investigated for PDT and have shown promising therapeutic effects in various types of cancer (Canti et al, 1990, Anderson et al, 1998). PC dyes have a well-defined chemical structure and are manufactured as pure compounds. They possess high triplet and singlet oxygen quantum yields, show insignificant toxicity in the absence of light, reach high tumor-to-tissue ratios 1 to 3 hours after intravenous administration, and absorb strongly in the 650 to 700 nm range, allowing deeper penetration of tissue by the activating light as compared with porphyrins (Spikes, 1986; Oleinick et al, 1993). Low accumulation levels in normal skin and rapid drug elimination result in minimal cutaneous photosensitivity. PC4, a silicon-based hydrophobic photosensitizer, is one of the most promising PCs in experimental use (Zaidi et al, 1993).

### A.2.4 Chlorine Derivatives

*Chlorines*, a heterogeneous group of porphyrin- or chlorophyll-derived compounds, show high extinction coefficients at wavelengths above 650 nm. The following chlorine-derived agents are used efficiently for the PDT of various cutaneous malignancies.

*Benzoporphyrin derivative-monacid ring A* (BPD-MA) is a lipophilic compound with maximal photoactivation at 690 nm (Pass, 1993). Basal cell (BCC) and squamous cell carcinomas (SCC) represent the main therapeutic indications for BPD-MA-based PDT in dermatology (Ochsner, 1997). Sufficient tumor-to-normal tissue ratios are already achieved 30 to 150 minutes after intravenous application at doses between 0.2 and 0.5 mg/kg b.w. (Richter et al, 1993). Because of the rapid clearance from tissues, skin photosensitivity lasts for only a few days.

*N-Aspartyl-chlorine e6* (NPe6), a highly water-soluble systemic photosensitizer with an absorption peak at 664 nm, enters the cells via endocytosis and accumulates predominantly in lysosomes (Spikes, 1990). Optimal photodynamic efficacy is achieved when light is applied 4 to 8 hours after the injection of NPe6 at a standard dosage of 0.5 to 3.0 mg/kg b.w. (Taber et al, 1998). Based on encouraging results obtained in preclinical studies, the drug has been utilized for the PDT of various cutaneous and subcutaneous malignancies, including recurrent adenocarcinoma of the breast as well as BCC and SCC (Taber et al, 1998; Nelson et al, 1987). To date mild skin photosensitivity is the only significant side effect reported (Taber et al, 1998).

*Tin etiopurpurin* ($SnET_2$) is a synthetic chlorine analogue with maximal excitation at 660 nm (Razum et al, 1996). The optimal time of irradiation lies within 24 to 72 hours after the infusion of 0.8 to 1.6 mg/kg b.w. (Ochsner, 1997). The sensitizer is cleared from the skin within a few days after treatment, causing mild photosensitivity; however, cutaneous reactions occurring 1 or more months after PDT have been reported (Garbo, 1996). $SnET_2$ has been used successfully for the photodynamic management of BCC, Bowen's disease (BD), cutaneous metastatic breast cancer, and AIDS-related Kaposi's sarcoma (Razum et al, 1996; Bisonette and Lui, 1997).

*Meso-tetra(hydroxyphenyl)-chlorine* (m-THPC; Foscan) is an extremely powerful photosensitizer showing up to 200 times the photodynamic activity of Photofrin in patients, in terms of drug/light dose. It is a pure compound that is 100 times more phototoxic at 652 nm and 10 times more phototoxic at 514 nm, has better selectivity for early carcinomas, and a shorter duration of skin photosensitivity (Savary et al, 1997).

### A.2.5 Lutetium Texaphyrin (Lu-Tex)

Texaphyrins are synthetic water-soluble compounds, which enrich in malignant lesions and atheromatous plaques (Young et al, 1996). Lutetium texaphyrin (Lu-Tex) is a highly fluorescent dye and absorbs strongly at 732 nm (Woodburn et al, 1996). The photosensitizer is administered systemically at doses ranging from 0.6 to 7.2 mg/kg b.w. (Ochsner, 1997). Rapid Lu-Tex accumulation in neoplastic tissues allows irradiation as early as 2 to 4 hours after drug administration. Preliminary results based on the therapy of various malignancies, such as recurrent breast cancer, invasive SCC, malignant melanoma, Kaposi's sarcoma, and BCC, have demonstrated best response rates in breast cancer lesions with complete response in 42% and partial response in 23% of the treated tumors (Renschler et al, 1997). The destruction of experimentally induced subcutaneous metastatic melanoma lesions has been achieved without significant damage of the overlying skin, demonstrating the excellent selectivity of the drug (Renschler et al, 1997). The lack of significant cutaneous phototoxicity is the most outstanding characteristic of this texaphyrin.

### A.2.6 Porphycenes

Porphycenes, synthetic isomers of porphines, are efficient generators of singlet oxygen, possess high fluorescence yields, and show a 10-fold higher light absorption at 630 nm compared with HpD (Kreimeier-Birnbaum, 1989).

### A.2.7 Other Photosensitizers

Further effective photosensitizing compounds include HPPH-23, bacteriochlorines, anthraquinones, hypericin and rhodamine 123 (Kreimeier-Birnbaum, 1989; Diwu and Lown, 1994; Kessel et al, 1993; Kessel et al, 1995; Pass, 1993). The chlorophyll A-derived photosensitizer HPPH-23 is cleared rapidly from normal skin and has an absorption maximum at 665 nm (Magne et al, 1997). Based on the successful PDT of SCC located on the nasal plane and facial skin of cats, HPPH-23 appears to be a potent photosensitizing drug for the management of skin cancer (Magne et al, 1997). The relevance of numerous novel drugs for PDT in dermatology is yet to be evaluated.

### A.2.8 Endogenous Porphyrins

*Topically applied* substances achieved increasing interest because they avoid generalized photosensitization as it is known from the systemically administered photosensitizers. This disadvantage could be overcome by a "tumor-selective" photosensitization, which was introduced 1990 by an Australian research group (Kennedy et al, 1990) using the topical application of the "non-photosensitizing" prodrug δ-aminolevulinic acid (ALA). This most important porphyrin precursor leads to an increased production of porphyrins preferentially in neoplastic and fast proliferating tissues.

ALA-induced *in vitro* – photosensitization was first demonstrated in 1987 (Malik and Lugaci, 1987). Subsequently, Kennedy, Pottier, and Pross (1990) introduced the use of ALA-PDT for successful treatment of various malignant skin lesions. During the last 10 years various research groups confirmed the efficacy of topical ALA-PDT in the treatment of superficial skin tumors (Cairnduff et al, 1994; Fijan et al, 1995; Fritsch et al, 1996; Szeimies et al, 1995; Wolf et al, 1993). In the last years, there were also reports on the successful use of *systemic ALA administration* in curative or palliative treatment of bronchial carcinomas, tumors of the gastrointestinal tract and bladder cancers in animal studies as well as in clinical trials (Kriegmair et al, 1996; Navone et al, 1988; Regula et al, 1995). Systemic administration of ALA is used predominantly for the management of gastrointestinal, bronchopulmonal, and cerebral tumors, whereas PDT with topical ALA formulations represents increasingly one of the most popular PDT techniques in dermatology. The main advantage of topical ALA-PDT is the absence of generalized cutaneous photosensitivity.

The standard procedure of topical ALA-PDT for skin tumors involves the application of 20% ALA in an oil-in-water emulsion, covered by an occlusive dressing to enhance the penetration of the drug into the tissue and to prevent undesired photodegradation of endogenously formed porphyrins by visible light. The optimal application time and concentration differ depending on the characteristics of the target cells.

## A.3 Definition of Fluorescence Detection with ALA-induced Porphyrins (FDAP)

Various diagnostic methods are used in daily dermatological practice to assess different types of skin diseases. Dermatoscopy is used to evaluate pigmented skin lesions mainly, the ultrasound measurement is applied to reveal the pathology of lymph nodes and to measure the thickness of skin lesions such as sclerodermiform or neoplastic ones. However, histopathological examination is the most important diagnostic procedure in dermatology to ensure the clinical diagnosis of any skin disease. Porphyrin mixtures such as HpD or Photofrin can be used as "tumor markers" in fluorescence detection techniques (Baumgartner et al, 1992). Although these substances allow a fluorescence description, e.g. in urothelial neoplasm, they have considerable disadvantages, such as a low tumor selectivity. Beyond this, the fluorescence-quantum-profit of the porphyrin mixture in the tissue is quite low and affords expensive techniques of photo-processing for the detection of fluorescence. Additionally, the systemic application of photosensitizers like Photofrin is always risky as far as phototoxic skin reactions are concerned.

Here, a novel diagnostic procedure is introduced, that is mainly used for tumor detection or for guidance of any subsequent tumor therapy – the fluorescence diagnosis with δ-aminolevulinic acid-induced porphyrins (FDAP). This diagnostic procedure enables the delineation of neoplastic (e.g., BCC, SCC) and inflammatory tissues (e.g. psoriatic skin lesions) from the surrounding normal skin. In FDAP, the diseased skin (e.g., tumor) produces and accumulates high amounts of porphyrins from the applied porphyrin prodrug ALA (Fig. 4). Consequently, a porphyrin-enriched tissue as such shows a specific red fluorescence when illuminated with Wood's light (UV-light).

The topical use of ALA, in particular in a 20% mixture in a cream base, for detection of neoplastic tissue has considerable advantages in dermatology:

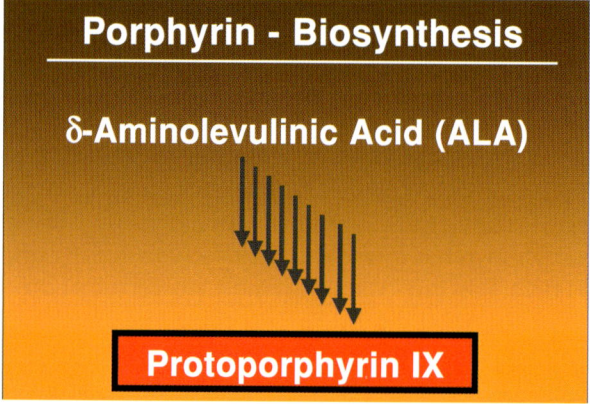

**Fig. 4.** In FDAP, ALA is the key compound. Exogenous administration of ALA leads to the formation of endogenous porphyrins. This pathway is catalyzed by the heme-associated enzymes. Protoporphyrin IX is the predominantly formed porphyrin after ALA treatment

**Table 1.** Termini used to describe the fluorescence diagnosis of tumors

| Tumors of the gastrointestinal tract | Reference |
| --- | --- |
| Endoscopic **fluorescence detection** | (Messmann et al, 1999) |
| Endoscopic **photodynamic diagnosis** | (Mayinger et al, 1999) |
| ALA-induced **protoporphyrin IX fluorescence for the detection** of GIT dysplasias | (Messmann et al, 2000) |
| Endoscopic **fluorescence diagnosis** | (Endlicher et al, 2001) |
| ALA for **laryngoscopic fluorescence diagnosis** of malignant intraabdominal tumors | (Gahlen et al, 2001) |
| **Bladder tumors** | |
| **Fluorescence photodetection** of neoplastic urothelial lesions | (Kriegmair et al, 1994) |
| **Fluorescence cystoscopy** following intravesical instillation of ALA | (Kriegmair et al, 1995) |
| **Light-induced fluorescence** of protoporphyrin IX following the topical application of ALA | (Jichlinski et al, 1997) |
| **Fluorescence detection** of bladder tumors with ALA | (Riedl et al, 1999) |
| **Photodynamic cystoscopy** for detection of bladder tumors | (Kriegmair et al, 1999) |
| **Photodetection** of early human bladder cancer | (Lange et al, 1999) |
| **Diagnosis** of bladder carcinoma **using** protoporphyrin IX **fluorescence** induced by ALA | (Koenig et al, 1999) |
| **Endoscopic detection** of transitional cell carcinoma with ALA | (Zaak et al, 2001) |
| **Other (experimental) tumors** | |
| **Photodynamic imaging** of pancreatic cancer with pheophorbide A | (Keller et al, 1996) |
| **Localization of transformed tissues** using pyropheophorbide-a | (Furukawa et al, 1996) |
| **Laser-induced fluorescence diagnosis (LIF)** of human renal cell carcinoma | (Pomer et al, 1995) |
| **Laser-induced fluorescence** in malignant and normal tissue in mice injected with two different carotenoporphyrins | (Nilsson et al, 1994) |
| **Computer-assisted fluorescence identification** of colon cancer in rats | (Jones et al, 1993) |
| **Photo detection** of carcinoma of the colon in a rat model | (von Rueden et al, 1993) |
| **Fluorescence detection** of tumours | (Mang et al, 1993) |
| Kidney preserving **tumor resection** in renal cell carcinoma **with photodynamic detection** | (Popken et al, 1999) |
| **Oral neoplasms** | |
| **Fluorescence spectroscopic identification** of hamster buccal pouch carcinogenesis | (Balasubramanian et al, 1995) |
| **Fluorescence imaging** of ALA-induced protoporphyrin IX for the detection of neoplastic lesions in the oral cavity | (Leunig et al, 1996) |
| **Fluorescence photography** as a diagnostic method of oral cancer | (Onizawa et al, 1996); |
| **Photodynamic diagnosis** of neoplasms of the mouth | (Leunig et al, 1996) |
| **Diagnosis** of early-stage oral cancer **by hematoporphyrin derivative-fluorescence technic** | (Wang, 1984) |
| **Visualizing carcinomas** of the mouth cavity **by stimulating synthesis of fluorescent protoporphyrin IX** | (Zenk et al, 1999) |
| **Carcinoma of the lung** | |
| Inhalation of ALA for **fluorescence detection** of early stage lung cancer | (Baumgartner et al, 1996) |
| **Fluorescence bronchoscopy** for detection and localization of early lung cancer | (Lam et al, 1993) |
| Fiberoptic bronchoscopic **laser photoradiation for tumor localization** in lung cancer | (Hayata et al, 1982) |
| Hematoporphyrin derivate as a **tumor marker in the detection and localization** of pulmonary malignancy | (King et al, 1982) |
| **Zervix neoplasms, breast tumors, endometriosis** | |
| Hematoporphyrin-derivative-fluorescence test colposcopy and colpophotography **in the diagnosis** of atypical metaplasia, dysplasia, and carcinoma in situ of the cervix uteri | (Kyriazis et al, 1973) |
| **Photodetection** of cervical intraepithelial neoplasia | (Hillemanns et al, 2000) |
| **Fluorescence diagnosis** of endometriosis | (Malik et al, 2000) |
| **Photodynamic diagnosis** of breast tumors | (Ladner et al, 2001) |
| **Cerebral tumors** | |
| **Fluorescence guided** resection of glioblastoma multiforme | (Stummer et al, 2000) |
| **Cutaneous Neoplasms** | |
| **Photodiagnosis** using endogenous photosensitization induced by ALA | (Marcus et al, 1996) |
| **Photodynamic diagnosis controlled** surgery | (Fritsch et al, 1996) |
| **Photodynamic diagnosis guided** $CO_2$-laser therapy | (Becker-Wegerich et al, 1997) |
| **Photodynamic diagnosis** in dermatology | (Fritsch et al, 1998) |
| *In vivo*-**detection** of BCC using imaging spectroscopy | (Wennberg et al, 1999) |
| **Fluorescence diagnostics** in head region | (Wang et al, 1999) |
| **Fluorescence diagnosis with ALA-induced porphyrins (FDAP)** | (Fritsch et al, 2000) |

the surrounding healthy skin is barely sensitized and there are no systemic side effects. In the past years, different descriptions (Table 1) and especially the term "photodynamic diagnosis" (PDD) were chosen for the detection of tumors using a photosensitizer and its fluorescence under UV-light.

Unfortunately, this term is not very suitable, because no reactive oxygen species, which would be necessary for a photodynamic reaction, are implicated in fluorescence detection techniques. For this reason, we decided to introduce the term FDAP.

### A.3.1 Physical Background of the Fluorescence in FDAP

Fluorescence detection is the basic principle of FDAP. Therefore the physical essentials of fluorescence and its attributes are explained. Fluorescence is a subsiding light emission by atoms or molecules, which are stimulated by absorption of energy.

*Absorption of light*: When light meets a medium, one part is reflected, one part is absorbed and one part penetrates the medium. The absorbed light will be transferred into heat or another form of energy (Doiron and Keller, 1985).

*Semi-stable condition of electrons*: In general, material can be stimulated by electricity, light or radio frequencies and transformed into a higher energy level of a stimulated electron level (semi-stable level). Collision of a molecule with other molecules leads to a quick transfer (approx. $10^{-11}$ sec) of its pulsation energy to the environment. The molecule (being in stimulated electron condition) moves step by step back to the ground condition (Fig. 5). The life span of the electron stimulation is sufficient to emit spontaneously energy as fluorescence (approx. $10^{-8}$ sec). By this mechanism the molecule turns into a higher pulsation level than that of the basic level (Frank-Condon principle). The intensity of the fluorescence $I\alpha$ is generally proportional to the intensity of the incoming radiation $Io$ and to the concentration of the fluorescing substance C. According to the law of Lambert-Beer, the intensity $\Delta I$ of the absorbed radiation of a substance is

$$\Delta I\alpha\ (\nu) = \alpha\ (\nu)\ Io\ (\nu)\ \Delta x,$$

if $\Delta I\alpha$ is smaller than $Io$.

$\Delta x$ means the thickness, $\alpha\ (\nu)$ the absorption coefficient of the substance at the frequency $\nu$ of the incoming radiation, which is proportional to the concentration C of the substance:

$$\alpha\ (\nu) = \varepsilon\ (\nu)\ C.$$

$\varepsilon\ (\nu)$ is the molar extinction coefficient of the substance at the light frequency $\nu$ (Bruls et al, 1984).

*Emission*: Electromagnetic radiation is released (emission) by the molecule's falling back to ground level. All those emission processes are summarized under the generic term *luminescence*. The radiation or the emission from the molecule can easily be demonstrated if the molecule's concentration in stimulated condition is very high or if the velocity of the radiationless deactivation is low in relation to the velocity of the radiation. The emission is termed *fluorescence* if the emission fades quickly ($10^{-9}$–$10^{-3}$ sec.) after light absorption. In contrast, in the case of *phosphorescence*, the emission is lasting longer, characteristically several seconds after absorption.

In most fluids and solutions at room temperature, the radiationless deactivating processes proceede so quickly that fluorescence or phosphorescence cannot be observed. However, there are compounds such as the fluorescein solution, which show a clear fluorescence. The range in which the fluorescence emission is a linear function of the concentration is used for the determination of the concentration of the respective substances. The following list gives examples for the use of fluorescence in photometry: Determination of riboflavin (vitamin B6) in cow milk, of thiamin (B1) in meat and cereals, and of porphyrins, enzymes, estrogens

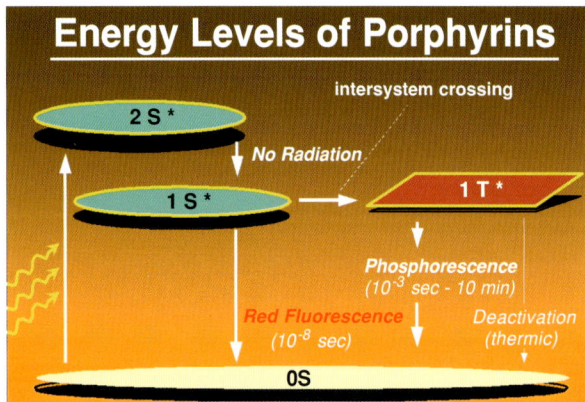

**Fig. 5.** Energy levels of porphyrin molecules as photosensitizers (PS). In general, the molecules are present in their ground state 0S. Light irradiation induces an elevation of the PS to its highly energetic but short living singlet states 2S* or 1S* states. PS decay back to the ground state by emitting fluorescence (= FDAP). Alternatively, PS are transfered to the highly energetic 1T* by intersystem crossing

and histidine in blood or urine. Fluorescence can exist at all wavelengths of the electromagnetic spectrum. The fluorescence follows the Stock's rule which postulates that the emitted radiation cannot be of a shorter wavelength than the exciting light (Whitaker, 1994).

## A.4 Mechanisms of Action in PDT

When ALA-treated tissues are exposed to light of appropriate wavelength and energy, the accumulated porphyrin metabolites (in particular protoporphyrin IX) (Fig. 4) produce a photodynamic reaction, a cytotoxic process dependent upon the simultaneous presence of light and oxygen (Fig. 6).

The initiating step of the photosensitizing mechanism is the absorption of a light photon by the sensitizer, causing a shift of the molecule from its ground state to the extremely unstable excited singlet state (Fig. 5). The excited photosensitizer molecule reverts to the ground state, resulting in the emission of light in form of fluorescence (which is used for FDAP). Alternatively, the excited photosensitizer undergoes intersystem crossing to the more stable triplet excited state by electron spin conversion. The interaction of the triplet sensitizer with surrounding molecules results in two types of photooxidative reaction. Type I pathway involves transfer of electrons or hydrogen atoms producing radical forms of the photosensitizer or the substrate. These intermediates may further react with oxygen to form peroxides, superoxide ions, and hydroxyl radicals, which initiate free

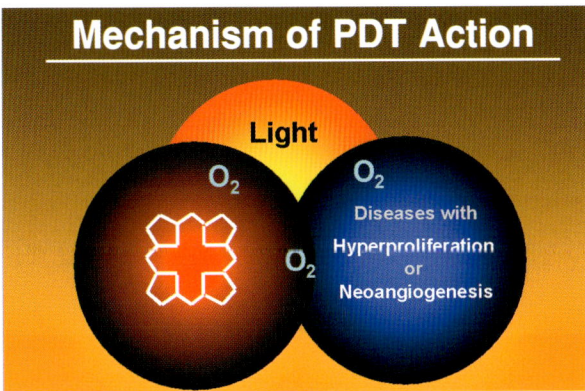

Fig. 6. For an effective photodynamic action the simultaneous presence of a vascularized neoplastic tissue, an intratumoral accumulated photosensitizer, light and oxygen is necessary

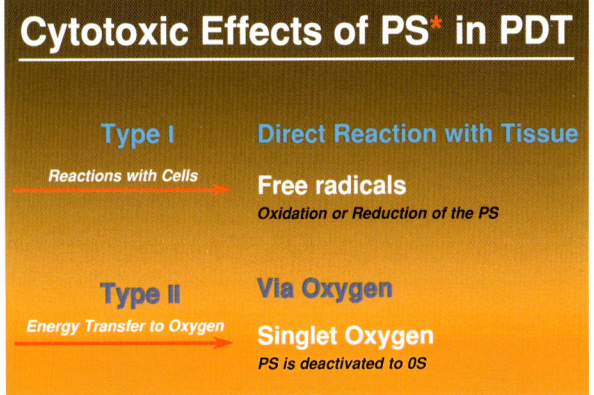

Fig. 7. In PDT, the energetic enriched porphyrin molecules transfer their energy to oxygen. Type I and type II reactions are responsible for the creation of reactive oxygen species

radical chain reactions. Type II mechanism is mediated by an energy transfer process with ground state oxygen, leading to the formation of singlet oxygen and the return of the sensitizer to its ground state (Fig. 7).

Singlet oxygen, generated by the Type II pathway, appears to play a central role in photodynamic cytotoxicity because of the highly efficient interaction of the singlet oxygen species with different biomolecules (Pass, 1993; Agarwal et al, 1992). Microscopically and biochemically detectable changes of cellular and organelle membranes can be observed as early events occurring after PDT (Pass, 1993). Lipid peroxidation and protein cross-linking affect the depolarization and inactivate membranous enzymes. The increased membrane permeability inhibits the transport of amino acids and nucleosides. The formation of blebs protruding from the plasma membrane, followed by cell lysis, occurs within hours after PDT. As nuclear damage does not seem to be an important factor of PDT-mediated cytotoxicity, PDT promises to include a low potential in inducing mutations or carcinogenesis. The response to photosensitization includes the activation of genes encoding for several stress proteins, such as heat shock proteins, heme oxygenase, and glucose-regulated proteins, as well as a transient induction of the early response genes (e.g., c-fos, c-jun, c-myc) (Kick et al, 1995; Luna et al, 1994; Klotz et al, 1998). Phosphorylation of p38 mitogen-activated protein kinase (MAPK) is enhanced to a similar extent after PDT. The effects of ALA-PDT on MAPKs are similar to stresses like UV irradiation or exposure to hydrogen peroxide with respect to activation of c-Jun-N-terminal kinase (JNK) and p38 MAPKs (Klotz et al, 1998). In addition to the direct damage of neoplastic cells, vascular injury plays an important role in the tumor destruction mediated by PDT. Oxygen radicals generated during the photodynamic process decrease the barrier function of endothelial cells. Arteriolar vessel constriction, thrombus formation in venules, and blood flow stasis cause indirect tumor cell kill due to long-term nutritional deprivation (Dellian et al, 1995). The degradation of phospholipids results in the release of various inflammatory mediators. Acute phase proteins, proteinases, peroxidases, complement factors, and cytokines are activated. The inflammatory signaling results in accumulation of immune effector cells, such as neutrophil granulocytes and macrophages.

# B  δ-Aminolevulinic Acid (ALA)

The role of ALA-PDT in precanceroses and epithelial tumors is steadily increasing and ALA has been shown to be the drug with the greatest clinical use in PDT. In dermatology, topical PDT with ALA is already being postulated to be the treatment of choice for solar keratoses (SK) and superficial BCC. Other indications for ALA-treatment are nontumoral applications, especially psoriasis, viral-induced diseases such as vulgar warts, or acne vulgaris.

## B.1  Chemistry of ALA and ALA Methylester

According to the JUPAC nomenclature, ALA is 5-Amino-4-oxopentanoic acid. Its molecular formula is $C_5H_{10}ClNO_3$ (Fig. 8) and the molecular weight is 167.61 g/mol. ALA is a white powder or crystals and is sensitive to light. In dermatology, 10–20% ALA is solved in an ointment. ALA is more soluble in hydrophilic ointments whereas skin penetration is higher from a lipophilic vehicle.

After the significant success of applying ALA externally as a precursor of intracellular porphyrins, a large number of derivatives of ALA have been synthesised and studied in order to develop compounds with even better efficacy. Since the active sensitiser for the photodynamic effect is not the precursor (prodrug), but the final metabolite(s), the aim was obvious:

1. To have quite high concentration of the precursor in a quite short time within the cells to synthesise the photoactive metabolites (**velocity**) and

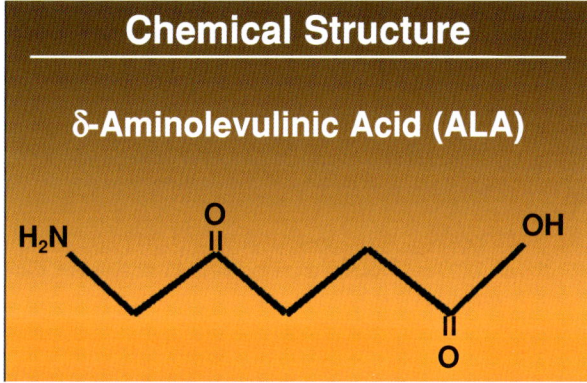

Fig. 8. Chemical structure of ALA

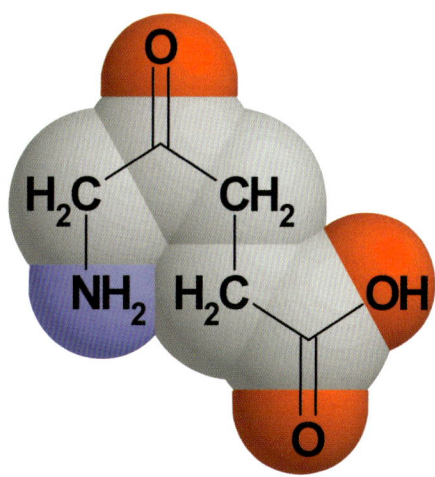

Fig. 8A. Formula of δ-aminolevulinic acid (ALA) with overlay of the space-fill model. The acidic COOH-group (lower right) prohibits passive diffusion into cells.

2. To achieve a concentration ratio between transformed, i.e. target cells and non involved cells as much in favour for target cells as possible (**selectivity**).

ALA, as the name indicates, is chemically a small organic acid Fig. 8A. The functional group of those acids is the polar carboxyl $-COO^-\ H^+$, thus the compound is not able to penetrate passively the lipid bilayer of the cell membrane and therefore cannot enter the cells by diffusion. The predominant avenue into the cells as for this type of amino acids is an active, ATP-dependent transport with saturation kinetics. This active carrier likely belongs to the family of the γ-amino butyric acid transporter and the sodium/potassium dependent β-amino acid transporter, the s.c. System-Beta-transporters (Döring et al, 1998). It shows a zero order kinetic and the uptake is therefore strictly limited by the turnover rate of the carrier.

In contrast, ALA-ME (aminolevulinic acid methylester, methyl aminolevulinate, methyl aminolevulinic acid, MALA), is not a free acid but an ester. The above mentioned polar COOH-group of ALA is masked by the esterification with an alcohol (methanol). This results in a fundamental change of the biophysical properties of the molecule (Fig. 8B).

Other than acids, esters can utilize both an additional active carrier for apolar amino acids and the diffusion pathway. Diffusion is charac-

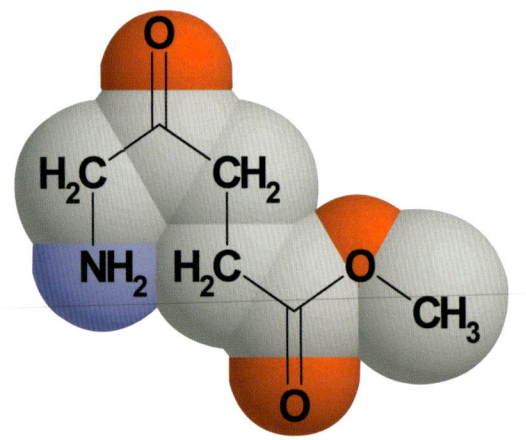

**Fig. 8B.** Formula of methyl aminolevulinate (ALA-ME, MALA) with overlay of the space-fill model. The acidic COOH-group of ALA (cf. Fig. 8A) is masked by the esterification with a methyl group –CH3 (lower right) enabling passive penetration through cell membranes as well as utilization of the carrier for apolar amino acids.

terised by a first order kinetic, depending directly upon the concentration gradient. This leads to a significant acceleration of the cellular uptake, mainly in the early beginning after application when the gradient is steep.

### Chemistry

ALA-ME is the methyl ester of the ALA. According to the JUPAC nomenclature the correct name is Methyl-[5-amino-4-oxopentanoate]. It is white crystalline powder, sensitive to light and since one molecule can easily build a cyclic dimer with another one, it is sensitive to temperature and other physical influences. This makes the galenical formulation for dermatological use difficult. Only highly controlled industrial production steps can guarantee the appropriate quality of the formulation, the brand of the industrial formulation is Metvix®. It is a rather small molecule, the hydrochloride which is used in the Metvix® formulation, has a molecular weight of 181,6.

### Metabolism

After cellular uptake, the ester partly dissociates to ALA and methyl alcohol. This ALA undergoes the same metabolic pathway as described above. But another parts remains as the ester and enters directly and fast the porphyrine synthesis. Our knowledge on this interesting part is still limited and subject to further research.

## B.2 Metabolism of ALA

ALA is an endogenous precursor of the highly photosensitizing porphyrin metabolites (Fig. 9) (Menon et al, 1989). *In vivo*, enzymatic condensation of ALA from glycine and succinyl-coenzyme A is the initial and rate-limiting step in the heme synthesis pathway. Subsequently four ALA molecules are condensed to porphobilinogen (PBG), the next pathway intermediate. The conversion from 4 PBG molecules to uroporphyrinogen I and uroporphyrinogen III (eight carboxyl groups) is catalyzed by PBG-deaminase. Only the III isomers can be further metabolized in the heme synthesis pathway. In steps, decarboxylation of uroporphyrino-

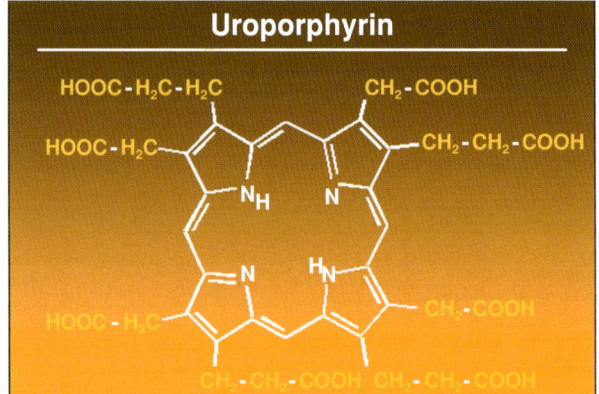

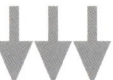

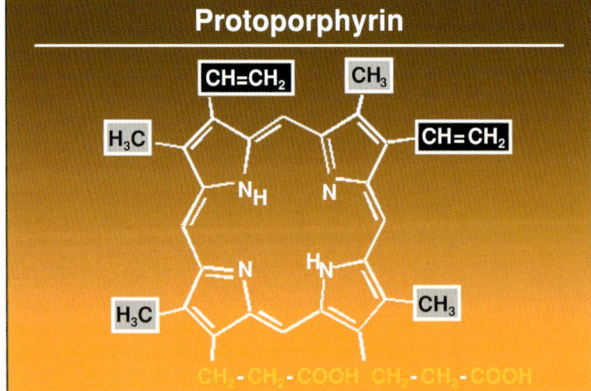

**Fig. 10.** Chemical structures of uroporphyrin and protoporphyrin IX. The molecule uroporphyrin presents 8 carboxyl groups (yellow). These groups undergo stepwise decarboxylation by the enzyme uroporphyrinogen decarboxylase. After six decarboxylation steps, the molecule protoporphyrin is formed. Protoporphyrin has two carboxyl groups

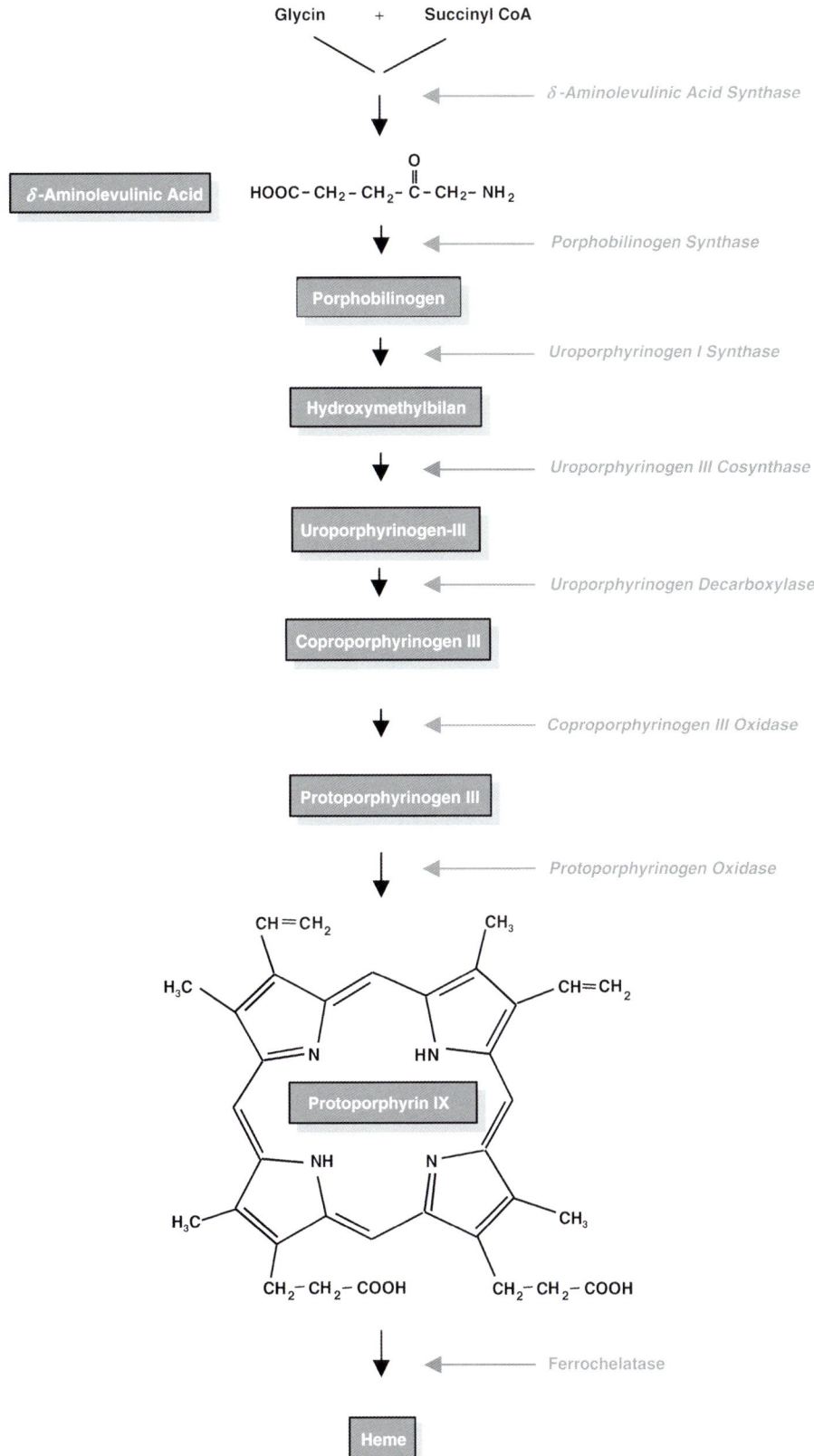

**Fig. 9.** Heme biosynthesis. ALA is synthetised from glycine and succinyl coenzyme A. 4 molecules ALA are the basis for the synthesis of uroporphyrinogen III. Stepwise decarboxylation leads to protoporphyrin. Heme is formed by insertion of iron into protoporphyrin

gen III leads to the formation of hepta-, hexa-, penta- and finally protoporphyrinogen (two carboxyl groups) (Fig. 10). Protoporphyrinogen is oxidized to protoporphyrin IX and the incorporation of iron into protoporphyrin IX to form heme, triggered by ferrochelatase, describes the final step of this pathway.

Under physiological conditions, ALA synthesis is tightly controlled by feedback inhibition of the enzyme aminolevulinic acid synthase (ALA-S), presumably by intracellular heme levels. Exogenous addition of ALA bypasses the inhibiting ALA-S and can therefore lead to higher formation of porphyrins in tumor cells and tissues.

## B.3 Pharmacodynamics of ALA

The application of ALA in PDT for cutaneous disorders was introduced in 1990 (Kennedy et al, 1990). Systemic administration of ALA is used predominantly for the management of gastrointestinal, bronchopulmonary, and cerebral tumors, whereas PDT with topical ALA formulations represents one of the most popular PDT techniques in dermatology. Little has been known about the systemic influence of systemically or topically administrated ALA or porphyrin metabolites in humans. ALA as the most important porphyrin precursor may be capable of inducing porphyria-like symptoms if administered in sufficient quantities (Medeiros et al, 1994; Onuki et al, 1994).

### B.3.1 Systemic Administration of ALA

The hemodynamic effects of orally administered ALA in doses used for PDT were examined in six patients with a significant history of cardiac disease (Herman et al, 1998). When compared to measurements made prior to ALA administration, all patients displayed a significant decrease in systolic and diastolic blood pressures, pulmonary artery systolic and diastolic pressures as well as pulmonary vascular resistance. Although no adverse sequels were appreciated as a result of the observed hemodynamic changes, this potential should be recognized in patients undergoing ALA-PDT. We measured the kinetics of ALA-induced porphyrins in hamsters bearing an amelanotic

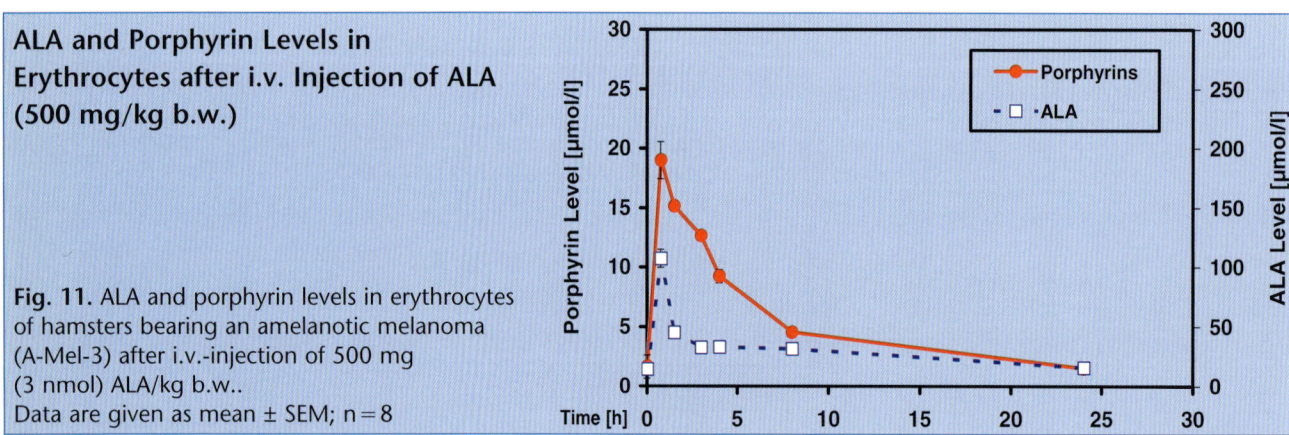

Fig. 11. ALA and porphyrin levels in erythrocytes of hamsters bearing an amelanotic melanoma (A-Mel-3) after i.v.-injection of 500 mg (3 nmol) ALA/kg b.w..
Data are given as mean ± SEM; n = 8

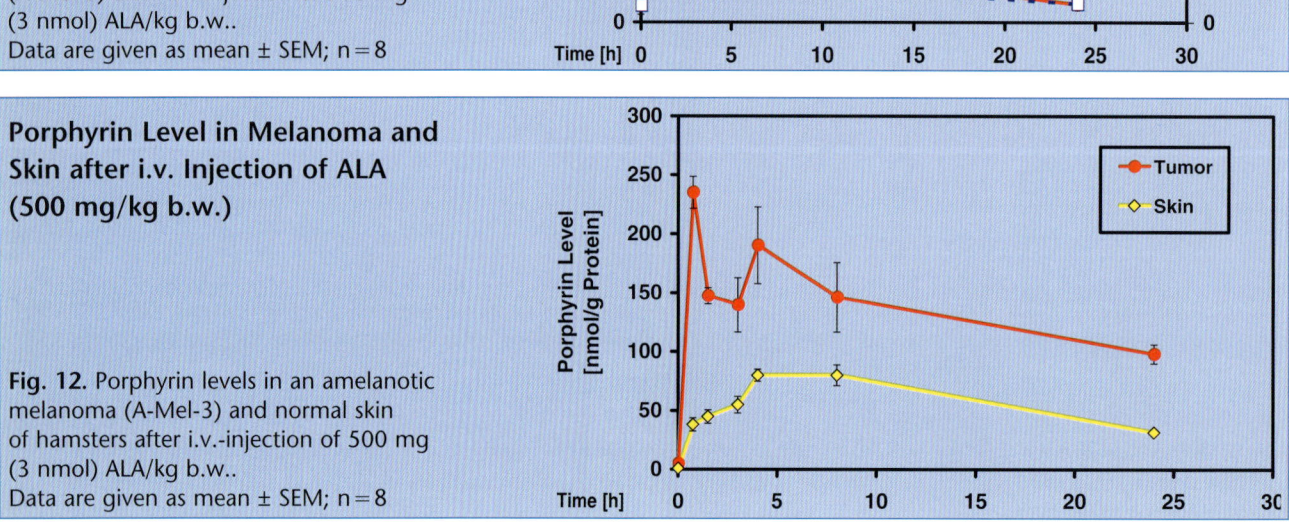

Fig. 12. Porphyrin levels in an amelanotic melanoma (A-Mel-3) and normal skin of hamsters after i.v.-injection of 500 mg (3 nmol) ALA/kg b.w..
Data are given as mean ± SEM; n = 8

melanoma (A-Mel3) up to 24 hours after i.v. administration of 500 mgALA/kg b.w. (Fritsch et al, 1997).

The basal levels of ALA and total porphyrins in erythrocytes were 15 ± 1 and 3 ± 1 µM, respectively. Intravenous injection of 500 mg/kgb.w. of ALA resulted in an increase of erythrocyte ALA and porphyrins with a maximum at 45 min (98 ± 8 and 19 ± 2 µM). Basal values were reached again 24 h after injection (Fig. 11).

ALA injection was followed by an accumulation of total porphyrins in tumor, skin, liver, and kidney. The porphyrin levels in tumor tissue showed maximum values at 45 min (228 ± 22 nmol/g protein) and 4 h (156 ± 32 nmol/g protein) and were still elevated after 24 h (Fig. 12). In skin, porphyrin accumulation was less pronounced, with maxima between 4 to 8 h (approx. 80 nmol/g protein) and still elevated levels detectable at 24 h. The highest ratio in tumor to normal skin was 6:1 already at 45 min.

In kidney, maximum levels were measured at 4 h (103 ± 12 nmol/g protein) which returned to basal values at 24 h. The highest porphyrin accumulation was measured in liver (106 ± 5) at 45 min, still increasing at 24 h (284 ± 32 nmol/g protein) (Fig. 13).

Protoporphyrin, coproporphyrin and the highly carboxylated porphyrins (= 5-8-COOH) were found in tumors in comparably high amounts, with maximum values at 45 min and 4 h (Fig. 14). In skin, the levels of protoporphyrin and the highly carboxylated porphyrins, but not coproporphyrin, showed a slight increase.

At the time point (45 min) of the maximal tumor/skin ratio of the porphyrin levels, coproporphyrin was the prevailing metabolite (Fig. 15). In liver tissue the predominant porphyrin metabolite was protoporphyrin with highest levels at 24 h. Protoporphyrin was also prevailing in kidney with maximum levels at 4 h followed by the highly carboxylated porphyrins.

The relatively high dose of 500 mg/kg b.w. was chosen because previous work on the dose-response relationship in the hamster revealed optimum porphyrin fluorescence tumor/skin ratios with this dose (Abels et al, 1994). Oral and intravenous administration of ALA (100 mg) to

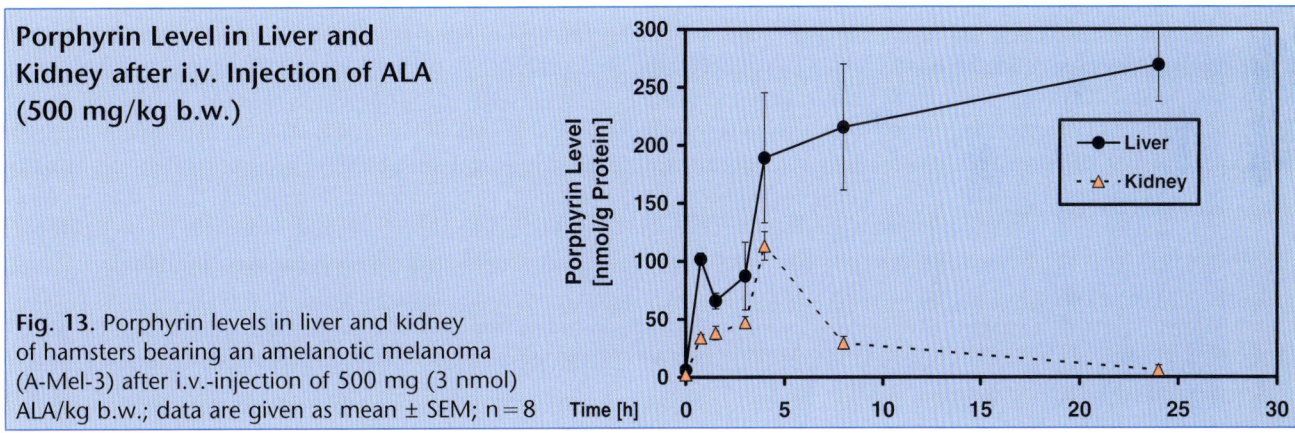

Fig. 13. Porphyrin levels in liver and kidney of hamsters bearing an amelanotic melanoma (A-Mel-3) after i.v.-injection of 500 mg (3 nmol) ALA/kg b.w.; data are given as mean ± SEM; n = 8

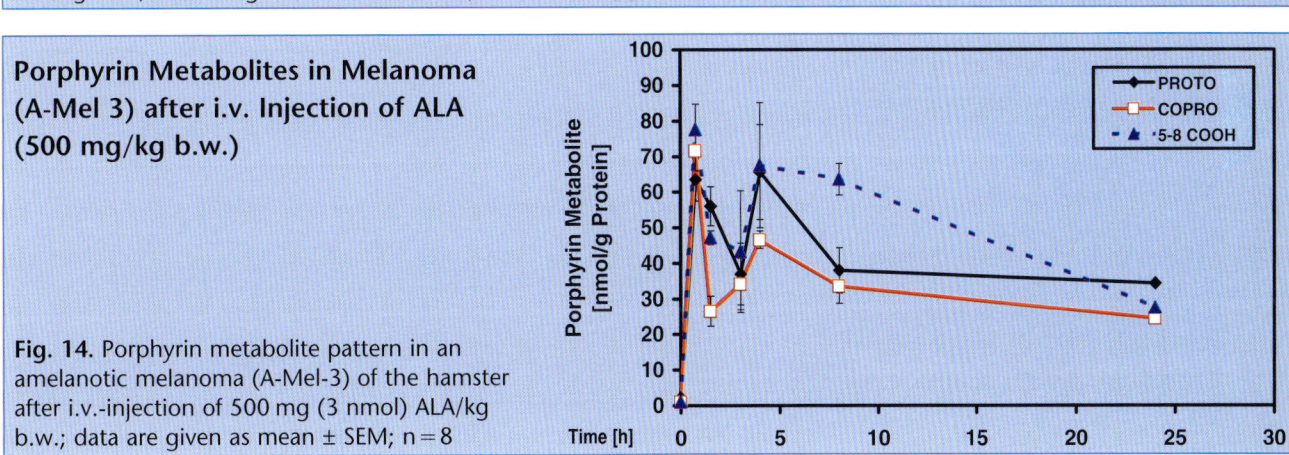

Fig. 14. Porphyrin metabolite pattern in an amelanotic melanoma (A-Mel-3) of the hamster after i.v.-injection of 500 mg (3 nmol) ALA/kg b.w.; data are given as mean ± SEM; n = 8

dogs was followed by a rapid decline of plasma ALA concentrations with a terminal half-life of 20 min (Dalton et al, 1999). Peak plasma concentrations of ALA after oral administration ranged from 1 to 9 μg/ml. Oral bioavailability in these animals averaged at 41 ± 15%. Two groups of rats were given 200 mg/kg b.w. ALA orally or intravenously (van den Boogert et al, 1998) and kinetics of ALA and porphyrins were measured. In both groups ALA concentrations were highest in kidney, bladder and urine. After oral administration, high concentrations were also found in duodenum and jejunum. Mild, short-lasting elevation of creatinine was seen in both treatment groups. Porphyrins, especially protoporphyrin IX, accumulated mainly in duodenal aspirate, jejunum, liver and kidney, less in esophagus, stomach, colon, spleen, bladder, heart, lung and nerve, and only slightly in plasma, muscle, fat, skin and brain. In mice, bearing a colon adenocarcinoma, which received intravenous injection of 50 mg ALA/kg b.w., the most intense porphyrin fluorescence was found in the tumor with maximum contrast to non-malignant organs of up to 30-fold at 4–6 h (Sroka et al, 1996). In mice bearing a mammary carcinoma, intraperitoneal injection of 250 mg ALA/kg b.w. also led to an early maximum tumor/skin ratio of porphyrin levels at 1 h (Peng et al, 1992). Intravenous injection of 300 mg ALA/kg b.w. into rats bearing a mammary adenocarcinoma induced maximum porphyrin ratios after 5 h. Protoporphyrin was the major intratumoral porphyrin metabolite (83%) and a low coproporphyrin level was reported (Hua et al, 1995). Taken together, systemic administration consistently results in a faster and higher intratumoral accumulation of porphyrins than topical application. When ALA was topically applied to humans or animals, maximum porphyrin fluorescence was detected after 4–6 hours (Peng et al, 1995).

In contrast to topical ALA application adverse effects are observed in systemic ALA-PDT. These include transient rises in serum aspartate aminotransferase, nausea, vomiting, headache, circulatory failure, and photosensitivity (Regula et al, 1995; Herrmann et al, 1998). This might be partly due to the 50-fold increase in the hepatic protoporphyrin level (Fig. 13). Systemic ALA administration for FDAP or PDT in humans has been performed using ALA doses between 10 and 60 mg/kg b.w. (Regula et al, 1995; Stummer et al, 1998). In 8 patients with a cerebral tumor undergoing FDAP using 10 mgALA/kg b.w., the porphyrin kinetics in blood and urine were measured (Fritsch et al, 1996).

The orally taken ALA induced an early peak (< 4 h) of ALA and porphyrin levels in erythrocytes and plasma. Baseline values were reached after 12 h (ALA) and 48 h (porphyrins) (Figs. 16 and 17).

These data clearly show that nearly all orally taken ALA is transported into plasma. Plasma levels of ALA rose more than ten times upon ALA ingestion. Porphyrins were accumulating up to ten-fold in plasma as well as in erythrocytes. These high initial peaks of ALA in the blood could be responsible for potential neurological or gastrointestinal side effects and hemodynamic disturbances. As many investigators administer ALA doses up to 60 mg/kg b.w. (we used 10), systemic ALA levels might be even much higher.

Urinary excretion of porphyrins and precursors upon oral ALA treatment shows normal values on day 3 after an increase on days 1 and 2 (Figs. 18 and 19).

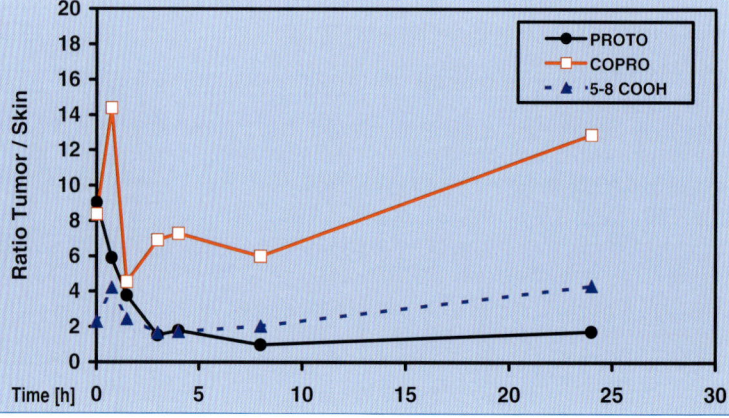

**Ratio Tumor / Skin of Porphyrin Metabolites after i.v. Injection of ALA (500 mg/kg b.w.)**

Fig. 15. Ratio of the porphyrin metabolites (tumor/skin) after i.v.-injection of 500 mg (3 nmol) ALA/kg b.w. to a hamster bearing an amelanotic melanoma (A-Mel-3). Data are given as mean ± SEM; n = 8. For coproporphyrin an even higher tumor selective capacity was found as compared to protoporphyrin or the highly carboxylated porphyrins

## ALA and Porphyrin Levels after Oral Administration of ALA (10 mg/kg b.w.)

**Fig. 16.** ALA and porphyrin kinetics in erythrocytes after oral administration of 10 mgALA/kg b.w. (mean ± SD; n=8). Six-fold levels of porphyrins were induced (4 h), reaching the upper limit of the physiologic range (<60 µg/dl). ALA levels did not change significantly (maximum normal level 51 µg/dl)

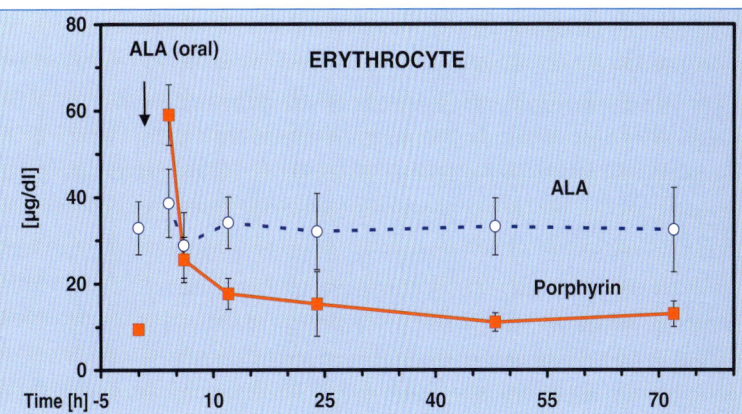

## ALA and Porphyrin Levels after Oral Administration of ALA (10 mg/kg b.w.)

**Fig. 17.** ALA and porphyrin kinetics in plasma after oral administration of 10 mg ALA/kg b.w. (mean ± SD; n=8). Ten-fold increase of ALA and porphyrins was measured (4 h). Maximum physiologic levels are 35 µg/dl (ALA) and 2µg/dl (porphyrins)

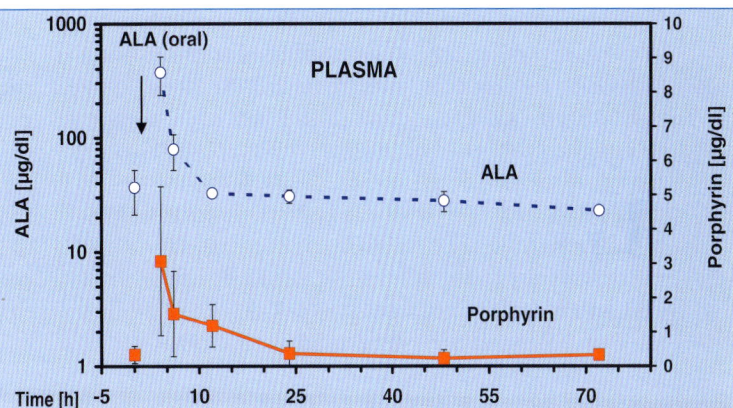

## Porphyrin Levels in Urine after Oral Administration of ALA (10 mg/kg b.w.)

**Fig. 18.** Porphyrin kinetics in urine after oral administration of 10 mg ALA/kg b.w. (mean ± SD; n=8). Porphyrin values were increased up to 40 times (12–24 h) as compared to baseline. Maximum individual concentration was 990 µg/l (normal range <150 µg/l). Values returned to baseline after 3 days

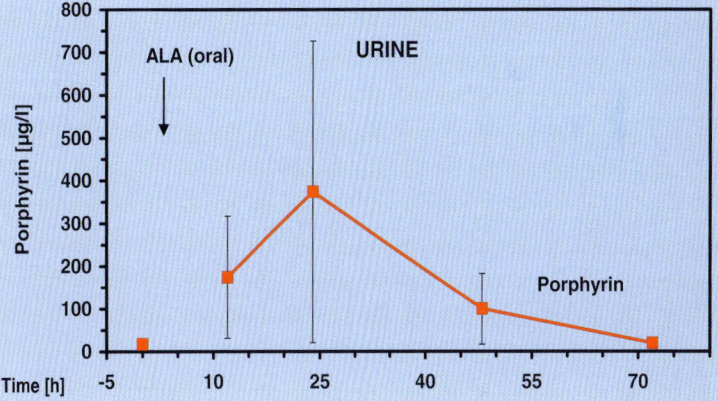

## Porphyrin Precursor Levels in Urine after Oral Administration of ALA (10 mg/kg b.w.)

**Fig. 19.** Kinetics of the porphyrin precursors ALA and porphobilinogen (PBG) in urine after oral administration of 10 mg ALA/kg b.w. (mean ± SD; n=8). Oral ALA supply induced an increase of ALA (two-fold) and PBG (six-fold) in urine. Baseline values were measured after 3 days

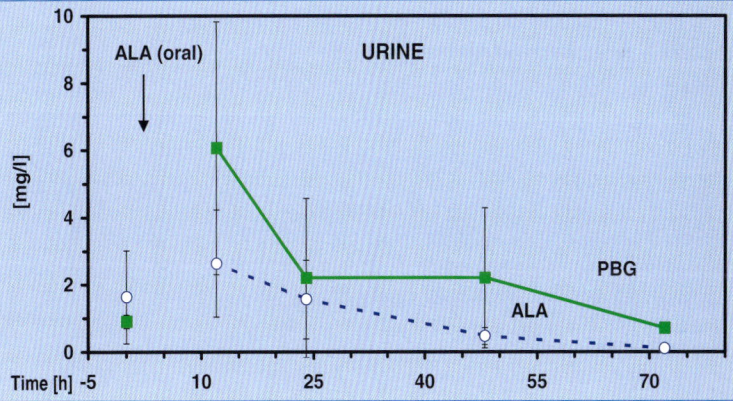

### B.3.2 Topical Application of ALA

The main advantage of topical ALA-PDT is the absence of generalized cutaneous photosensitivity. We investigated the porphyrin metabolism in blood and urine upon topical ALA treatment to exclude any systemic effects of topical FDAP or PDT (Fritsch et al, 1996).

The study confirmed that topical application of ALA in amounts from 0.05 to 0.2 g/cm$^2$ (total amounts of ALA: 0.02 to 7 g) did not induce significant systemic accumulation of porphyrins (Figs. 20–23).

Numerous attempts have been made to potentiate the efficacy of ALA-based PDT with the use of penetration enhancers or additive compounds to induce or inhibit certain enzymes of the heme synthesis pathway. Desferrioxamine has been shown to enhance the ALA-induced protoporphyrin accumulation (Fijan et al, 1995). The combination of dimethyl sulfoxide (DMSO) and ethylendiaminetetraacetic acid (EDTA) with ALA increased the protoporphyrin production in the depth of the lesions and enhanced the complete response rate of nodular BCC (Peng et al, 1995; Soler et al, 2000).

Lipophilic ALA ester derivatives show weaker porphyrin fluorescence but higher tumor selectivity, most likely because of alternate penetration through cellular membranes compared with the hydrophilic ALA (Rud et al, 2000). PDT with ALA methylester resulted in high response rates of nodular BCC, indicating that this photosensitizer-prodrug may be useful for the cure of thicker tumors (Braathen et al, 2000; Basset-Seguin et al, 2000).

### Pharmacodynamics

The above mentioned aims for the development of ester derivatives of ALA were:

1. Acceleration of the uptake to shorten the time between topical application of the drug and commence of the irradiation and
2. A better ratio of de-novo porphyrin synthesis in healthy cells versus transformed cells resulting in a better selectivity.

Both aims could be reached. The American regulatory authority for the application authorisation of drugs (FDA) declares a time between application of the registered ALA Cream Levulan® 2 of

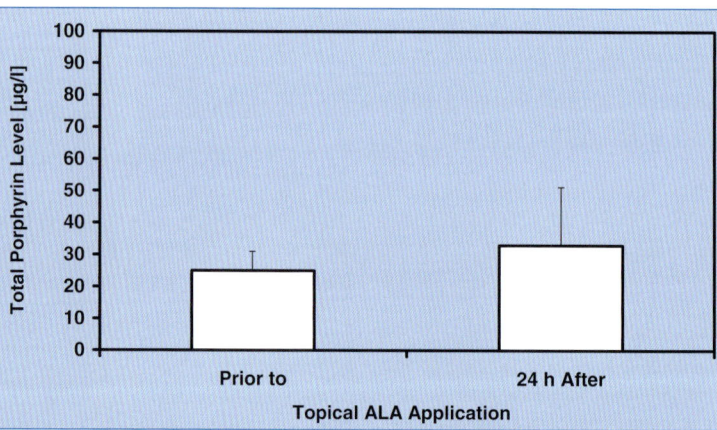

Fig. 20. Total porphyrin level in urine prior to and 24 h after PDT with topically applied ALA (n = 20; mean ± SEM). In some patients, there seemed to be a week correlation between the total amount of ALA applied and the amount of porphyrins excreted. However, urinary porphyrin excretion was not significantly changed (normal value: <150 µg/l)

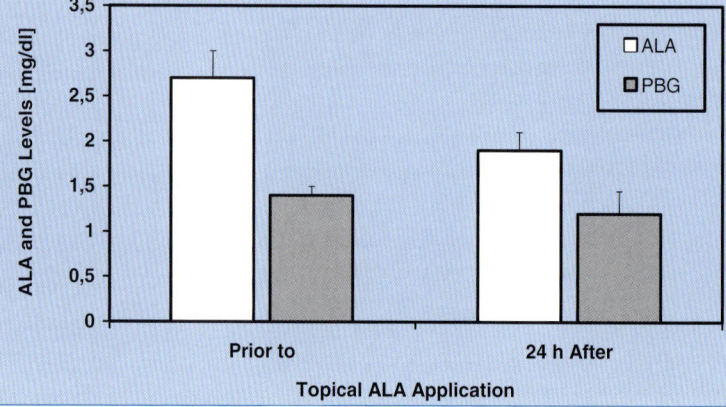

Fig. 21. ALA (open bars) and PBG (filled bars) levels in urine prior to and 24 h after PDT with topically applied ALA (n = 20; mean ± SEM). No significant changes were detected (normal values: ALA 4.5 mg/l; PBG 2.5 mg/l)

## Porphyrin Levels in Red Blood Cell and Plasma after Topical Application of 20% ALA

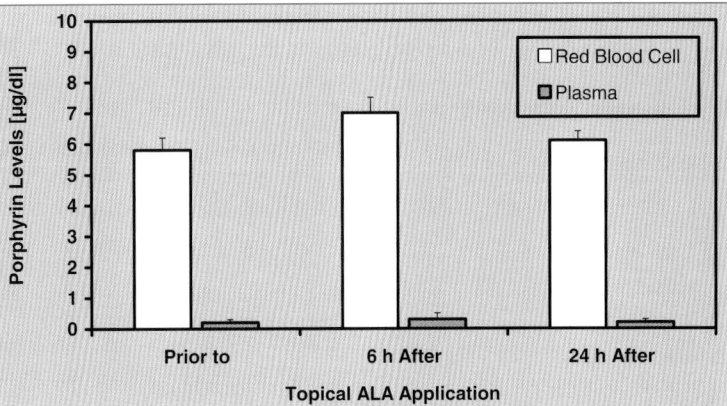

**Fig. 22.** Total porphyrin levels in red blood cells (open bars) and plasma (filled bars) prior to and 24 h after PDT with topically applied ALA (n=20; mean ± SEM). After PDT no significant changes in porphyrin levels were measured either in red blood cells or in plasma, although there seemed to be a slight increase in several patients 6 h after ALA application (normal values: RBC 60 µg/dl; plasma 2 µg/dl)

## ALA Level in Red Blood Cell after Topical Application of 20% ALA

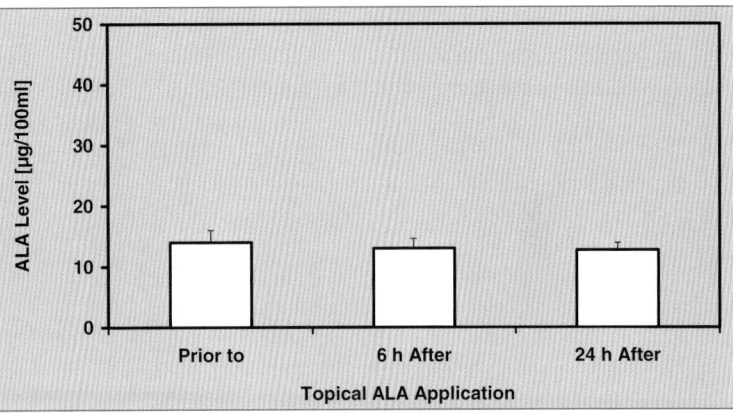

**Fig. 23.** ALA level in red blood cells prior to and 6 and 24 h after PDT with topically applied ALA (n=20; mean ± SEM). No significant differences were demonstrated (normal value: 50 µg/100ml)

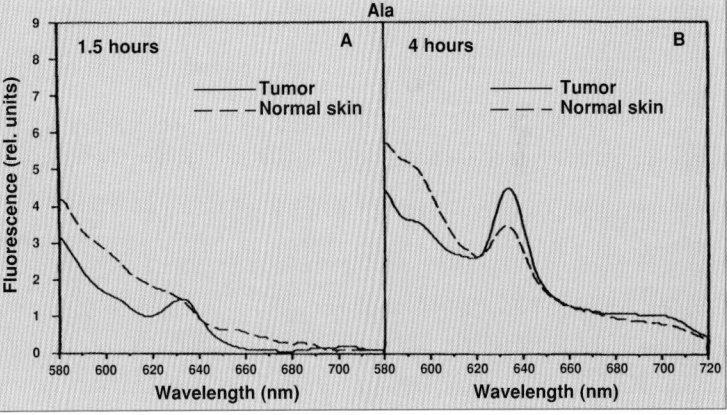

**Fig. 23A.** 634 nm Fluorescence of human BCCs after 1.5 and 4.0 hours after application of ALA. The ratio between the fluorescence of normal skin and tumor skin is a measure for selectivity

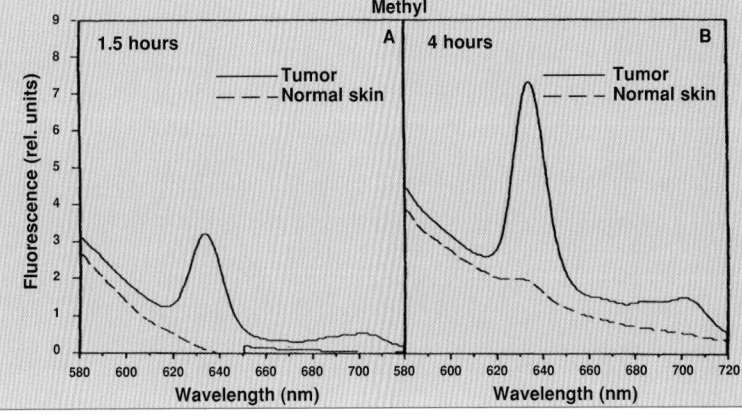

**Fig. 23B.** 634 nm Fluorescence of human BCCs after 1.5 and 4.0 hours after application of MALA. The ratio between the fluorescence of normal skin and tumor skin is a measure for selectivity

16 hours whereas the time for the MALA Cream Metvix® is only 3 hours. This is an advantage not only in terms of patient compliance but also in terms of office management.

Selectivity has been studied very carefully with different esters other than the methyl ester. It depends on the molecular length of the ester and the –methyl seems to show an optimum similar to –hexyl but by far better than e.g. –heptyl or –octyl. The fact of this very high selectivity could be clearly demonstrated by comparing the 634 nm fluorescence of human BCCs after application of ALA or MALA after different times after application of the respective drugs (Fig. 23A and Fig. 23B).

## C  Light Used in FDAP and PDT

The absorption spectrum of porphyrins exhibits a maximum in the Soret band ranging from 360 to 400 nm, followed by 4 smaller peaks between 500 and 635 nm (Q-bands) (Fig. 24) (Soret, 1883).

The drug is activated by light corresponding to the absorption spectrum of the compound. The depth of tissue penetration depends on the wavelength of this spectrum. Significant tissue penetration is achieved with light at 630 to 635 nm, which corresponds to the weakest of the absorption peaks. 630 nm light penetrates the first 5 mm of most tissues, whereas photons at 700 to 800 nm reach cells as deep as 1 to 2 cm (Driver et al, 1991; Wilson, 1986; Frazier, 1996). Light at wavelengths longer than 850 nm does not yield enough energy to produce sufficient photochemical response.

In dermatology, performing FDAP, Wood's light systems (370–405 nm) are used (Fig. 25). Wood's light extends into the absorption maximum of the porphyrins revealing highest fluorescence yield. For PDT, the lesions are exposed to light at 635 nm 3 to 6 hours after ALA application. However, photodynamically active products are also generated at wavelengths beyond the activation spectrum of PpIX, indicating that broad-band illumination may be most effective (Dietel et al, 1996).

The irradiation sources used most frequently include: incoherent light sources comprising red (570–750 nm) (Fritsch et al, 1998), green (545 nm) (Fritsch et al, 1997) or blue light (417 nm) (Omrod and Jarvis, 2000), (400–410 nm) (Marcus et al, 1996) and laser systems (e.g., argon pumped dye lasers). UVA (blue light)-irradiation was shown to be superior in cytotoxic mechanisms as compared to green or red light (Buchczyk et al, 2001). Concerning the cure rate and the cosmetic outcome, there is no statistically significant difference between an incoherent lamp (570–740 nm) and laser (630 nm) (Soler et al, 2001).

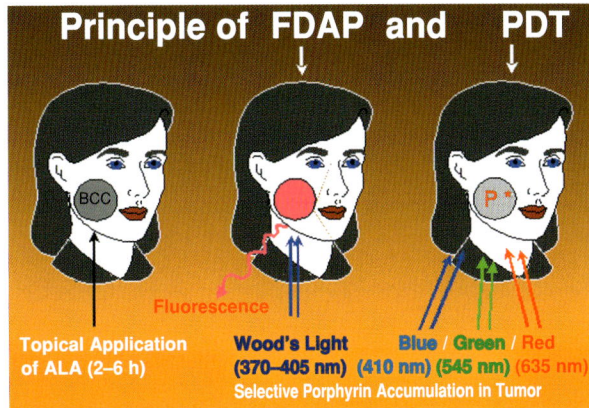

Fig. 25. ALA ointment is applied topically to e.g. a basal cell carcinoma (BCC) under an occlusive foil. After 2–6 h, the rest of the substance is removed. In FDAP, the BCC is irradiated by Wood's light with the effect that red intralesional porphyrin fluorescence is emitted. To induce a photodynamic action (PDT), the porphyrin-enriched tissue is irradiated by green, red or blue light

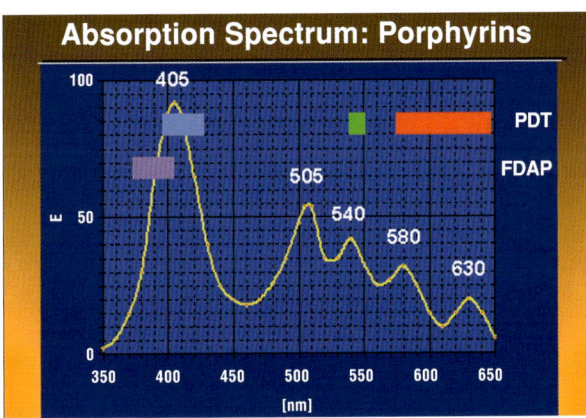

Fig. 24. Absorption spectrum of porphyrin molecules. Porphyrins show five strong absorption peaks. Maximum of absorbance is around the so-called Soret band at 405 nm. This maximum is followed by additional 4 peaks with decreasing intensity. For FDAP, light around 405 nm, for PDT green, yellow, red or recently also blue light is used

# D  Unresolved Issues in FDAP and PDT

FDAP techniques have already been developed in urology, gastroenterology or recently also neurosurgery. In dermatology, this technique has been used since 1997, however, a statistically relevant number of clinical and histopathological trials was still lacking. Several indications were tried to be treated by this technique. Response rates ranged from 0 up to 100% depending on the lesion selected, the follow up time and the treatment parameters. The FDA granted approval for the application of ALA in December 1999. Although FDAP and PDT are presently approved as officially legalized techniques and are increasingly included as routine strategies by dermatologists, there are still no defined guidelines.

The following chapters comprise relevant clinical data on FDAP and PDT allowing the optimum use of these diagnostic and therapeutic modalities.

## Concerning FDAP studies on the following topics will be discussed in detail:

- Evaluation of the ALA-induced fluorescence in skin diseases;
- Biochemical measurement of the ALA-induced porphyrins in skin tumors and psoriasis lesions;
- Course of FDAP in relation to the number of PDT sessions;
- Correlation of the macroscopic fluorescence with histopathology;
- Evaluation of the optimum photosensitizing substance or its prodrug;
- Evaluation of the optimum exciting light source;
- Course of FDAP in relation to the number of PDT sessions.

## Concerning the efficacy of PDT in dermatology studies on the following topics will be discussed in detail:

- Evaluation of the efficacy in solar keratoses;
- Evaluation of the efficacy in Bowen's disease;
- Evaluation of the efficacy in basal cell carcinoma;
- Evaluation of the efficacy in squamous cell carcinoma;
- Evaluation of the efficacy in psoriatic lesions;
- Evaluation of the efficacy in selected cutaneous diseases;
- Evaluation of the optimum photosensitizing substance or its prodrug;
- Evaluation of the optimum exciting light source.

# E  Fluorescence Detection of ALA-induced Porphyrins (FDAP)

## E.1. FDAP: Evaluation of the ALA-induced Fluorescence in Skin Diseases

**Material and Methods**

In the period from April 1998 to March 2001, FDAP was performed in 212 basal cell carcinomas (BCC), 158 squamous cell carcinomas (SCC), 498 solar keratoses (SK), 47 cases of Bowen's diseases (BD), 8 cases of Paget's disease (PD), 20 lesions of mycosis fungoides (MF), 17 Kaposi's sarcomas (KS), 30 malignant melanomas (MM), 13 cases of lentigo maligna (LM), 35 nevus cell nevi (N), 42 lesions of lupus erythematosus (LE), 85 psoriatic lesions (PS), 25 areas of atopic eczema (AE), 32 areas of acne vulgaris (AV) and 240 areas of normal skin (NS). Additionally, follow up studies of FDAP were performed in 50 cases of SK and 35 BCC treated by PDT.

*Selection of the ALA and preparation of the ALA mixture.* ALA (hydrochloride form) is provided by different chemical companies (Merck Darmstadt Germany, Fluka or Sigma-Aldrich, Deisenhofen, Germany) as a chemical drug (Table 26). Since 1998 the company Medac GmbH (Wedel, Germany) offers ALA with the highest degree of purity of all providers and beyond that as a medical product. The companies Schering AG (Berlin, Germany) PhotoCure ASA (Oslo, Norway), and Galderma (Freiburg, Germany) are presently introducing medical products, which contain ALA Kerastick® or ALA methylester (Metvix®) in a solution or a cream, respectively. In general, ALA can be mixed in an ointment or a cream. We use either Neribas® ointment (Asche AG, Hamburg, Germany) or aqueous hydrophilic ointment (DAB 10; unguentum emulsificans aquosum). Advantages of an ointment – in comparison to the cream – are the better adhesion to the skin surface and improved percutaneous penetration of the substrate. On the other hand, the cream offers a stronger hydrophilicity and thus a more homogeneous solution of ALA.

*Pretreatment of the examined tissue.* Prestudies showed that FDAP loses effectiveness if the ALA mixture is applied on a dry, crusty lesion (e.g., SK, BD, or BCC) whereas in skin areas colonized by bacteria FDAP appears more intensive (e.g., intertriginous areas or facial skin). The following pretreatments were found to work satisfactorily in the different indications:

*SK, MF, KS, LE, MM, LM, N, AE, AV without or with only fine crusts:*
- Gentle abrasion of the fine crusts with isopropanol-soaked gauze.

*SK on the scalp with hyperkeratoses, superficial BCC (Fig. 26), SCC, BD with (hemorrhagic) crusts:*
- Rigorous abrasion of the crusts with isopropanol-containing gauze.
- Removal of all visible and gropable crusts with a curette and/or tweezers. Local anesthesia is generally not required.
- Treatment of any bleeding areas by application of gauze and pressure.

*SK with strong hyperkeratoses, PS with hyperkeratotic plaques:*
- Pre-treatment with salicylic acid (5%) containing ointments twice daily for 5 days.

*Solid BCC or SCC, e.g., in the face:*
- Abrasion of fine crusts with isopropanol-containing gauze.
- Generous debulking of the exophytic tumor part as well as removal of superficial epithelial layers of the adjacent, clinically healthy skin with a curette. Local anesthesia is recommended.
- Control of any bleeding by local pressure using gauze.

*Application of the ALA mixture.* ALA (Medac GmbH, Wedel, Germany) was mixed in aqueous hydrophilic ointment (DAB 10; unguentum emulsificans aquosum). For FDAP, we applied approx. 0.2 g ointment/cm$^2$ with ALA concentrations from 10% (SK) to 20% (all other lesions) (approx. 20–40 mg ALA/cm$^2$) (Fig. 27). The treated area was covered with a foil (Tegaderm®, 3M) (Fig. 28) and an aluminum foil (Fig. 29), in order to enhance the tissue penetration of the substance and to avoid any photobleaching. After an application period of 4–6 hours tape and ointment were removed.

*Fluorescence diagnosis procedure.* In a completely darkened room Wood's light irradiation was performed. A fluorescence standard (adhesive tape) was fixed to the skin surface in proximity of the fluorescent lesion (Fig. 30) to allow later correlation of fluorescence intensities. For fluorescence excitation we used Fluotest forte® (370–405 nm, Atlas material Testing Technology) or Fluolight® (370–400 nm, Saalmann GmbH, Herford, Germany). Fluorescence patterns were photographically documented. For the documentation of fluorescent lesions a very sensitive film (e.g., Ektachrom P 1600, Kodak) was selected and developed like 1600 ASA. The necessary exposure duration depends on the intensity of the Wood's light source. Using the Fluolight® lamp exposure times from 0.25 to 1.5 seconds are recommendable (personal communication, diplom photo designer Wilfried Neuse, department of dermatology, Düsseldorf). After FDAP, the treated lesions were covered by a light-protecting tape to avoid any further irritation due to room or sun light. This measure was necessary because porphyrin kinetic studies showed a sensitization of the normal skin up to 24 hours after topical ALA application (Fig. 72).

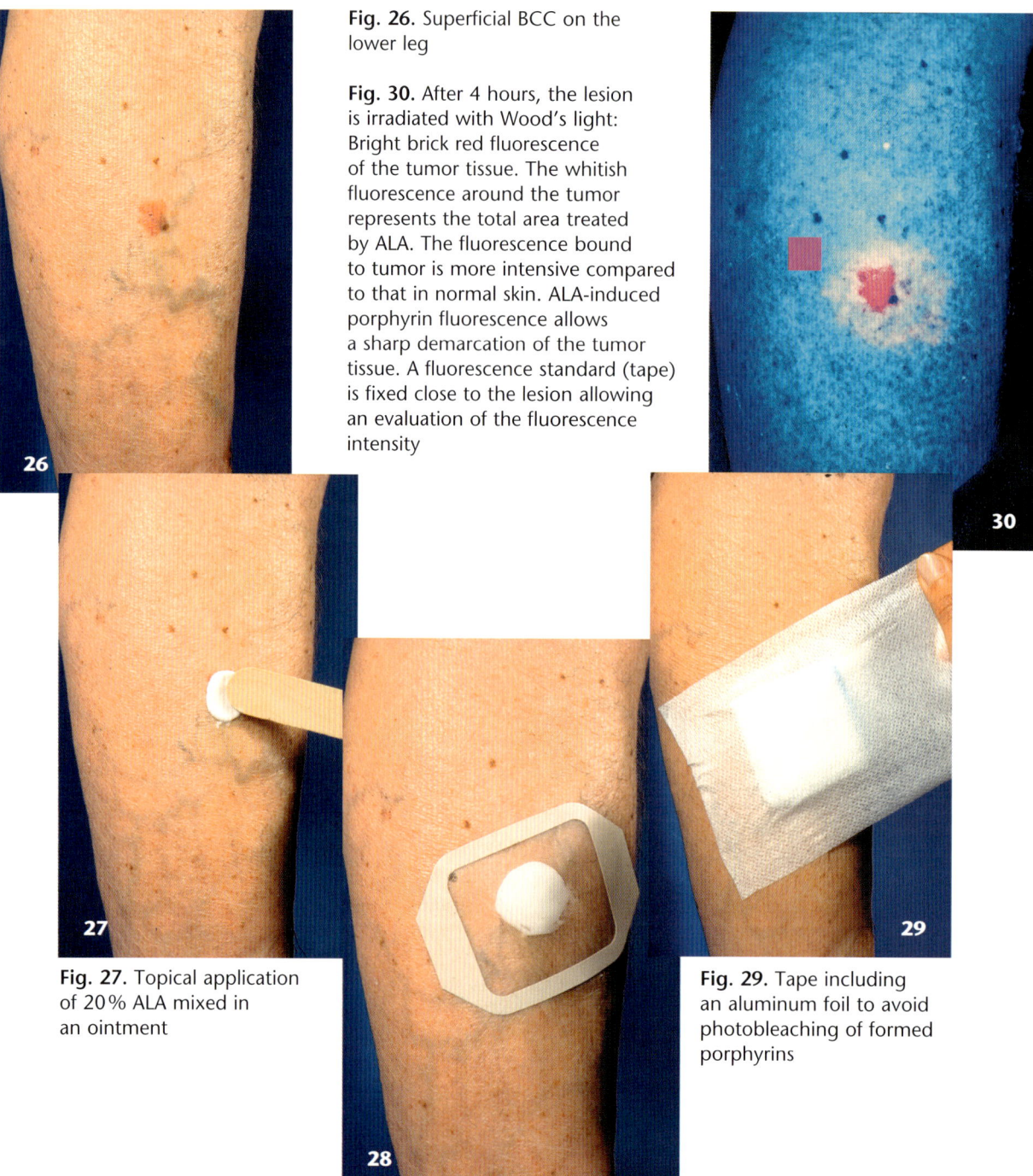

**Fig. 26.** Superficial BCC on the lower leg

**Fig. 30.** After 4 hours, the lesion is irradiated with Wood's light: Bright brick red fluorescence of the tumor tissue. The whitish fluorescence around the tumor represents the total area treated by ALA. The fluorescence bound to tumor is more intensive compared to that in normal skin. ALA-induced porphyrin fluorescence allows a sharp demarcation of the tumor tissue. A fluorescence standard (tape) is fixed close to the lesion allowing an evaluation of the fluorescence intensity

**Fig. 27.** Topical application of 20% ALA mixed in an ointment

**Fig. 29.** Tape including an aluminum foil to avoid photobleaching of formed porphyrins

**Fig. 28.** Occlusive tape to enhance penetration of the substance

## Results

All derived fluorescence intensities are listed in Fig. 31:

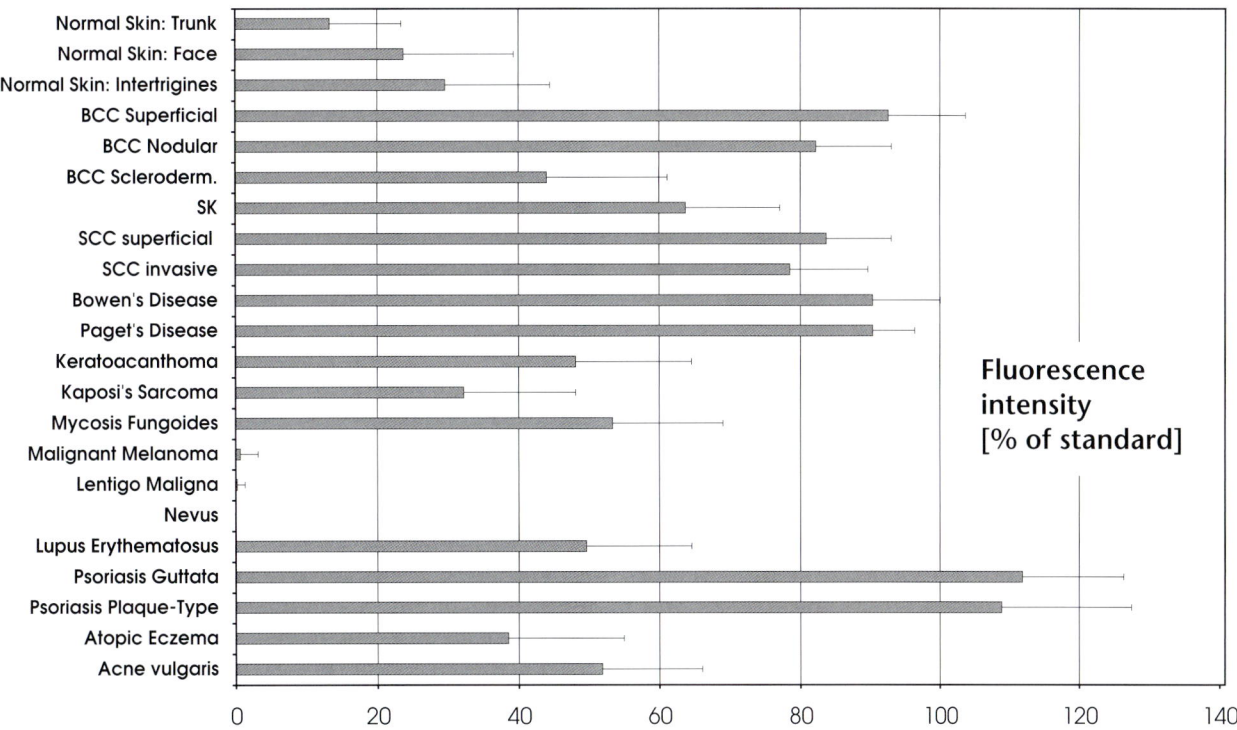

Fig. 31. Fluorescence intensities

Six hours after application of ALA all epithelial neoplasms, such as BCC (Figs. 32 and 33), SCC, Bowen's disease (Figs. 34 and 35), SK (Figs. 36–39) and extramammary Paget's disease (Figs. 40 and 41), showed a strong red fluorescence under Wood's light.

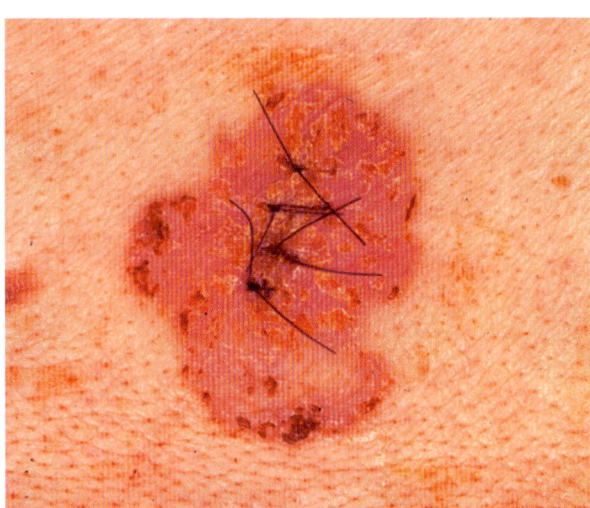

Fig. 32. BCC on the back. The lesion is sharply demarcated

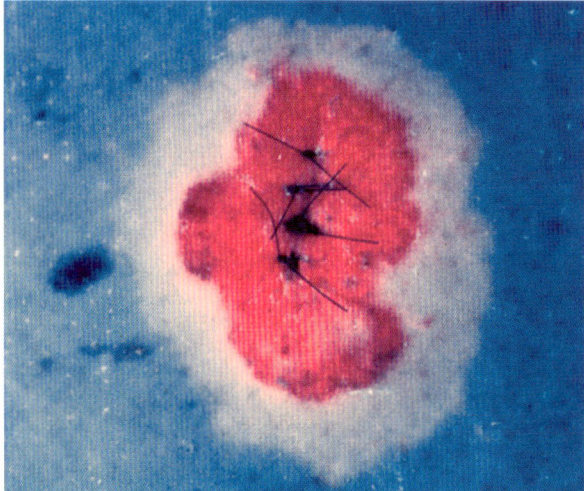

Fig. 33. In FDAP, the lesion shows a bright fluorescence with sharp demarcation. Tumor surrounding skin also reveals a fluorescence, which is, however, of weak intensity. The fluorescent area correlates well with the clinical picture of the tumor

# Fluorescence Detection of ALA-induced Porphyrins (FDAP)

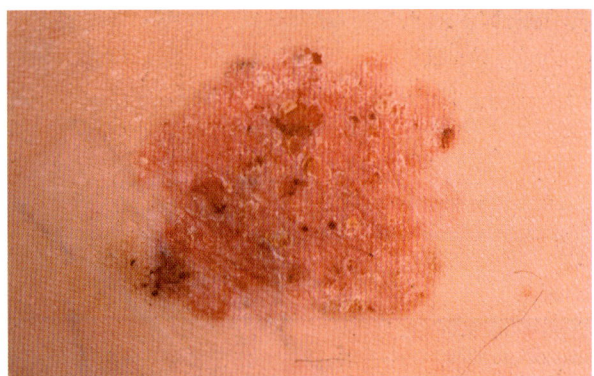

Fig. 34. BD at gluteal area

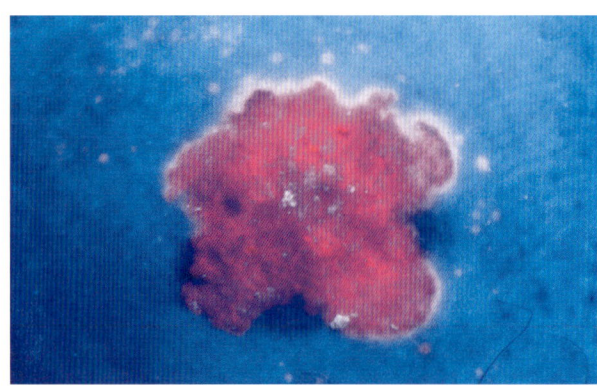

Fig. 35. FDAP: Sharp bright fluorescence of the tumor

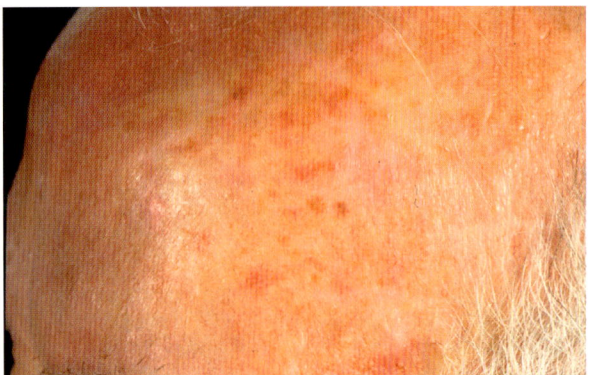

Fig. 36. SK on the front left appearing as erythematous macules

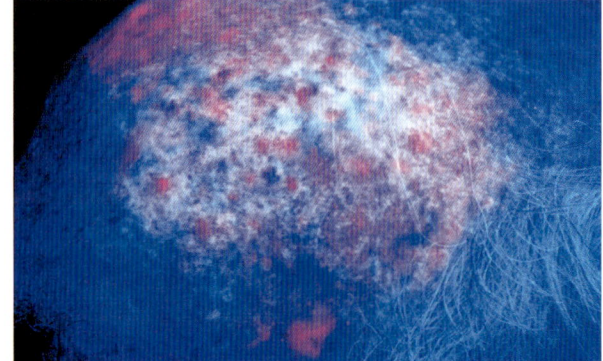

Fig. 37. FDAP: Spotty fluorescence pattern. There are many more lesions detectable by FDAP than by clinical appearance alone

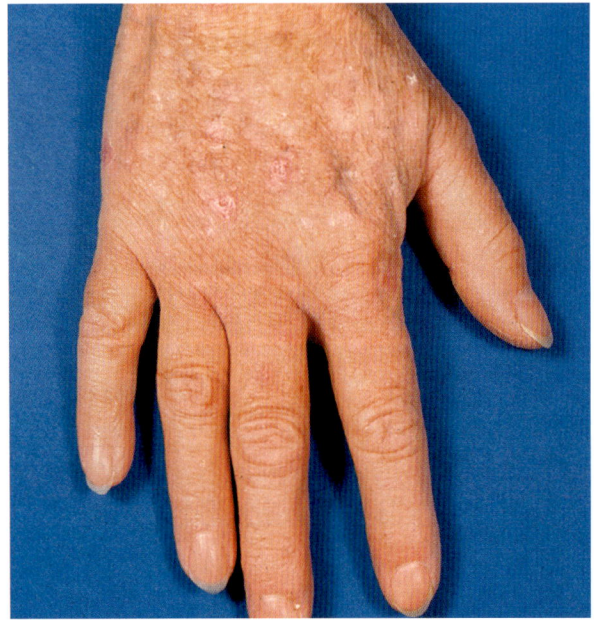

Fig. 38. SK on the back of the hand. The lesions are better gropable than visible

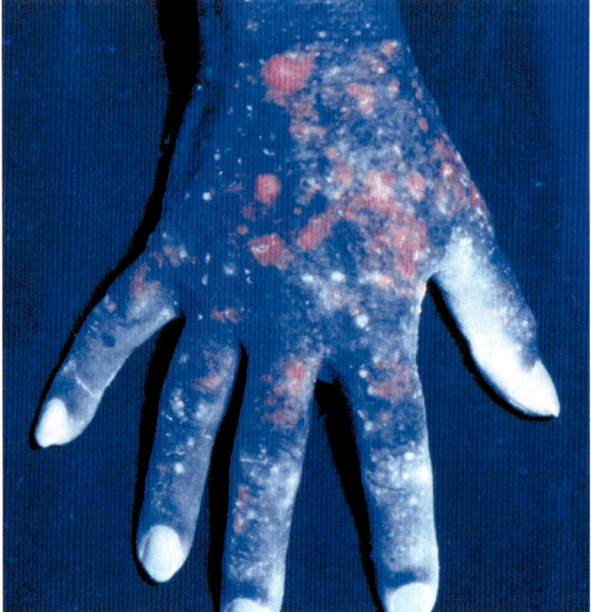

Fig. 39. FDAP: Fluorescence detection of multiple lesions

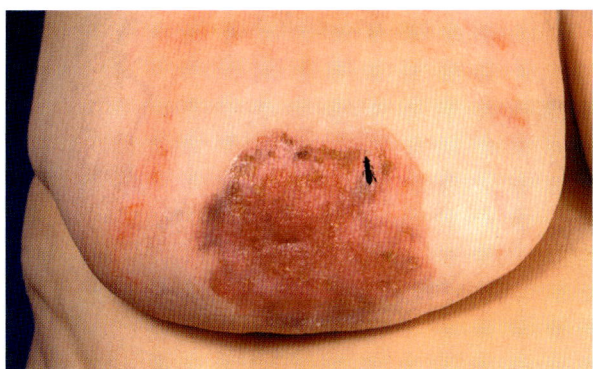

**Fig. 40.** Paget's disease. Erythemato-squamous plaque on the right breast

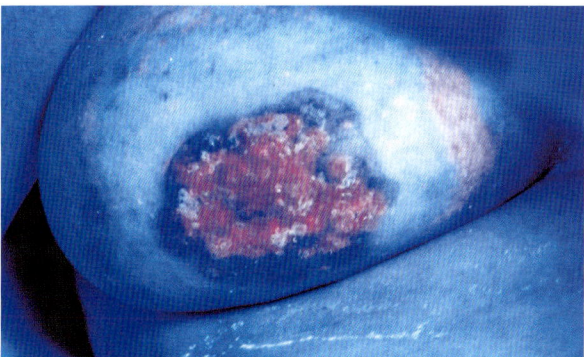

**Fig. 41.** FDAP: Bright fluorescence, presenting, however, a nonhomogeneous pattern in the outer part of the lesion

There was a medium intensity fluorescence in Kaposi's sarcoma, the lesions of lupus erythematosus, and in the plaques of cutaneous T-cell lymphoma (mycosis fungoides) (Figs. 42 and 43) and only a slight or no fluorescence in the pigmented benign and malignant skin changes such as nevocytic nevus, lentigo maligna and malignant melanoma (Figs. 44 and 45).

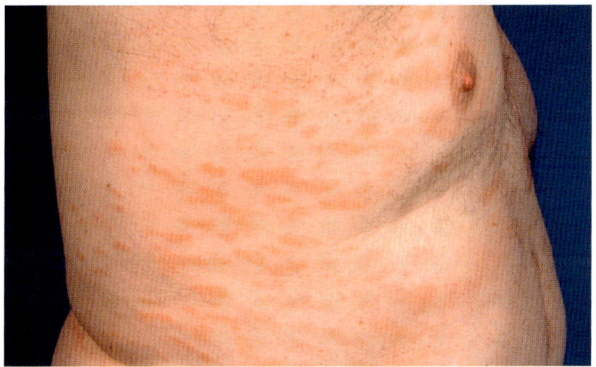

**Fig. 42.** Mycosis fungoides. The typical digitiform patchy pattern of flat erythematous plaques is presented on the lateral trunk

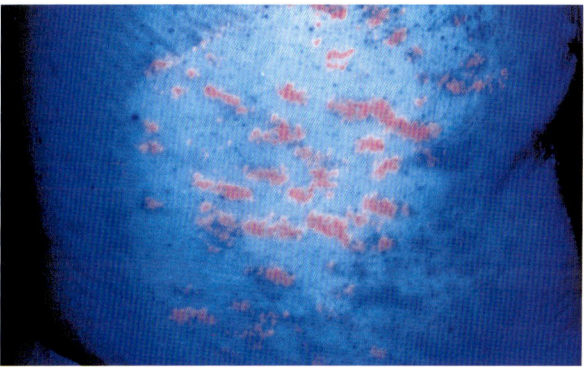

**Fig. 43.** FDAP: Most of the plaques accumulate porphyrins and show a bright fluorescence

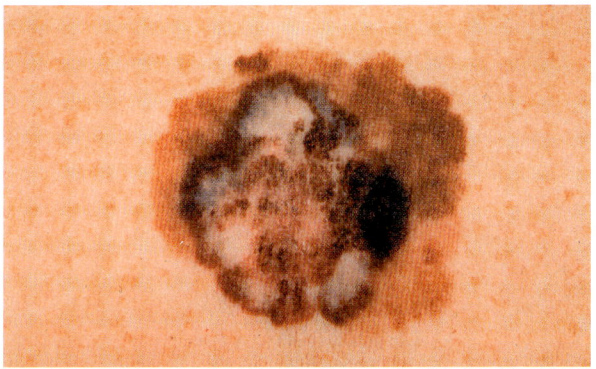

**Fig. 44.** Malignant melanoma (superficial spreading type). Asymmetric lesion, multiple colors, diameter of 4.7 cm. Histopathology proved level IV and tumor thickness of 2.2 mm

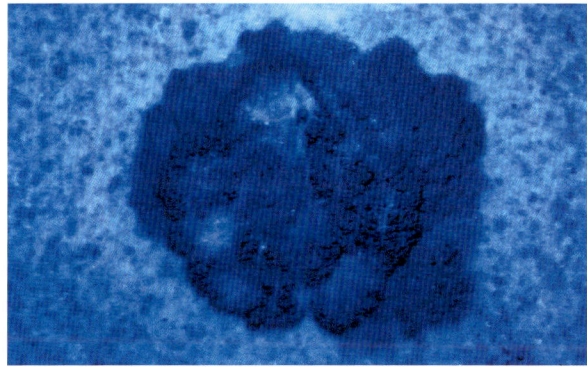

**Fig. 45.** FDAP: There is no fluorescence at all

All examined verrucae vulgares (Figs. 46–48) did not show any fluorescence at all.

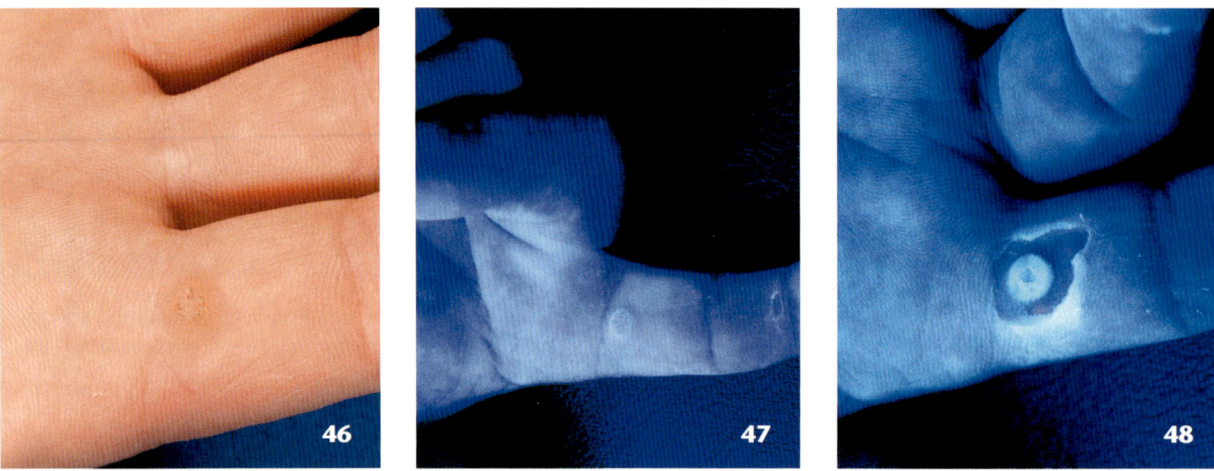

Fig. 46. Vulgar wart on the index finger of the right hand. Hyperkeratotic nodule. Pre-treatment was performed with salicylic acid (5%) containing ointment; Fig. 47. FDAP: The wart does not show any fluorescence. There are reports on the effective use of ALA-PDT in the treatment of warts [Stender et al, 2000]. Speculating that the superficial hyperkeratotic tissue was limiting the penetration of ALA, a more profound curettage was performed; Fig. 48. FDAP: After topical application of salicylic acid containing tapes (Guttaplast®) for 2 weeks and removal of the upper part of the lesion by curettage. There is still no fluorescent tissue detectable indicating that warts do not form sufficient porphyrins after topical ALA treatment

In psoriatic lesions, strong fluorescence intensities were detectable (Figs. 49–52).

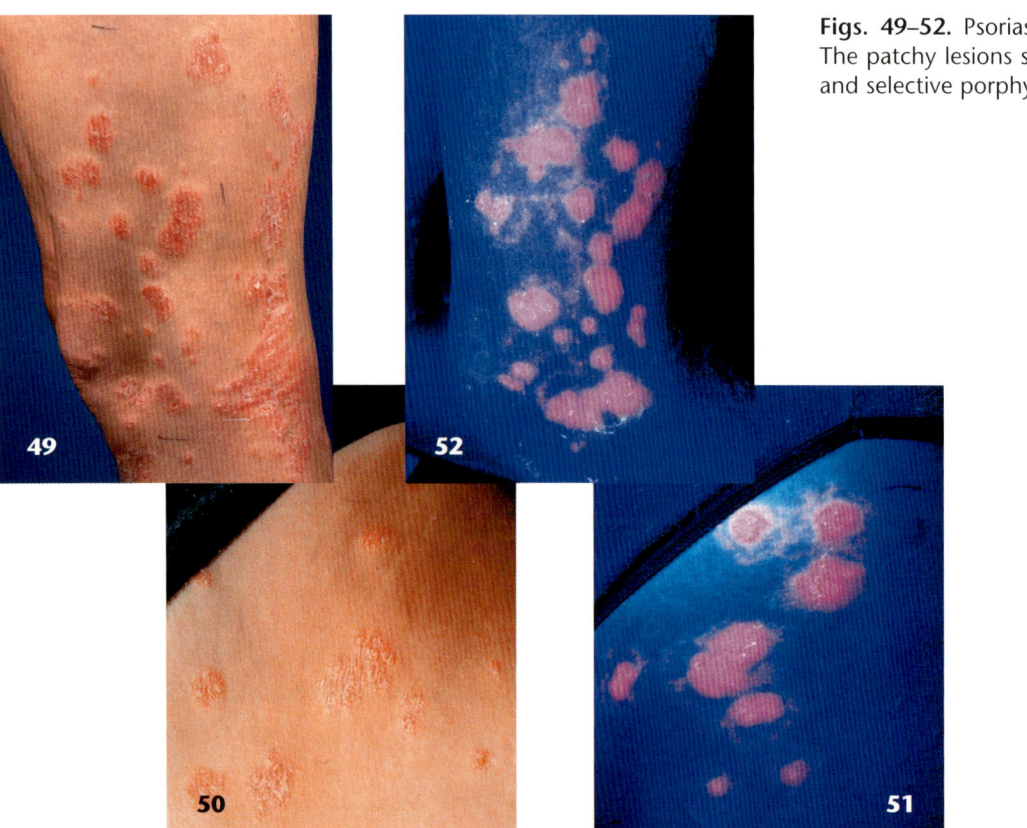

Figs. 49–52. Psoriasis vulgaris. FDAP: The patchy lesions show a very bright and selective porphyrin fluorescence

*Fluorescence patterns in FDAP.* In most epithelial skin tumors, cutaneous precanceroses, PD, and KS the fluorescence patterns were homogeneous. In MF, LE, AE and AV, the fluorescences were partly nonhomogeneous (Figs. 53 and 54).

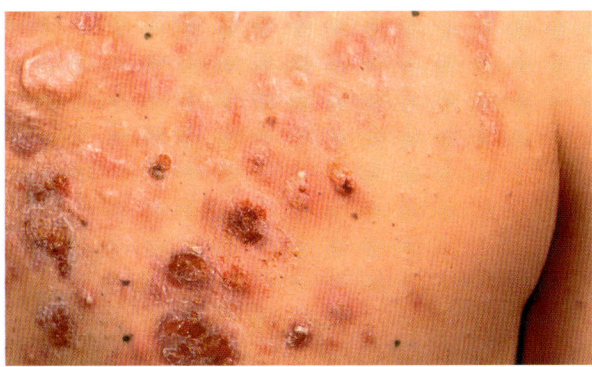

**Fig. 53.** Acne conglobata on the back of a 21-year-old patient. The skin in the right corner was treated by ALA

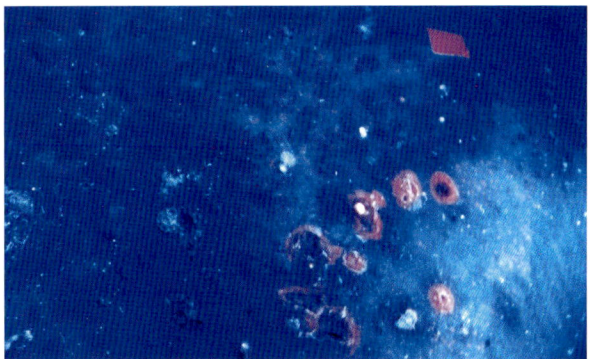

**Fig. 54.** FDAP: Within the treated area the papules reveal bright red fluorescence. Untreated lesions are not fluorescing

Psoriasis showed the lowest homogenicity of all tissues examined (Figs. 55–58).

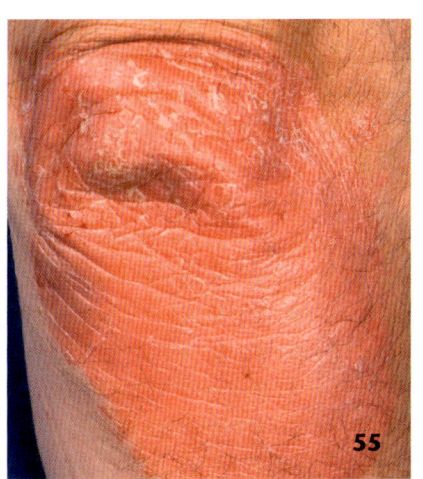
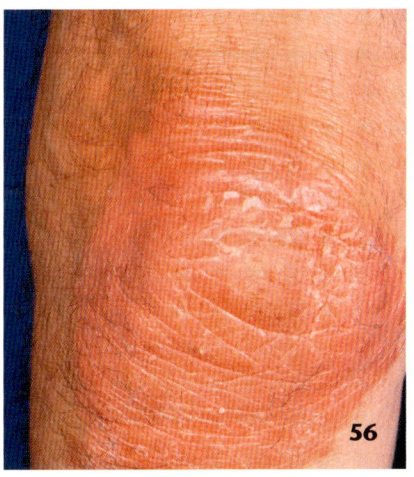

**Figs. 55 and 56.** Psoriatic plaques over the ellbow on both sides. Pre-treatment with an ointment containing 5% salicylic acid was performed twice a day for 7 days. Skin lesions show a symmetrical pattern on both arms

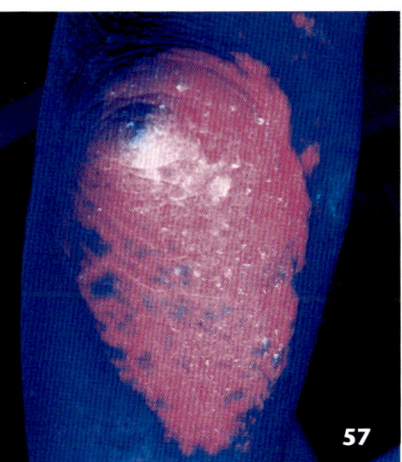
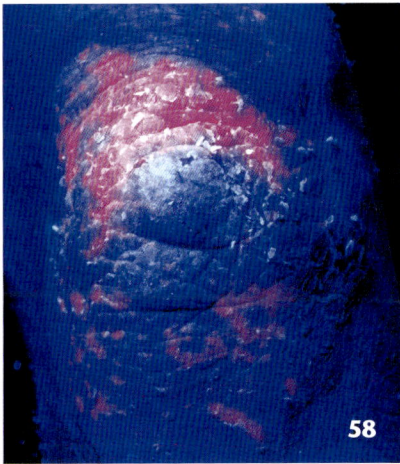

**Figs. 57 and 58.** FDAP: Both plaques display fluorescence of comparable intensity. However, in the lesion on the right ellbow only approximately 20% of the clinically visible lesion area were fluorescing. The reason for this nonhomogeneous fluorescence pattern in psoriatic plaques is still not clarified. Remaining hyperkeratotic tissue or different stages of disease activity might be responsible for this phenomenon

## Chapter Discussion

As presented in Fig. 31, FDAP can be effectively used as a diagnostic tool for detection or delineation in various epithelial precanceroses and tumors. In all cutaneous neoplasms here examined (BCC, SCC, BD, SK, Paget's disease), we measured an intensive, strong and sharply bordered red fluorescence under Wood's light 4–6 h after topical application of ALA. These results illustrate that tumors and psoriasis plaques offer an increased porphyrin biosynthesis in comparison to the adjacent "normal" skin. The increased porphyrin biosynthesis seems to be dependent on a damage of the stratum corneum and an increased proliferating rate of the tissue, which is mainly present in neoplastic or inflammatory processes.

The high fluorescence intensities in psoriatic lesions suggest that psoriasis may also be amenable to treatment by PDT. However, the partly nonhomogeneous fluorescence pattern (Figs. 59 and 60) may give a limitation to PDT in psoriasis.

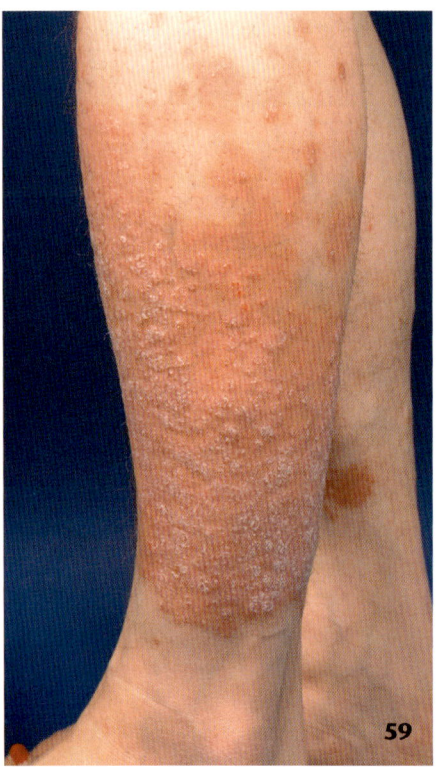
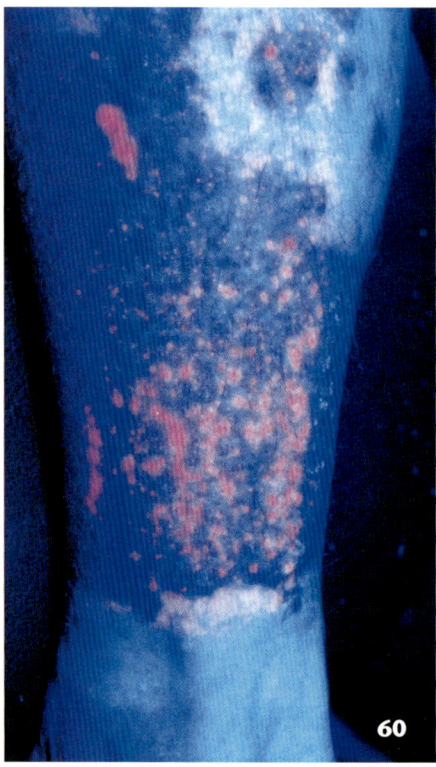

**Figs. 59 and 60.** Psoriatic plaques on the lower leg. FDAP: Nonhomogeneous fluorescence of the psoriatic skin

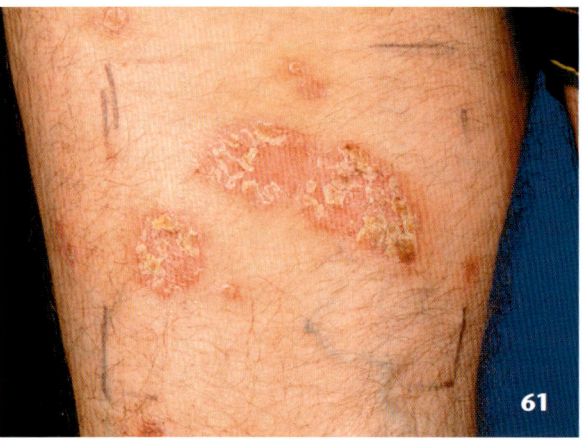
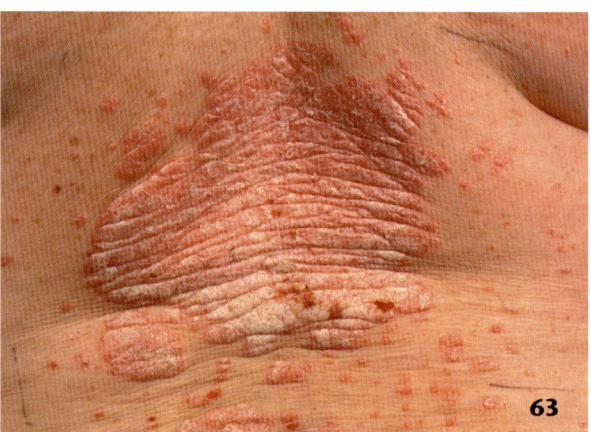

**Figs. 61 and 63.** Psoriatic plaques on the lower leg and on the back

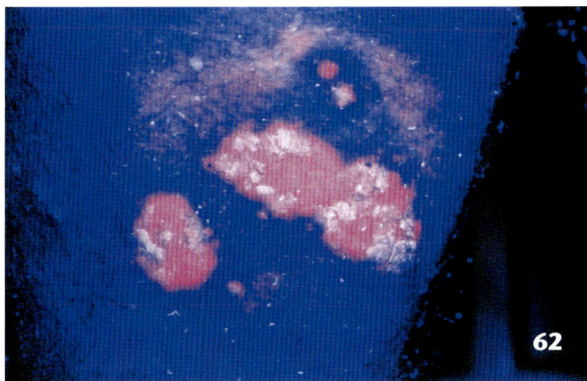
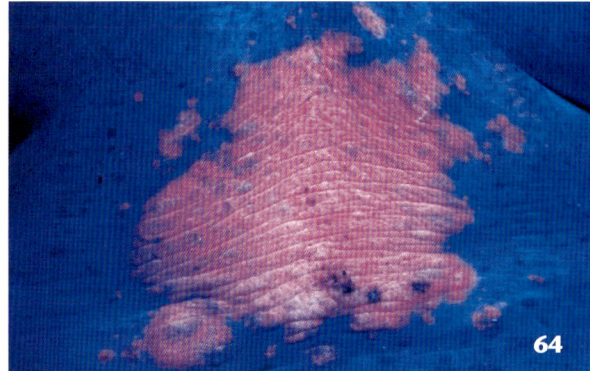

**Figs. 62 and 64.** FDAP: Scales are limiting the fluorescence detection (Fig. 62). After treatment with salicylic acid (5%) ointment, fluorescence is more homogeneous (Fig. 64)

To achieve best results in FDAP, it is recommendable to remove any hyperkeratotic crusts (Figs. 61–64).

The medium strong fluorescence in lesions of lupus erythematosus and in patches of mycosis fungoides supports the idea that these diseases could be approachable to PDT. Even cutaneous B-cell lymphoma displayed high fluorescence in FDAP (Figs. 65 and 66).

There may be several reasons for the slight fluorescence intensity in malignant melanomas. On the one hand, it is well proven by *in vitro* – experiments that melanoma cells can synthesize high levels of porphyrins if ALA is added to the culture medium (Fig. 67) (Bolsen et al, 1997). However, the intact surface of most malignant melanomas may limit the penetration of ALA as compared to, e.g. BCC which present an ulcerated surface. Disturbed skin surface is one postulated key reason for increased ALA penetration in epithelial skin cancers. Physical factors may also take part in the FDAP behavior of malignant melanomas: the melanin-dependent reduced stimulation or emission of the porphyrin fluorescence. These physical factors may also be responsible for the relatively low fluorescence yield in Kaposi's sarcoma. The lack of fluorescence in common warts might be due to comparable physical reasons and, in addition, to the thick epithelial layer.

The brick red fluorescence, typical for porphyrins, is also demonstrated in teeth, urine-soaked diapers and bones of patients with severe porphyrias (Fritsch et al, 1998).

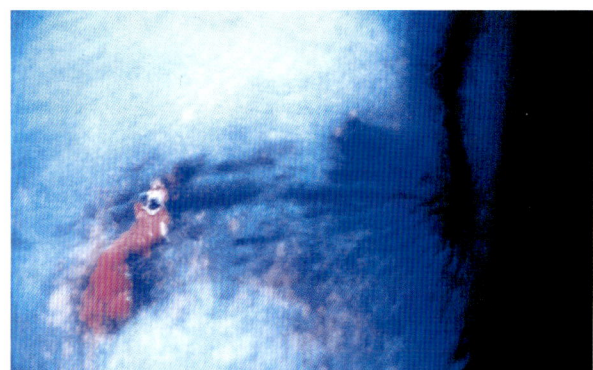

**Fig. 66.** FDAP: The tumorous area shows an intensive fluorescence

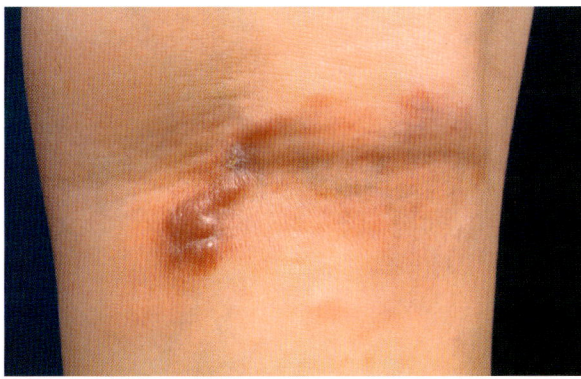

**Fig. 65.** Erythematous brownish tumor in the left knee of a 54-year-old woman. Histopathology proved a B-cell lymphoma. The tumor was classified as B-cell lymphoma of the lower leg

# F  Ex vivo – Investigations on ALA-induced Porphyrins

## F.1 Porphyrin Accumulation in Cells (*in vitro*)

### Material and Methods

ALA-induced porphyrin accumulation was measured in different cells: normal fibroblasts, liver carcinoma cells (HepG2) and melanoma cells (SK-Mel-28). Cells were floated in 10 ml Dulbecco's modified Eagle's medium (DMEM; ICN-Flow, Irvine Scotland), supplemented with 10% fetal calf serum (FCS), penicillin (400 µg/ml/), streptomycin (50 µg/ml) and glutamine (300 µg/ml). Cells were incubated with 1 mM ALA (16.76 mg in 100 ml DMEM) for 36 hours. Incubation was performed in an atmosphere of humidified air with 5% $CO_2$ and 95% air in the dark. Porphyrin analysis was performed prior to, and at 1, 2, 4, 8, 16, 24 and 36 h of incubation. Cell viability was controlled by MTT-Test.

### Results

All cells showed an increased porphyrin synthesis upon ALA-treatment. Maximum porphyrin accumulation was measured after 24 hours (fibroblasts, SK-Mel-28) or 36 hours (HepG2). Porphyrin enrichment in melanoma cells was almost 4-fold as compared to normal fibroblasts (24/36 h) (Fig. 67).

### Chapter Discussion

Thus far the obtained experimental findings do not allow a decision whether the tumor cells in skin accumulate more ALA and/or show an increased porphyrin biosynthesis in comparison to normal cells. The mechanisms of ALA uptake and accumulation in malignant and regenerative cells are not completely understood. Major responsibility for the tumor selectivity of ALA or syntesized porphyrins is the increased permeability of abnormal keratin layers in epithelial skin tumors. The active transport of the compound through plasma membranes was demonstrated in micro-organisms and in cell culture (Rud et al, 2000; Langer et al, 1999). Based on the fact that ALA is synthesized from glycine and succinyl-CoA and is a relatively small molecule like other amino acids it could penetrate the cell membranes. Recent studies showed that active as well as passive transport mechanisms are involved in the uptake of ALA into cells and that the ALA uptake can be competitively inhibited by the amino acid alanine (Kalka et al, 1997; Rud et al, 2000). Probably, with regard to FDAP and PDT, not only the uptake of the amino carbon acid in cells is the limiting and selective step, but the synthesis and the accumulation of the formed porphyrins preferentially in tumor cells are also relevant factors.

Other *in vitro* – studies using different cell cultures (K562 leukemia cells, endothelial cells, HaCaT, fibroblasts, melanoma cell lines: Sk-Mel 23 and Bro) also showed an increased and specific porphyrin synthesis in all cells by application of ALA to the incubation medium. The amount of synthesized porphyrins, however, did not correlate with the malignancy of the cell line (Hananina et al, 1992; Lim et al, 1994; Malik and Lugaci, 1987; Bolsen et al, 1996; Kalka et al, 1997; Ortel et al, 1993).

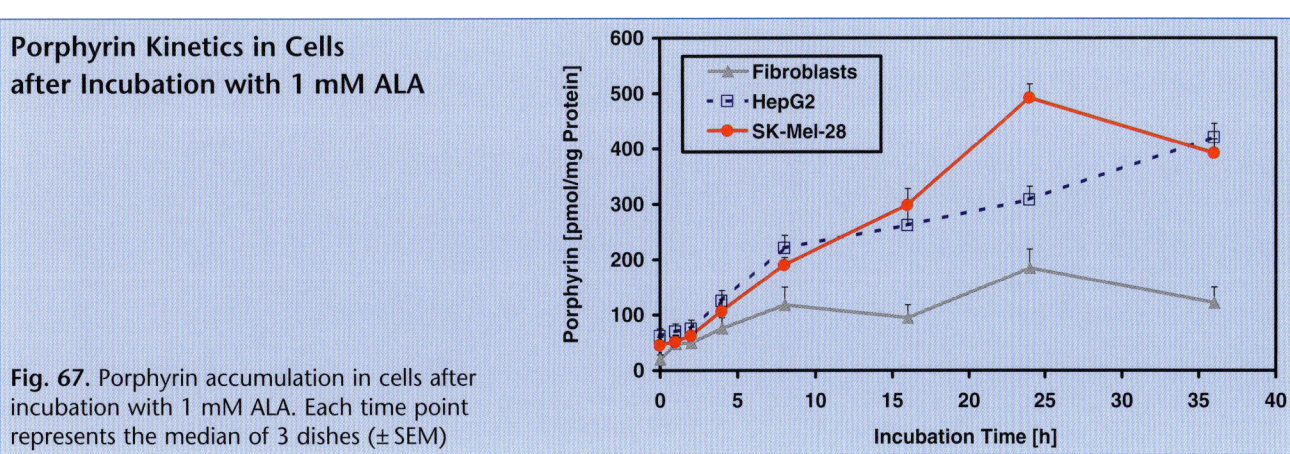

Fig. 67. Porphyrin accumulation in cells after incubation with 1 mM ALA. Each time point represents the median of 3 dishes (± SEM)

## F.2 Porphyrin Accumulation in Skin Tumors, Colon and Bronchial Carcinomas after Administration of ALA (*ex vivo*).

Many authors speculate that the reason for the preferred accumulation of porphyrins in tumors after ALA application is due to differences in the activities of enzymes associated with porphyrin biosynthesis. We found protoporphyrin to be the major porphyrin metabolite, supporting other investigations which postulated this specific porphyrin metabolite as the most active compound in ALA-PDT (Szeimies et al, 1995, Grant et al, 1993, Peng et al, 1992).

### Material and Methods

Using an organic culture model, tissue samples of normal skin, keratoacanthoma, BCC, colon and bronchial carcinoma were incubated with 1 mM ALA as described in Sect. F.1.

### Results

Enrichment of culture medium with ALA as the precursor of porphyrins led to porphyrin formation in all samples with lower amounts in tissues than in supernatants (Fig. 68). Tissues of neoplastic and normal skin accumulated comparable amounts of porphyrins with $0.05 \pm 0.04$ (normal skin), $0.7 \pm 0.1$ (KA) and $0.8 \pm 0.1$ nmol/g tissue (BCC). However, profound differences of porphyrin levels were shown in the corresponding supernatants with six- to seven-fold higher values in the samples of neoplasms (KA: $21.2 \pm 2.1$ and BCC: $17.3 \pm 2.2$ porphyrin/g tissue) than of normal skin ($2.9 \pm 0.3$ nmol/g tissue).

In the supernatant of all samples the predominant metabolite was uroporphyrin followed by coproporphyrin in KA and normal skin ($p < 0.05$: KA vs normal skin), and by protoporphyrin in BCC ($p < 0.05$: BCC vs normal skin) (Fig. 69). However, most important differences in ALA-induced porphyrin patterns were found in tissues. Normal skin and KA showed a marked predominance of uro-

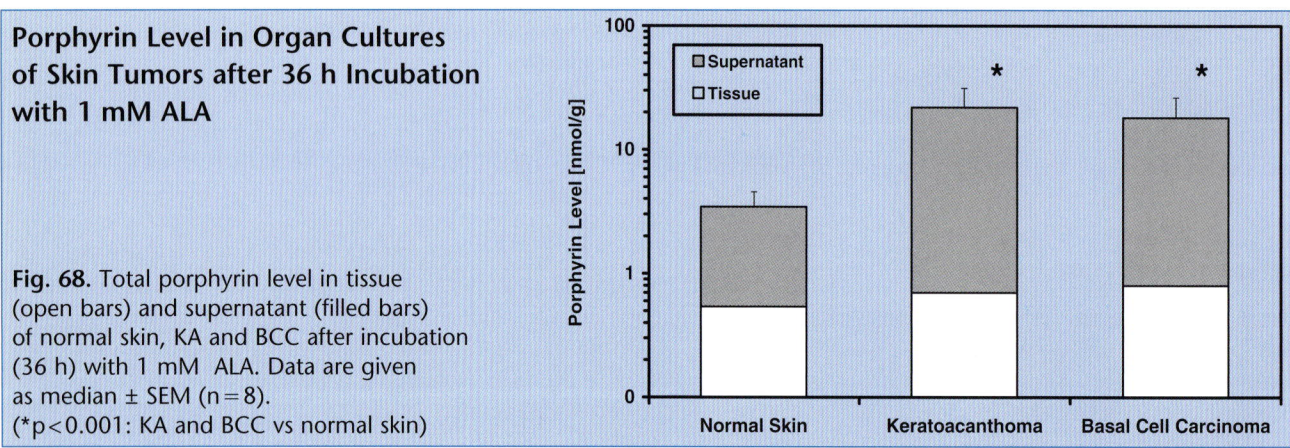

**Porphyrin Level in Organ Cultures of Skin Tumors after 36 h Incubation with 1 mM ALA**

Fig. 68. Total porphyrin level in tissue (open bars) and supernatant (filled bars) of normal skin, KA and BCC after incubation (36 h) with 1 mM ALA. Data are given as median ± SEM (n=8). (*$p<0.001$: KA and BCC vs normal skin)

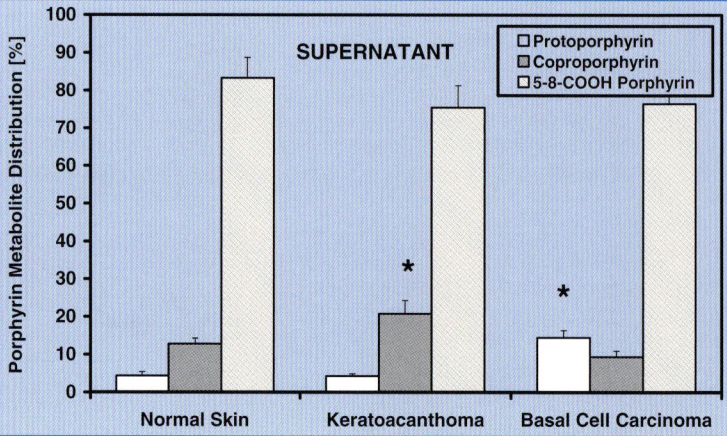

**Porphyrin Metabolites in Organ Cultures of Skin Tumors after 36 h Incubation with 1 mM ALA**

Fig. 69. Porphyrin metabolite distribution in the supernatant of normal skin, KA and BCC after incubation (36 h) with 1 mM ALA. Protoporphyrin, coproporphyrin and the highly carboxylated metabolites (= 5-8-COOH) are presented. Data are given as median ± SD (n=8). (*$p<0.05$ vs. normal skin)

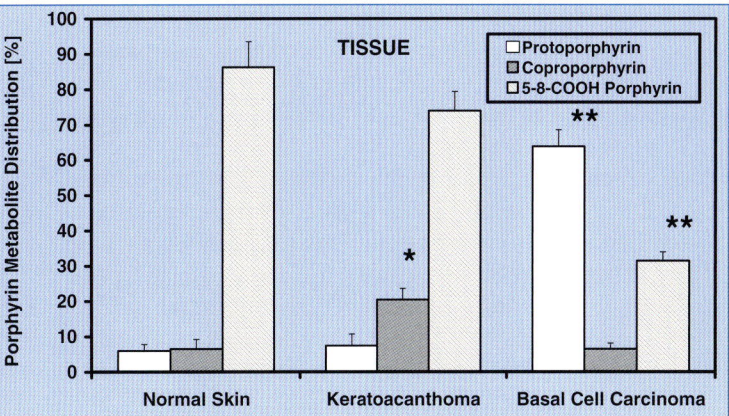

**Porphyrin Metabolites in Organ Cultures of Skin Tumors after 36 h Incubation with 1 mM ALA**

**Fig. 70.** Porphyrin metabolite distribution in tissues normal skin, KA and BCC after incubation (36 h) with 1 mM ALA. Protoporphyrin, coproporphyrin and the highly carboxylated metabolites (=5-8-COOH) are presented. Data are given as median ± SD (n = 8). (*p < 0.05; **p < 0.01 vs. normal skin)

porphyrin in normal skin and KA (p < 0.01: BCC vs normal skin) and coproporphyrin (p < 0.01: KA vs normal skin). In contrast, protoporphyrin was the prevailing metabolite in BCC (p < 0.05: BCC vs normal skin and KA) (Fig. 70).

The biochemical *ex vivo* – measurements showed that bronchial and colon cancers bring the prerequisites for an effective FDAP or PDT. In both tumor tissues, 1,5 to 2 fold higher porphyrin levels than in the tumor surrounding normal tissues were found (Fig. 71).

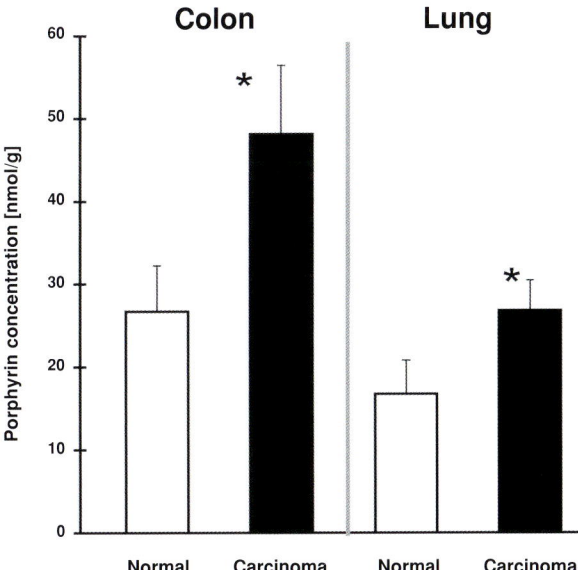

**Fig. 71.** Total porphyrin concentrations in colon and bronchial carcinoma versus normal tissues after *ex vivo*-incubation (36 h) with 1 mM ALA (mean ± SEM; n = 12). Profound differences were found with 26.7 ± 5.6 in colon, 48.2 ± 8.3 in colon carcinoma, 16.8 ± 4.0 in lung and 26.8 ± 3.7 nmol/g tissue in bronchial carcinoma (*p < 0,001 colon carcinoma vs normal colon and bronchial carcinoma vs normal lung)

## Chapter Discussion

The data show that skin tumors as well as other neoplastic tissues such as colon and brochial carcinomas synthesize more porphyrins upon incubation with ALA than normal skin or healthy tumor-surrounding tissue. Although protoporphyrin IX is generally believed to be the photosensitive molecule upon which the technique of PDT depends, present *ex vivo* (Figs. 69 and 70) and *in vivo* data (Fig. 14) suggest the presence of additional tumor-specific photosensitizers such as copro- or uroporphyrin. Photosensitizing efficacy of coproporphyrin is intermediate between protoporphyrin IX and uroporphyrin (Menon et al, 1989).

The obstacle of the mitochondrial ferrochelatase, which catalyzes the iron insertion into protoporphyrin, would lead to a lowered heme concentration with a diminished negative feedback. This could justify the accumulation of protoporphyrin in tumor tissue in analogy to fibroblasts (Bloomer et al, 1977) or lymphocytes (Sassa et al, 1979) of patients with erythropoietic protoporphyria (EPP; congenital defect of the ferrochelatase). The relevance of the heme biosynthesis associated enzymes for porphyrin accumulation in skin was indicated by testing skin biopsies of patients with various porphyrias: patients with acute intermittent porphyria (AIP; defect of the uroporphyrinogen decarboxylase) showed approximately 50% less porphyrin formation in skin in comparison to healthy persons. In contrary, in the skin of patients with porphyria cutanea tarda (PCT; autosomal dominant defect of uroporphyrinogen decarboxylase) increased basal porphyrin amounts and a further induction of porphyrin biosynthesis after application of ALA were found (in comparison with the skin of healthy persons or of AIP patients) (Bickers et al, 1977).

Accordingly, it is conceivable that there is a defect in one or several enzymes of the heme biosynthesis, which leads to the accumulation of heme precursors such as porphyrins. Other enzymes of the porphyrin biosynthesis, such as ALA dehydratase, which was found to be lower in certain tumors (murine mammary carcinoma, human mammary adenocarcinoma) and in liver of tumor-carrying animals, could also contribute to an altered porphyrin synthesis in tumors (Navone et al, 1988; Tschudy and Collins, 1957). The ALA synthase is accepted as being the limiting enzyme of the heme biosynthesis (Kappas et al, 1988).

In erythrocytes, the ALA synthase and the ferrochelatase are limiting steps in the heme biosynthesis due to special circumstances: the ALA synthase is regulated by an X-chromosomal located gene. In all other cells, the chromosome-13 located gene of a different ALA synthase controls the heme biosynthesis (Kappas et al, 1989). Although erythrocytes and tumor cells are profoundly different, it may be assumed that in tumor cells or rapidly proliferating cells in addition to ALA synthase also ferrochelatase is limiting. This is indicated by fluorescence measurements and biochemical findings, demonstrating an enrichment of protoporphyrin in tumor models (*in vivo*, *ex vivo*) after treatment with ALA (Grant et al, 1993; Peng et al, 1992; Szeimies et al, 1995, Fritsch et al, 1999).

# G  *In vivo* – Investigations on ALA-induced Porphyrins/FDAP

Up to now studies on porphyrin biosynthesis in human skin are scarce (Bickers et al, 1977; Goerz et al, 1995; Navone et al, 1988). Examinations were predominantly done to study the pathomechanism of porphyria diseases, but recently porphyrin studies have been increasingly used to measure the effect of PDT with ALA-induced porphyrins. The main questions are, why tumor cells display increased uptake of ALA and why tumors predominantly transform ALA into porphyrins, accumulate them and do not metabolize porphyrins to heme.

The ALA concentrations (1–20%) and vehicles (ointment) used in our department as well as those mentioned in the literature show sufficient efficacy in FDAP and PDT. It is not yet clarified which mechanism is relevant for the penetration of ALA into the skin. The stratum corneum is the main barrier for substances applied topically to the skin. As the keratin layers of superficial skin tumors and precanceroses are pathologically changed, ALA is able to penetrate quickly into these lesions in contrast to normal skin where the ALA uptake is lower due to an intact surface (Peng et al, 1995; Szeimies et al, 1994). The uptake of ALA or ALA-induced porphyrins in skin can be fortified by treating the skin with dimethylsulfoxide (DMSO), which leads to a destruction of the skin barrier (Peng et al, 1995). This is another hint for the implication of a damaged stratum corneum for enhanced ALA penetration.

## G.1 FDAP: Kinetics of ALA-induced Porphyrins in Human Cutaneous Tumors, Psoriasis Lesions and Normal Skin

### Material and Methods

Tissue samples used were: basal cell carcinomas (BCC; n = 32), squamous cell carcinomas (SCC; n = 32), psoriatic lesions (PS; n = 32), normal skin (NS; n = 160). Tumor samples were obtained from patients who underwent surgery. Psoriatic tissue samples were taken from punch biopsies that were excised for histopathological examination. Patients received detailed information according to the declaration of Helsinki.

Normal skin was examined: (a) from patients with tumors or psoriasis which were treated with ALA, and (b) from subjects free of tumor or psoriasis. Tissue samples of normal skin from patients with tumors or psoriasis were either taken from the tumor- or psoriasis-adjacent site (NS-A) or from locations distant from the lesions (NS-D) = individual controls. Additionally, normal skin samples (NS) were obtained from patients free of BCC, SCC or PS = interindividual controls. This study design was chosen to investigate the influence of the proximity of normal skin to neoplastic or psoriatic skin on ALA-induced porphyrin accumulation. Each patient received comprehensive information about the scope of the study.

*ALA-treatment and FDAP.* Pilot studies on topical ALA application (up to 80 mg/cm$^2$) to normal skin revealed plateau porphyrin levels (approximately 4 nmol/g protein) > 40 mg ALA cm$^2$ (data not shown). Based on these data and due to clinical experience in ALA-PDT (Calzavara-Pinton et al, 1995; Wolf et al, 1993) an ALA (hydrochloride) mixture of 20% was prepared in an ointment (Neribas®, Schering, Berlin, Germany). Of the 20% ALA mixture, 0.2 g (40 mg ALA cm$^2$) were applied to a 1 cm$^2$ skin area of BCC, SCC, psoriatic lesions, and all normal skin lesions. Treated skin was covered with an occlusive foil (Tegaderm®, 3M Healthcare, Borken, Germany), gauze, aluminum foil and tape to enhance tissue penetration and avoid photobleaching of the formed porphyrins. After defined incubation times (1, 2, 4, 6, 9, 12 and 24 h) the tape and the ointment were removed and the treated area was illuminated with Wood's light (Fluotest®, Xenotest, Hanau, Germany; 370–405 nm). Basal values were obtained from untreated skin areas. Fluorescence intensity was measured and expressed semiquantitatively according to a fluorescence standard as 0 (no), 1 (low), 2 (medium) and 3 (strong fluorescence). The fluorescent area was marked. According to our clinical experience, BCC and SCC revealed a strong, homogeneous, ALA-induced porphyrin fluorescence under Wood's light (Figs. 33 and 35) (Fritsch et al, 1996, Fritsch et al, 1997), whereas about 20–40% of psoriatic lesions showed areas with nonhomogeneous or even lacking fluorescence (Figs. 58, 60 and 62). For better comparison of intralesional porphyrin formation in PS and tumors, only uniform fluorescing psoriatic areas were selected for the study. Biochemical analysis was also performed in nonfluorescing psoriatic areas (n = 8) which were treated with ALA for 6 h.

*Preparation of skin samples.* Only superficial layers of skin samples (<1 mm) were included in the study due to the limited penetration of topically applied ALA (Szeimies et al, 1994; Martin et al, 1995; Peng et al, 1995). Immediately after excision tissue samples were frozen in liquid nitrogen and stored at –80°C until further examination.

*Determination of total porphyrin and protein levels in tissues.* Tissue samples were weighed and cut into small pieces. After homogenization with an Ultraturrax and centrifugation at 3000 U/min for 10 min, porphyrins were isolated with 1.0 N perchloric acid/methanol (1/1, v/v). In the supernatant, the total porphyrin level was assessed by fluorescence spectroscopy (Perkin Elmer LS-5, Uberlingen, Germany); emission was recorded in a range of 520–700 nm at an excitation wavelength of 405 nm (Soret band). For quantification a protoporphyrin standard (Porphyrin Products Inc., Logan, Utah, USA) was used (Fritsch et al, 1999). Protein levels were determined in the pellet according to (Lowry et al, 1951).

*Determination of porphyrin metabolites in tissues.* The supernatant was adjusted with acetic acid to pH 3–4, porphyrins were bound to talcum, esterified and metabolites were identified by HPLC with fluorescence detection (L-7480, Merck Hitachi, Darmstadt, Germany) using a porphyrin standard mixture (Porphyrin Products Inc., Logan, Utah, USA) for quantification (Seubert and Seubert, 1982). The following metabolites were analyzed: protoporphyrin, tricarboxylic porphyrin, coproporphyrin, pentacarboxylic porphyrin, hexacarboxylic porphyrin, heptacarboxylic porphyrin and uroporphyrin. The last four porphyrin metabolites are designated as highly carboxylated porphyrins (5-8-COOH-porphyrins); data are given as the sum of these compounds.

*Statistical calculation.* Statistical analysis of the data was performed by Student's t-test. Data are reported as mean ± SEM. Changes were considered statistically significant when $P < 0.05$.

## Results

*Fluorescence intensities of treated tissues.* The highest macroscopic fluorescence intensities were found in BCC, SCC and PS 4–6 hours after ALA application. At all time-points normal skin (NS) revealed only slight fluorescence intensities compared with neoplastic and psoriatic skin (Table 2).

*Porphyrin levels.* In untreated tissues (basal values), the levels of total porphyrins were similarly low in normal skin, tumors and psoriasis (Fig. 72). ALA application induced porphyrin synthesis in all tissues. The porphyrin levels in BCC and SCC showed maximum values between 2 hours (53.8 ± 19.3 and 46.8 ± 17.3) and 6 hours (60.0 ± 13.4 and 49.4 ± 13.1 nmol/mg protein).

The highest porphyrin accumulation was measured in psoriatic lesions with 91.7 ± 14.4 nmol/mg protein at 6 h. Normal skin samples: in NS and NS-D, the accumulation of ALA-induced porphyrins was comparably low with a maximum at 24 hours (15.6 ± 6.6 nmol/mg protein) (Fig. 72); at 6 h, NS-A close to tumors or PS showed higher porphyrin levels (23.8 ± 4.0 and 19.1 ± 4.1 nmol/mg protein) than NS or normal skin distant from lesions (NS-D).

The ratio of porphyrins measured in BCC vs NS (BCC/NS) showed maximum values between 1 and 6 hours (4.8–5.5) (Fig. 72). The maximum ratio of porphyrins SCC/NS (4.8–5.1) was observed 1–4 h after ALA application. In PS, there was the most distinct maximum of the porphyrin ratio to NS with 7.0 after 6 hours. However, using normal skin adjacent to tumors of PS (NS-A) as reference, the ratios of porphyrin levels in lesions vs skin were lower: maximum values were measured after 2 h for BCC (3.7), after 4 h for SCC (3.3) and after 6 h for PS (4.8).

*Porphyrin metabolites.* The pattern of porphyrin metabolites was comparable in all untreated tissues with protoporphyrin as the predominant metabolite (82.9–92.3%) followed by uropor-

**Table 2.** Fluorescence intensities of tissues treated with 20% ALA

| | Application time of ALA | | | | | | |
|---|---|---|---|---|---|---|---|
| | 1 h | 2 h | 4 h | 6 h | 9 h | 12 h | 24 h |
| NS | 0.8 ± 0.2 | 0.8 ± 0.2 | 0.8 ± 0.2 | 1.3 ± 0.2 | 1.5 ± 0.3 | 1.5 ± 0.3 | **1.5 ± 0.3** |
| BCC | 2.8 ± 0.2 | 2.6 ± 0.2 | 2.8 ± 0.2 | **2.9 ± 0.2** | 2.6 ± 0.2 | 2.8 ± 0.2 | 2.5 ± 0.2 |
| SCC | 2.8 ± 0.2 | 2.5 ± 0.3 | **3.0 ± 0.2** | 2.8 ± 0.2 | 2.5 ± 0.3 | 2.5 ± 0.3 | 2.3 ± 0.2 |
| Psoriasis | 1.3 ± 0.2 | 1.8 ± 0.4 | **2.8 ± 0.2** | **2.8 ± 0.2** | 2.5 ± 0.3 | 2.5 ± 0.3 | 1.5 ± 0.3 |

Fluorescence intensities of ALA-treated skin irradiated by Wood's light (370–405 nm, 10 cm distance, 5 mW/cm$^2$). Values are given semiquantitatively according to a fluorescence standard: 0 = no fluorescence, 3 = maximum fluorescence (n = 4; mean ± SEM). Fluorescence of normal skin (NS) was measured in patients free of tumors and psoriasis. NS, BCC, SCC or PS not treated by ALA did not show any fluorescence

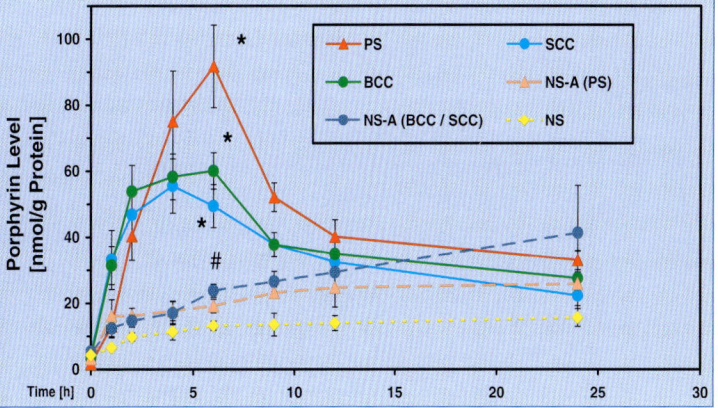

**Porphyrin Level after Topical Aplication of 20% ALA**

**Fig. 72.** Porphyrin levels in BCC, SCC, PS, NS adjacent to tumors [NS-A (BCC and SCC)], NS adjacent to PS [NS-A (PS)] and NS of patients with tumor or psoriasis but not treated by ALA. In all tumor and psoriatic tissues, the maximum porphyrin accumulation was detected at 2–6 h after ALA application (*$p < 0.005$ BCC, SCC, PS vs NS). NS-A showed higher porphyrin levels than NS obtained from patients free of lesions, respectively (#$p < 0.05$). Porphyrin levels in NS distant from lesions (NS-D) were not different from those measured in NS (data are not included in this figure). Mean ± SEM [n = 4; except NS-A (BCC, SCC): n = 8 for each data point]

phyrin (all tissues) (4.6–6.2%), heptacarboxylic porphyrin (NS: 0.9% and PS: 1.5%), and coproporphyrin (BCC: 2.7% and SCC: 3.9%). The pattern of metabolites was not changed following ALA treatment. Protoporphyrin was still the predominant metabolite and accumulated in all tissues over a period of 24 hours. Only at 1 h there was a slight decrease in protoporphyrin and a slight increase in the highly carboxylated porphyrins. At the timepoint of the maximum ratio of porphyrins in BCC/NS, SCC/NS or PS/NS (1–12 h, 6 h), protoporphyrin was the prevailing metabolite in all lesions.

## Chapter Discussion

In normal human tissues (liver, fatty tissue, skin), the basal porphyrin levels were shown to be low with 0.2–1.2 nmol/g (Goerz et al, 1995). Basal porphyrin concentrations in human tumors such as bronchial carcinoma, carcinomas of the gastrointestinal tract (Fig. 71), epithelial skin tumors such as BCC and SCC (Fig. 72) (Fritsch et al, 1999), or precancerous lesions such as SK (Fig. 73) (Fritsch et al, 1998) were also low with <1 nmol/g. Skin tumors and normal skin showed comparable basal porphyrin levels. This finding refutes the theory that tumors may have altered activities of one or more enzymes associated to the hemebiosynthesis. The increased permeability through the damaged keratin layer by ALA seems to be the major responsible factor for the tumor selective enrichment. This phenomenon contributes to the greatest limitation of topical ALA-PDT; the poor ALA-drug penetration through intact keratinized surface layers of nodular tumors may be the reason for the therapeutic refractoriness of these malignancies.

Treatment of cutaneous tissues *ex vivo* (Figs. 68–71) (Fritsch et al, 1997) or *in vivo* (Fig. 72) (Fritsch et al, 1999) with exogenous ALA led to an increased synthesis of porphyrins. In addition, the biochemical studies proved that the increased fluorescence intensity correlated with the concentrations extracted of porphyrin in the tumor tissues (Fritsch et al, 1997; Grant et al, 1993; Hua et al, 1995, Peng et al, 1992). However, reports on FDAP, so far, only concerned experiences with bladder cancers (Kriegmair et al, 1994; Steinbach et al, 1994) and intracerebral tumors (Stummer et al, 1998). The biochemical studies on ALA-induced porphyrins presented here were the first which clearly defined the time points of maximum (optimum) porphyrin enrichment in BCC, SCC and psoriatic lesions. According to these data, we recommend the performance of FDAP or PDT in SCC or BCC at 2–4 hours and in psoriatic lesions at 4–6 hours after ALA application. As the kinetics of the visible fluorescence (Table 2) corresponds well with biochemically measured porphyrin metabolites, it can be stated that FDAP gives a valid representation of intralesionally accumulated porphyrins. Therefore, FDAP can be recommended a use as a diagnostic tool for the detection of epithelial skin cancers and to evaluate if a specific dermatological disease is suitable for an effective PDT.

## G.2 FDAP: Kinetics of Porphyrin Accumulation in Solar Keratoses: ALA versus ALA Methylester

### Material and Methods

Tissues samples of solar keratoses (SK) and normal skin (NS) adjacent to the lesions (each n = 40) were obtained from patients who underwent surgery. Tissue samples were taken as follows: without substrate application (n = 8), 1 h after application of ALA (n = 8) or ALA methylester (ALA-ME) (n = 8) and 6 h after application of ALA (n = 8) or ALA-ME (n = 8). One part of the excised tissue was examined histopathologically. Each patient received comprehensive information about the scope of the study (Fritsch et al, 1998).

*ALA treatment and FDAP.* Based on pilot studies of topical ALA application (Fritsch et al, 1999) and on clinical experience in ALA-PDT (Fritsch et al, 1998; Wolf et al, 1993, Fijan et al, 1995), 20% ALA hydrochloride (Merck, Darmstadt Germany) or the short-chain methyl ester (Sigma Aldrich Chemie, Deisenhofen, Germany) were mixed in an ointment (Neribas®, Schering, Berlin, Germany) and 0.2 g of this mixture was applied to a 1 cm² skin area (= 40 mg/cm²) of SK or NS. Treated skin was covered with an occlusive foil (Tegaderm®, 3M Healthcare, Borken, Germany), gauze, aluminum foil and tape to enhance tissue penetration and avoid photobleaching of porphyrins. After 1 or 6 h, the ointment was removed and the treated area was illuminated with Wood's light (Fluotest®, Xenotest, Hanau, Germany; 370–405 nm). Detected fluorescence intensity was expressed semiquantitatively relative to a fluorescence standard. The fluorescent area was marked. Basal values were obtained from untreated controls.

*Preparation of skin samples.* Only superficial layers of skin (<1 mm) were included in the study because of the limited penetration of topically applied ALA (Martin et al, 1995, Peng et al, 1995; Szeimies et al, 1994). Immediately after excision, tissue samples were frozen in liquid nitrogen and stored at −80°C.

*Determination of total porphyrin and protein levels.* Tissue samples were weighed and cut into small pieces. After homogenization with an Ultraturrax and centrifugation at 3000 U/min for 10 min, porphyrins were isolated with 1.0 N perchloric acid/methanol (1/1, vol/vol). In the supernatant, the total porphyrin level was assessed by fluorescence spectroscopy (Perkin Elmer LS-5, Überlingen, Germany); emission was recorded between 520 and 700 nm at an excitation wavelength of 405 nm (Soret band). A protoporphyrin standard was obtained from Porphyrin Products (Logan, UT, USA) (Fritsch et al, 1997). Protein levels were determined in the pellet (Lowry et al, 1957). The relative porphyrin enrichment was expressed by the ratio of porphyrin levels in SK versus adjacent NS.

*Porphyrin metabolites.* The supernatant was adjusted with acetic acid to pH 3–4, porphyrins were bound to talcum, esterified and metabolites were identified by HPLC with fluorescence detection (L-7480, Merck Hitachi, Darmstadt Germany) using a porphyrin standard mixture (Porphyrin Products) for quantification (Seubert and Seubert, 1982). The following metabolites were analyzed: protoporphyrin, tricarboxylic porphyrin, coproporphyrin, pentacarboxylic porphyrin, hexacarboxylic porphyrin, heptacarboxylic porphyrin and uroporphyrin. The latter four porphyrins are designated as highly carboxylated porphyrins (5-8-COOH-porphyrins).

*Statistical calculation.* Statistical analysis was performed by Student's T-test. Data are reported as means ± SEM. Changes were considered statistically significant when the p value was < 0.05.

## Results

*Fluorescence intensities of treated tissues.* In SK, fluorescence intensity was higher using topical treatment with ALA than ALA-ME for 6 h. In normal skin, fluorescence was weaker for ALA-ME than for ALA (Table 3).

**Table 3.** Fluorescence intensities of tissues treated by ALA or ALA methylester

|  | ALA | | ALA methylester | |
| --- | --- | --- | --- | --- |
|  | 1 h | 6 h | 1 h | 6 h |
| Normal skin | 1.1 ± 0.2 | 1.9 ± 0.3 | 0.5 ± 0.2 | 0.8 ± 0.2 |
| Solar keratoses | 1.9 ± 0.2 | 2.9 ± 0.1 | 1.4 ± 0.2 | 1.9 ± 0.2 |

Fluorescence intensities of skin treated by ALA or ALA methylester irradiated by Wood's light (370–410 nm, 10 cm distance, 5 mW/cm²). Values are given semiquantitatively according to a fluorescence standard: 0 = no fluorescence, 3 = maximum fluorescence (n = 8; mean ± SEM).

*Basal total porphyrin levels.* In untreated tissues, the levels of total porphyrins were similarly low: 1.2 ± 0.1 in normal skin and 1.3 ± 0.1 nmol/g protein in SK (Fig. 71).

*Total porphyrin levels after topical application of ALA or ALA-ME.* Topical application of both compounds led to increased porphyrin levels in SK compared to NS. Highest levels were detected at 6 h. The ALA treatment induced highest porphyrin values: 36.4 ± 4.0 in SK and 7.2 ± 0.5 nmol/g protein in NS adjacent to the lesions (Fig. 73). Using ALA-ME as substrate, porphyrin levels in SK were 14.9 ± 2.2 nmol/g protein, which is less than 50% of the amount induced by ALA. Furthermore, lowest porphyrin levels were detected in NS treated with ALA-ME (1.7 ± 0.2 nmol/g protein), which is four times less than for ALA (Fig. 74).

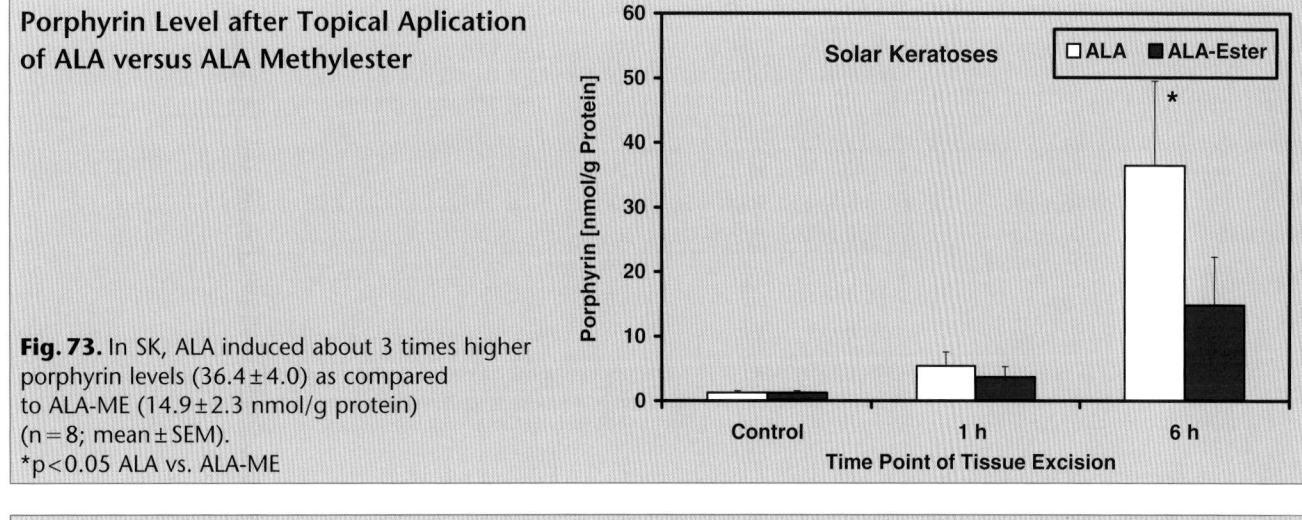

**Fig. 73.** In SK, ALA induced about 3 times higher porphyrin levels (36.4 ± 4.0) as compared to ALA-ME (14.9 ± 2.3 nmol/g protein) (n = 8; mean ± SEM).
*p < 0.05 ALA vs. ALA-ME

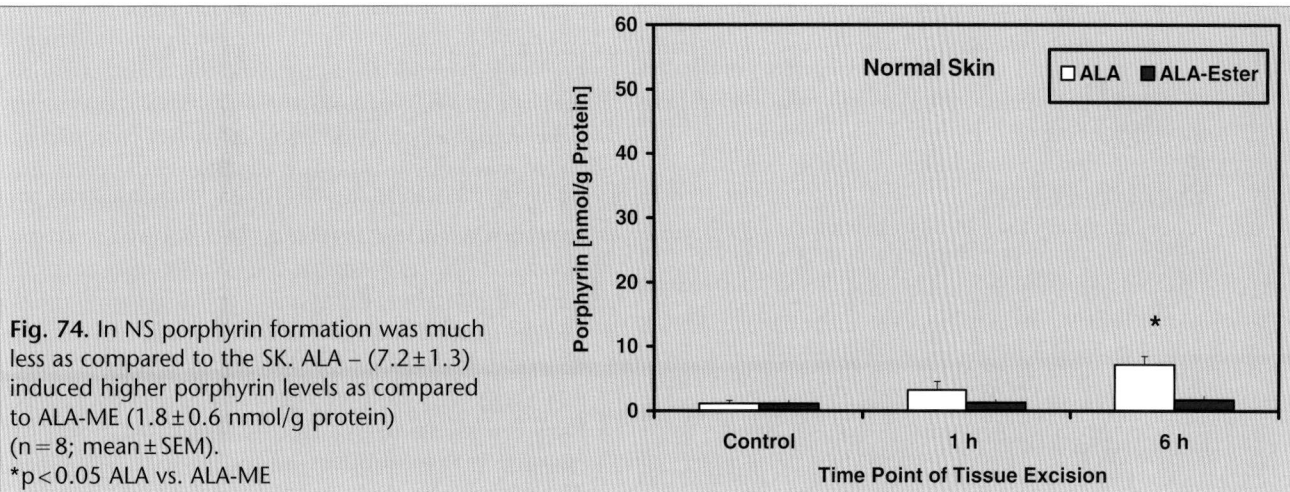

**Fig. 74.** In NS porphyrin formation was much less as compared to the SK. ALA – (7.2 ± 1.3) induced higher porphyrin levels as compared to ALA-ME (1.8 ± 0.6 nmol/g protein) (n = 8; mean ± SEM).
*p < 0.05 ALA vs. ALA-ME

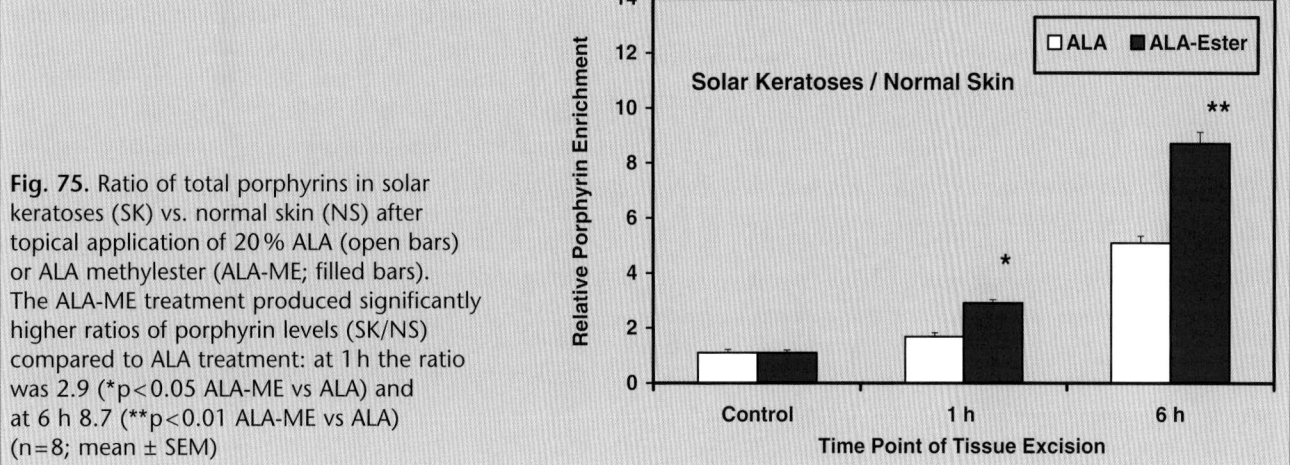

**Fig. 75.** Ratio of total porphyrins in solar keratoses (SK) vs. normal skin (NS) after topical application of 20 % ALA (open bars) or ALA methylester (ALA-ME; filled bars). The ALA-ME treatment produced significantly higher ratios of porphyrin levels (SK/NS) compared to ALA treatment: at 1 h the ratio was 2.9 (*p < 0.05 ALA-ME vs ALA) and at 6 h 8.7 (**p < 0.01 ALA-ME vs ALA) (n = 8; mean ± SEM)

The relative porphyrin enrichment, i.e., the ratio of the level in SK vs. NS (SK/NS), showed maximum values at 6 h: 5.1 for ALA and 8.7 for ALA-ME (Fig. 75).

*Porphyrin metabolite levels in SK and normal skin.* The basal pattern of porphyrin metabolites was comparable in both untreated tissues with protoporphyrin as the predominant metabolite

Table 4. Porphyrin metabolites in skin and SK after topical application of ALA or ALA-ME

|  | Substrate | Total porphyrins | Proto-porphyrin | Copro-porphyrin | Penta-carboxylic porphyrin | Hexa-carboxylic porphyrin | Hepta-carboxylic porphyrin | Uro porphyrin |
|---|---|---|---|---|---|---|---|---|
|  |  | (nmol/g protein) | (%) | (%) | (%) | (%) | (%) | (%) |
| Normal skin | No | 1.2 ± 0.1 | 91 ± 7 | 3 ± 1 | 1 ± 1 | 0 ± 1 | 0 ± 4 | 1 ± 3 |
|  | ALA | 7.2 ± 0.5 | 90 ± 2 | 0 ± 1 | 0 ± 0 | 0 ± 0 | 4 ± 1 | 7 ± 1 |
|  | ALA-ME | 1.7 ± 0.2 | 89 ± 2 | 0 ± 0 | 0 ± 0 | 1 ± 0 | 4 ± 0 | 6 ± 1 |
| Solar keratoses | No | 1.3 ± 0.1 | 89 ± 7 | 3 ± 3 | 0 ± 0 | 0 ± 1 | 1 ± 1 | 7 ± 9 |
|  | ALA | 36.4 ± 4.0* | 90 ± 1 | 1 ± 1 | 0 ± 0 | 2 ± 1 | 2 ± 0 | 3 ± I |
|  | ALA-ME | 14.9 ± 2.2† | 82 ± 4 | 8 ± 2 | 0 ± 1 | 2 ± 1 | 5 ± 1 | 5 ± 1 |

Data are given as nmol porphyrin/g protein and percent of total porphyrins (n = 8; mean ± SEM; *P < 0.005, †P < 0.01: solar keratoses vs. normal skin). Porphyrin patterns showed no significant differences between solar keratoses and normal skin

(89–91%) followed by uroporphyrin and coproporphyrin (Table 4). The pattern of metabolites remained unchanged upon treatment. Protoporphyrin was still the predominant metabolite (82–91%) and accumulated in SK and normal skin over the period of 6 h.

## Chapter Discussion

Highest levels of porphyrins are achieved after 6 h in SK and normal skin. The study was focused on the application times of 1 and 6 h, because of the evaluated time course of ALA-induced porphyrin formation in epithelial skin tumors with maximum intralesional porphyrin levels between 1 and 6 h (Fritsch et al, 1999) (Fig. 72).

Porphyrin accumulation was more intense using ALA than ALA-ME, suggesting that ALA may penetrate the epidermal barrier with subsequent conversion into porphyrins more efficiently than ALA-ME, which requires hydrolysis after penetration. Using ALA the lesion-adjacent normal skin also accumulated relatively high porphyrin amounts. In contrast, the topical application of ALA-ME diminishes porphyrin sensitization in normal skin. Regarding the relative enrichment in porphyrin levels for SK/NS, ALA-ME seems to penetrate preferentially the damaged skin of SK (Fig. 75). The low levels of porphyrins in perilesional NS might be primarily due to weak penetration of ALA-ME through intact skin, less formation of porphyrins from the ester form due to slower de-esterification in normal keratinocytes or lower leakage of intralesionally formed porphyrins into the perilesional tissue as postulated for ALA (Fritsch et al, 1999).

The formation of porphyrins after topical application of ALA esters was recently investigated in murine skin (Peng et al, 1996). All ALA derivatives studied there (methylester, ethylester and propylester) showed higher induction of porphyrin fluorescence than free ALA, particularly after a prolonged application time of 14 h. In contrast, our human *in vivo* data show that NS is less sensitized with porphyrins using ALA-ME when compared with ALA. The use of different species and the lack of neoplastic tissue in mice used might explain the different results. It is known that perilesional NS, as examined in our study, accumulates about three times more porphyrin than NS distant from lesions such as SCC when treated topically by ALA (Fig. 72) (Fritsch et al, 1999). Thus, it is surprising as well as encouraging that the NS localized close to the SK accumulated only low porphyrin levels upon treatment with ALA-ME. The specificity of ALA-ME versus ALA may also differ depending on the time of application.

The porphyrin metabolite pattern shows normal activity of the heme-biosynthesis-associated enzymes in human SK. The accumulation of higher total porphyrin levels appears to be the major effect responsible for intralesional photosensitization.

The penetration depth of porphyrin fluorescence induced by topical ALA was shown to be nonhomogeneous (Martin et al, 1995; Szeimies et al, 1994; Peng et al, 1995; Warloe et al, 1992; Stringer et al, 1996, Malik et al, 1995). Further studies have to show whether ALA esters are superior to free ALA with respect to homogeneous porphyrin formation, especially in the deeper parts of neoplastic lesions.

In topical ALA-PDT, local photosensitivity commonly lasts for a maximum of to 48 h (Fig. 72) (Lang et al, 2001). The higher lesional selectivity of ALA-ME-induced porphyrins leads to reduced cutaneous light sensitivity, particularly in perilesional NS. Based on *in vitro* data it might be speculated that long-chain ALA esters are even more efficient in PDT than ALA or short-chain ALA esters (Gaullier et al, 1997). Optimum efficacy of topical PDT may be expected if irradiation of SK is performed 3 h after treatment with ALA-ME. For FDAP however, using ALA or ALA-ME, application times of 5–6 h are recommendable to achieve an optimum fluorescence contrast (Fritsch et al, 1996; Fritsch et al, 1998; Lang et al, 2001). The use of ALA esters in PDT and FDAP seems to be a promising modality with highly selective intralesional porphyrin formation.

## G.3 FDAP: Use of the *in vivo* – Fluorescence for Surgical Planning

### Material and Methods

*FDAP – procedure*. Sixtyfour lesions clinically suspicious to be epithelial skin tumors were treated by FDAP-guided surgery from March 1998 until December 2000 (Table 5). After a slight debulking procedure, ALA (20% in an ointment) was topically applied. The treated area was covered by an occlusive foil. After 4 h application time the foil and the rest of the mixture were removed. Lesions were illuminated by Wood's light (370–405 nm; Fluolight®, Saalmann, Herford, Germany). Clinical and fluorescence pictures were documented (Figs. 76).

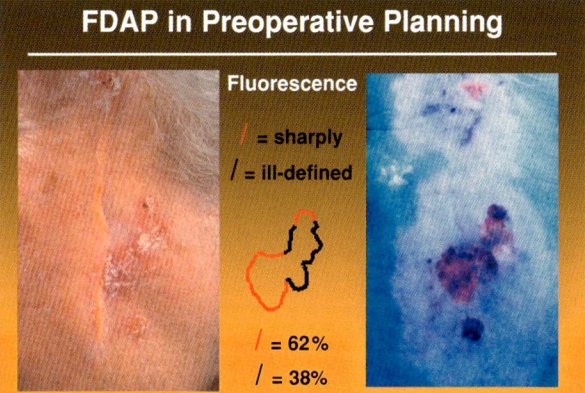

**Fig. 76.** SK on the left cheek, demonstrating the image analysis on the hand of one of the most difficult cases. Clinical picture (left) and FDAP (4 h ALA) (right) are evaluated concerning the delineation of tumor borders. Well-defined fluorescing area was marked by red lines, ill-defined by black ones. Sharply demarcated fluorescence was expressed as percent of the total marked area

*Computer assisted measurement of the fluorescence pattern*. Fluorescence intensity was characterized according to a fluorescence standard (Fig. 30). Values were given semi-quantitatively as 0 = no, 1 = weak, 2 = intermediate, and 3 = strong fluorescence. In addition, the borders of the fluorescent area were analyzed concerning the criteria of sharp demarcation. By means of image analysis (Power Point, Microsoft; Image Access, Imagic) the entire fluorescent area was measured by marking a line. Ill-defined areas were marked in a different color. Percentage of sharply demarcated tumor area was calculated (Fig. 76).

*Clinical demarcation of the macroscopic fluorescence*. While performing the FDAP-procedure, the outer borders of the fluorescence pattern of each lesion were delineated by a surgical pen. Excision of the lesions was performed according to the markings. Histopathological examination was performed to demonstrate whether the excision margins were free of tumors.

### Results

All lesions examined revealed middle-strong and strong fluorescent patterns (values 2 to 3) and histopathological examinations proved BCC, SCC or SK (except two cases). One lesion (dermatitis) showed a weak false positive fluorescence.

*Fluorescence pattern*. Lower fluorescence intensity was found in sclerodermiform BCC and SK. For clinically well-defined lesions, the area of the fluorescence correlated well with the clinical extension as well as with the histopathological borders of the tumors. In the case of clinically ill-defined lesions, mostly sclerodermiform BCC, the correlation with the fluorescence pattern was limited.

*Fluorescence demarcation and histopathological correlation*. Best demarcation of fluorescence was achieved for superficial and nodular BCC, Bowen's disease and SK. Histopathology proved that FDAP was excellently correlating with an *in toto*-excision for superficial BCC (100%), Bowen's disease (100%) and SK (94%). For nodular BCC (86%) and SCC (91%) also an encouraging result was achieved. However, in the case of the sclerodermiform type of BCC, FDAP did not correctly indicate the real extension of the tumor area.

### Chapter Discussion

The promising results of this particular study proved that FDAP is very useful to delineate and demarcate neoplastic cutaneous tissues prior to a

Table 5. Fluorescence intensities in tissues treated by 20% ALA

| | Type of lesion | | | | | | |
|---|---|---|---|---|---|---|---|
| | BCC Superf. | BCC Nodular | BCC Sclerod. | BD | SCC | SK | No Tumor |
| | [n] | [n] | [n] | [n] | [n] | [n] | [n] |
| | Diagnosis | | | | | | |
| Clinical | 18 | 7 | 3 | 4 | 14 | 18 | 0 |
| Histological | 20 | 7 | 3 | 5 | 11 | 16 | 2 |
| | FDAP | | | | | | |
| Fluorescence | 20 | 7 | 2 | 5 | 11 | 16 | 1 |
| Intensity | 2.6 ± 0.5 | 2.7 ± 0.5 | 1.0 ± 0.8 | 2.6 ± 0.5 | 2.6 ± 0.5 | 2.3 ± 0.7 | 1.0 ± 1.0 |
| Demarcation | 96 ± 5 | 92 ± 6 | 56 ± 12 | 96 ± 7 | 95 ± 6 | 91 ± 12 | 100 ± 0 |
| | Histopathology | | | | | | |
| Excision in toto | 100% | 86% | 33% | 100% | 91% | 94% | 0% |

Fluorescence intensities of ALA-treated skin irradiated by Wood's light (370–405 nm, 10 cm distance, 5 mW/cm$^2$). Superficial, nodular and sclerodermiform BCC, BD, SCC, and SK were examined. Values are given semiquantitatively according to a fluorescence standard: 0 = no fluorescence, 3 = maximum fluorescence (total n = 64; mean ± SEM). Histopathology of the two nontumoral lesions showed spongiotic dermatitis. Most of the lesions were completely excised. For the sclerodermiform type of BCC, the FDAP-guided surgery was shown to be of low efficacy only

surgical intervention. Excision was done according to the outer borders of the visible fluorescence and most tumors were primarily excised *in toto*. As an exceptional, the sclerodermiform type of BCC was completely excised in only one of three cases (33%).

These results encouraged us to perform detailed histopathological studies on FDAP-guided tumor excision to clarify the exactness of FDAP (see Sect. G.6.).

## G.4 FDAP: Evaluation of the Optimum Photosensitizing Substance or its Prodrug

### Material and Methods

First experiences with tumor fluorescence detection were made using hematoporphyrin (Figge et al, 1948). In carcinoma patients intravenous injection of hematoporphyrin led to a characteristic red porphyrin fluorescence during UV-illumination. However, only since the introduction of the topical use of ALA (Kennedy et al, 1990) a selective intratumoral porphyrin accumulation could be guaranteed and visualized without the support of a high technical image analyzing computer unit. ALA treatment leads to excellent results in FDAP and the compound can be recommended as the substance of choice for PDT at the present moment. However, in certain lesions, e.g., BCCs in the facial skin, nodular BCC, nodular SCC or sclerodermiform BCC, FDAP has limitations due to high fluorescence levels in the tumor-surrounding skin or due to weak fluorescence in the defined lesion.

For this reason, we investigated if other porphyrin prodrugs such as ALA methylester might increase the selectivity of induced porphyrins in certain lesions. Thirty six superficial BCC were treated topically by either ALA (medac GmbH, Wedel, Germany; 20% in Neribas® ointment, Schering, Germany), ALA methylester (20%, Metvix® PhotoCure ASA, Olso, Norway) or TPPS$_4$ (tetraphenylporphine sulphonate) for 2 or 5 hours (Table 6). TPPS$_4$ was chosen as a synthetic porphyrin because its high efficacy in topical PDT of epithelial skin cancers had already been proven (Santoro et al, 1990). In all lesions, all three substances were tested. The order of the substance application was changed within the three groups to avoid the influence of a certain sequence.

*Definition of the fluorescence pattern* and *clinical demarcation of the macroscopic fluorescence* was performed as described above (Sect. G.3.).

### Results

*Clinical demarcation of all tumors.* All BCC were of the superficial type. The BCCs localized on the trunk could be clinically nicely demarcated (range: 95–99% of the total lesion areas). In the case of the facial BCCs the lesions showed partly a weaker definition (range: 92–94% of the total lesion areas) (Table 6).

*Fluorescence intensity.* Using ALA, the fluorescence intensities were highest (2.9–3). Topical

Table 6. Fluorescence in BCC depending on the photosensitizer or its progrug

| FDAP | | 1st week | | 2nd week | | 3rd week | |
|---|---|---|---|---|---|---|---|
| | | n = 6 | n = 6 | n = 6 | n = 6 | n = 6 | n = 6 |
| | | trunk | face | trunk | face | trunk | face |
| **ALA** | Order | 1 | | 2 | | 3 | |
| Applic. time | [h] | 5 | 5 | 5 | 5 | 5 | 5 |
| Clinical borders | [%] | 97 ± 2 | 93 ± 4 | 95 ± 5 | 93 ± 5 | 95 ± 5 | 92 ± 6 |
| Fluor. intensity | [1–3] | **3** | **2.9** | **3** | **3** | **3** | **2.9** |
| Fluor. borders | [%] | **98** ± 3 | 88 ± 6 | 92 ± 6 | 91 ± 9 | **97** ± 4 | 92 ± 3 |
| Correl. with clinic | [%] | 97 ± 3 | 94 ± 4 | 97 ± 2 | 91 ± 6 | 96 ± 4 | 93 ± 4 |
| Excision *in toto* | [%] | **100** | 83 | 83 | 66 | **100** | **100** |
| **ALA methylester** | Order | 2 | | 3 | | 1 | |
| Applic. time | [h] | 5 | 5 | 5 | 5 | 5 | 5 |
| Clinical borders | [%] | 97 ± 3 | 93 ± 4 | 99 ± 2 | 94 ± 4 | 96 ± 5 | 92 ± 7 |
| Fluor. intensity | [1–3] | 2.2 | 2.3 | 2.7 | 1.9 | 2 | 2.1 |
| Fluor. borders | [%] | **98 ± 2** | **97 ± 2** | **96 ± 3** | **96 ± 4** | **97 ± 3** | **96 ± 3** |
| Correl. with clinic | [%] | 98 ± 2 | 95 ± 3 | 98 ± 2 | 95 ± 2 | 98 ± 3 | 97 ± 2 |
| Excision *in toto* | [%] | **100** | **100** | **100** | 83 | **100** | **100** |
| **TPPS** | Order | 3 | | 1 | | 2 | |
| Applic. time | [h] | 2 | 2 | 2 | 2 | 2 | 2 |
| Clinical borders | [%] | 97 ± 2 | 94 ± 6 | 98 ± 3 | 95 ± 3 | 97 ± 2 | 93 ± 4 |
| Fluor. intensity | [1–3] | 0.7 | 1 | 0.8 | 0.7 | 1 | 0.6 |
| Fluor. borders | [%] | 54 ± 14 | 40 ± 15 | 59 ± 10 | 35 ± 12 | 42 ± 15 | 30 ± 11 |
| Correl. with clinic | [%] | 34 ± 18 | 36 ± 15 | 42 ± 16 | 37 ± 15 | 31 ± 13 | 26 ± 12 |
| Excision *in toto* | [%] | 83 | 66 | 66 | 66 | 66 | 50 |

All data concerning the fluorescence pattern are given as mean ± SD (n= 6). Concerning the clinical borders, facial lesions showed less sharp demarcation as compared to the lesions on the trunk. Using ALA, highest levels of fluorescence intensities were achieved (highlighted green numbers). Demarcation of the lesions' borders by fluorescence was easiest after topical application of ALA-ME (highlighted blue numbers). Most effective complete excision of the BCC was achieved performing surgery according to the borders of ALA-ME-induced porphyrin fluorescence (highlighted red numbers)

application of ALA methylester led to an approximately 30% reduced fluorescence yield (1.9–2.7) as compared to the lesions treated with ALA. For TPPS$_4$, the fluorescence values were the lowest.

*Demarcation of the fluorescence and surgical success.* Fluorescing areas could be best delineated by the use of ALA methylester. In particular, for the facial BCC, ALA methylester was superior to ALA in fluorescence demarcation (96–98% *vs.* 91–94%). These results correlated with the histopathological data. Nearly all tumors (even those in the facial skin; 94%) were excised *in toto* if surgery was performed according to the porphyrin fluorescence induced by ALA methylester. For ALA, the results were also rather good, however, several (n = 3; 16%) facial BCCs were not completely excised.

## Chapter Discussion

ALA and ALA methylester are both very effective substances to induce a porphyrin fluorescence for delineating cutaneous tumor tissue. Topical TPPS$_4$ also leads to a certain tumor sensitization, however, the efficacy in fluorescence detection and PDT is much less as compared to ALA or its ester. Topical TPPS$_4$ induces a high porphyrin fluorescence in normal skin increasing the risk of local photosensitization and diminishing the contrast to the tumor tissue and is thus ineffective in skin cancer delineation. Topical TPPS$_4$ was reported to be highly effective in treating BCC by PDT (Santoro et al, 1990), but there was an intensive local photosensitivity. In additional own experience, the photosensitizing quality of other porphyrin compounds such as protoporphyrin IX and uroporphyrin was investigated. The effects of these compounds in tumor destruction (BCC) were encouraging (Table 19). However, there was local photosensitivity with an induction of erythema, burning and also partly blister formation upon irradiation with red light.

Therefore, the extraordinary advantage of the endogenous porphyrin accumulation by the use of porphyrin precursors such as ALA or ALA-ME favors these substances. Further investigations should focus on the potential efficacy of selected ALA ester compounds such as ALA hexylester (Peng et al, 1996).

## G.5 FDAP: Evaluation of the Optimum Exciting Light Source

**Material and Methods**

Although FDAP has been a routine technique in e.g., urology for several years, in dermatology a specific light source for FDAP has not been developed yet. The optimum parameters for such a lamp are quite clear theoretically. The light source has to emit wavelengths around the absorption maximum of the porphyrin metabolites, the so-called Soret band at 405 nm (Soret, 1883). In general, all available Wood's lamps on the market do emit light around or close to the Soret band. Most problematic point is, however, that most or even all of these industrially available lamps emit only low intensity light, specifically most of the small hand Wood's light systems. Such light sources do not lead to clear bright porphyrin fluorescence even if large amounts of porphyrins accumulate intratumorally. Therefore all available light sources developed for Wood's light irradiation were tested.

**Results and Discussion**

We found that the Fluotest® (Xenotest, Hanau, Germany) was the most effective light source. This lamp was originally produced for the textile industry to control the quality and purity of a certain cloth material. According to the physical data of this lamp and performing several modifications, the German company Saalmann constructed the prototype Fluolight®, which is now available on the market for FDAP. Fluolight® is the most powerful Wood's light source suitable for FDAP, which is available in the international market at present. All other available Wood's light systems, particularly the hand devices, emit insufficient energy to excite the fluorescence of the intratumorally accumulated porphyrins.

## G.6 FDAP: Correlation of *in vivo* – Tumor Fluorescence and Histopathology

**Material and Methods**

The previous studies revealed the optimum drug and light source for FDAP. Consequently, the specificity of FDAP was evaluated. The histopathological results as mentioned in chapter G.4. (*in toto* or not) do still not give any information on the precision of the fluorescence in correlation to the exact tumor extension. The fluorescence could be much larger than the tumor tissue. Therefore, a study was designed that allows the correlation of the histopathological borders of e.g., a BCC with the macroscopic fluorescence pattern (borders) of the lesion.

*Study design.* Twenty BCC (10 on the face, 10 on the trunk) were included (Table 7). Three spots painted by a surgical pen were placed close to the lesion to allow a later overlaying of all taken pictures and an exact image processing. All lesions were photographically documented (Fig. 77).

ALA methylester (20%, Metvix®, PhotoCure ASA, Oslo, Norway) was applied for 24 h. Fluorescence pictures including a fluorescence standard were taken prior to (Fig. 78) and 3 (Fig. 79), 5 (Fig. 80), and 24 h (Fig. 81) after the application of the substance. After each photo (at 3 and 5 h), the ALA methylester mixture was freshly applied.

*Surgical treatment.* 24 hours after ALA methylester application, the last fluorescence documentation was performed. The lesion was locally anaesthetized (Xylonest 1%). During Wood's light irradiation (Fluolight®, Saalmann, Herford, Germany), the outer borders of the fluorescence were marked by gentle incisions using a scalpel. The entire lesion was excised with a certain safety margin, including all relevant data – the incised area and the three marked spots.

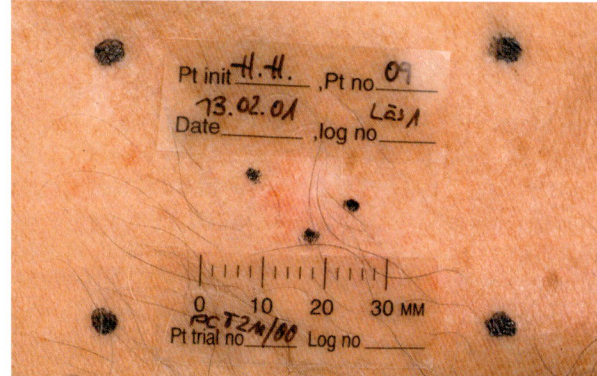

Fig. 77. BCC of superficial type on the trunk. Diagnosis was verified by histopathology. Three spots were marked with a surgical pen close to the clinically visable tumor borders. The marking remained during the entire following FDAP procedure. Therefore, it was guaranteed, that all pictures taken during FDAP could be compared by image analysis. The four large spots on the edges of the picture were used to photograph always the same part of the body

**Table 7.** FDAP: Fluorescence kinetics in BCC using ALA methylester

| FDAP | Trunk | | | | Face | | | |
| --- | --- | --- | --- | --- | --- | --- | --- | --- |
| | n = 10 | | | | n = 10 | | | |
| | Back | 3 h | 5 h | 24 h | Back | 3 h | 5 h | 24 h |
| ALA methylester | [%] | [%] | [%] | [%] | [%] | [%] | [%] | [%] |
| Intensity | 0 | 81 ± 10 | 97 ± 14 | 113 ± 14 | 0 | 83 ± 12 | 99 ± 13 | 113 ± 10 |
| Demarcation | 0 | 92 ± 4 | 97 ± 4 | 96 ± 9 | 0 | 88 ± 4 | 95 ± 3 | 89 ± 6 |
| Excision *in toto* | – | – | – | 100 | – | – | – | 100 |
| Fluo vs. clinic | – | 90 | 95 | 90 | – | 90 | 95 | 85 |
| Fluo vs. histo | – | 85 | 95 | 75 | – | 70 | 90 | 70 |
| Clinic vs. histo | – | – | 95 | – | – | – | 90 | – |

All data are given as mean ± SD. Fluorescence intensity is given as percentage according to a fluorescence standard. Demarcation represents the percentual part of the total length of the outer bordes of the fluorescence which could be clearly delineated (all 165 sections of all 20 lesions are summarized). Perfect correlation of the clinical borders with the histopathological extension of the tumor was defined if the distance between both lines was less than 2 mm (supposed that the clinical area is > than the histopathological extension of the tumor tissue). All lesions were completely excised 24 h after ALA methylester treatment. Good correlation of fluorescence with the histopathological borders of the tumor was defined if the distance between both lines was less than 2 mm (supposed that the fluorescent area was > than the histopathological extension of the tumor tissue)

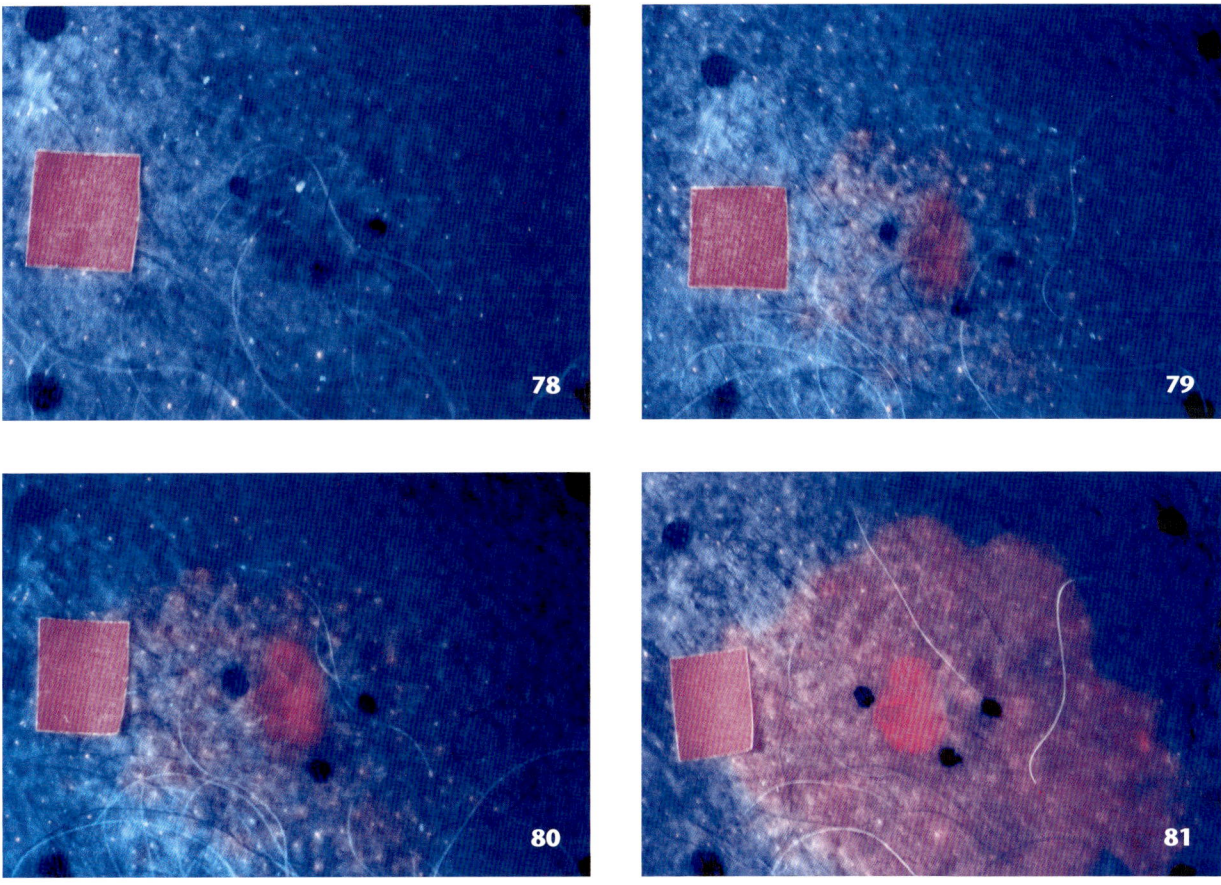

**Figs. 78–81.** BCC of superficial type on the trunk (same lesion as in Fig. 77). 20% ALA methylester (Metvix®) was topically applied. After 3 h (Fig. 79), 5 h (Fig. 80) and 24 h (Fig. 81), fluorescence photographs were recorded. Prior to ALA methylester application, there was no fluorescence detectable. After 3 h, the tumor tissue was already fluorescing, however intensity was still weak. At 5 h, fluorescence intensity was rather high and the lesion could be well demarcated by the flurescence pattern. At 24 h, the fluorescence intensity was still very good, however, the tumor surrounding normal skin also revealed bright fluorescence. Therefore, it is more difficult to delineate the tumor 24 h than 5 h after topical ALA-ME treatment. Scalpel incision was performed according to the fluorescence borders at 24 h

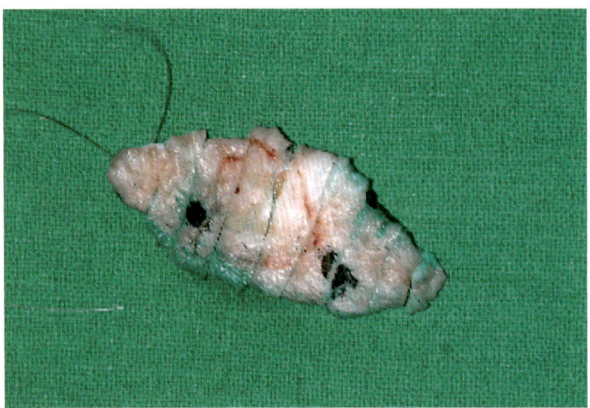

Fig. 82. BCC of superficial type on the trunk after surgical excision. The 3 markings are still included. The inner circle of incised tissue represents the fluorescence borders at 24 h (Fig. 81). The tissue was cut into thin slices (approximately 2 mm). Every single slice represents an own histopathological block, which was separately examined, in detail one section per tissue block)

*Histopathological evaluation.* The excidate was sliced into pieces of approximately 2 mm width. The sliced tissue cake was photographically documented (Fig. 82) to allow a later exact correlation of a certain section with its localization in the tumor tissue.

*Image analysis.* All clinical, fluorescence, and histopathological pictures were scanned and digitally stored using the image processing programs Power Point (Microsoft, USA) and Image Access (Imagic, Germany). The clinically visible area of the tumor was evaluated. Total fluorescence areas were measured. Fluorescence intensities were given in percent in relation to a fluorescence standard (= 100%). In all histopathological sections, the distance from the tumor cells to the scalpel incisions was measured (left and right side separately) (Fig. 83).

## Results

All tumors included into the study were histopathologically proven as BCC.

*Fluorescence intensity.* Untreated lesions did not reveal any fluorescence at all (Fig. 78). Topical application of ALA methylester led to increasing fluorescence kinetics with maximum levels at 24 h (trunk: 87 and face: 94% of standard) (Fig. 81).

*Demarcation of the fluorescence.* Although the fluorescence quantity was highest 24 h after ALA methylester application, the optimum delineation of the fluorescence area from the tumor surrounding skin was measured at 5 h (trunk: 97%, face 95%).

*Histopathological evaluation.* The number of total sections varied from 5 to 11 per lesion (mean ± SD; 8.4 ± 1.3). Histopathological measurement of the distance from the incisions to the borders of the tumor tissue allowed the correlation of all evaluated borders (clinical, FDAP 3 h, FDAP 5 h, FDAP 24 h) with the real extension of the tumor. According to the clinically visible borders, 90% of all BCC on the trunk and 60% of all facial BCC would have been completely excised. Distances measured ranged from 0.1 ± 0.83 (left), 0.3 ± 0.12 (right) to 1.33 ± 0.96 (left), 1.49 ± 0.12 mm (right). One lesion on the trunk (no. 4) (Fig. 84) showed tumor extension (left: –0.13 ± 0.26; right: –0.26 ± 0.25 mm) that was clinically not visible. On the face, even more lesions (no. 11, 13, 15, 19) (Fig. 84) were histologically verified to be larger than their clinical

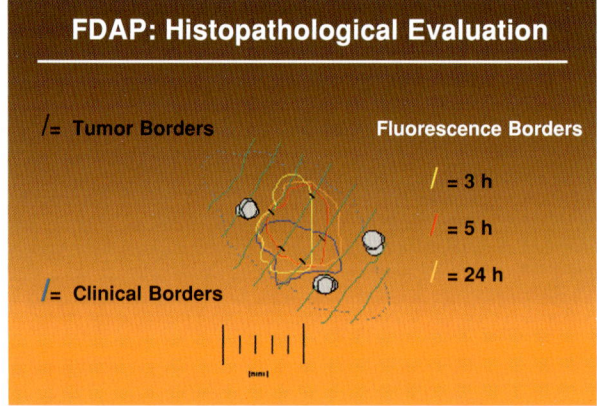

Fig. 83. Clinical, FDAP and histopathological data of one selected case are summarized in this graphical illustration. The following photographic documentation was performed: Clinical picture prior to ALA methylester treatment (blue line) and FDAP pictures at 3 (yellow), 5 (red) and 24 h (orange line) after application of the substance. At the time point of 24 h, scalpel incision was performed according to the fluorescence pattern. The excised tissue was cut into thin small slices (width: approx. 2 mm) (green lines) and the distance of the incisions to the borders of the tumor was microscopically measured. In all histopathological sections, there were totally 5 incisions detectable (3 on the left, 2 on the right side of the tumor). These "real" borders of the tumor are included into the illustration as small black lines. By means of this evaluation technique it was possible to measure all false negative and false positive distances from clinically estimated or in FDAP detected borders to the exact position of the tumor tissue

## Histopathological Correlation of Tumor Cells with Clinical Size of BCC

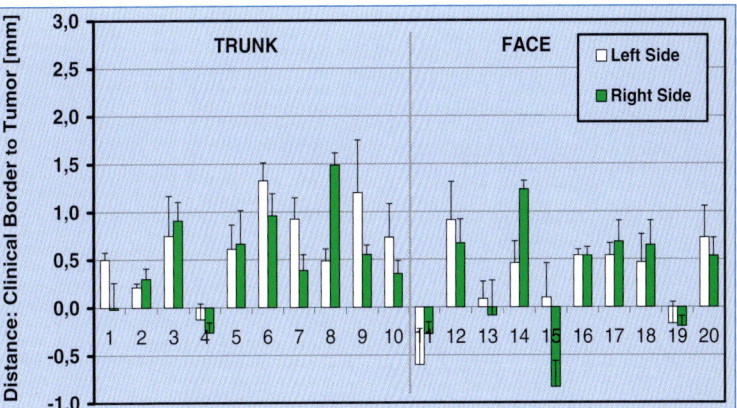

**Fig. 84.** Distance of the clinically visible borders to the tumor edges as measured by histopathology. For each lesion mean ± SD is given for all histopathological sections (varying from 5–11). Empty bars represent the left side, filled bars the right side of the lesion

## Histopathological Evaluation of FDAP in BCC after Topical Application of 20% ALA Methylester for 3h

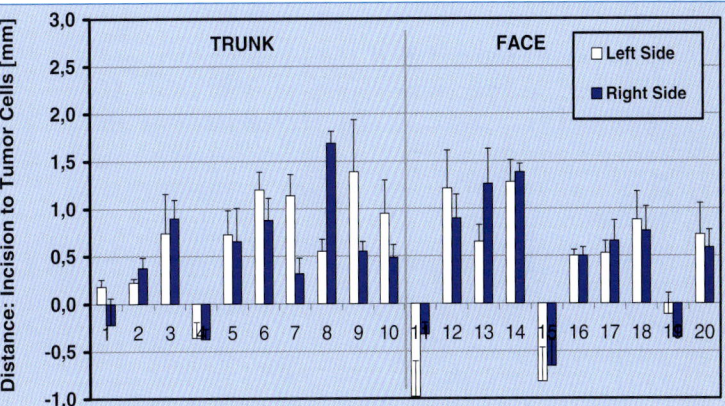

**Fig. 85.** Distance of the clinically visible borders to the tumor edges as measured by histopathology. For each lesion mean ± SD is given for all histopathological sections (varying from 5–11)

## Histopathological Evaluation of FDAP in BCC after Topical Application of 20% ALA Methylester for 5h

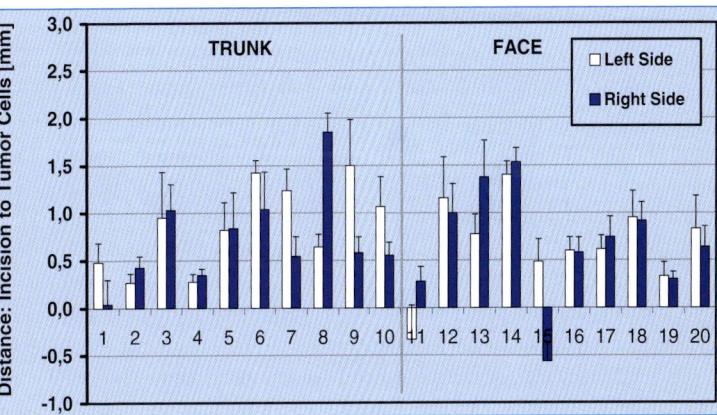

**Fig. 86.** Distance of the clinically visible borders to the tumor edges as measured by histopathology. For each lesion mean ± SD is given for all histopathological sections (varying from 5–11)

## Histopathological Evaluation of FDAP in BCC after Topical Application of 20% ALA Methylester for 24h

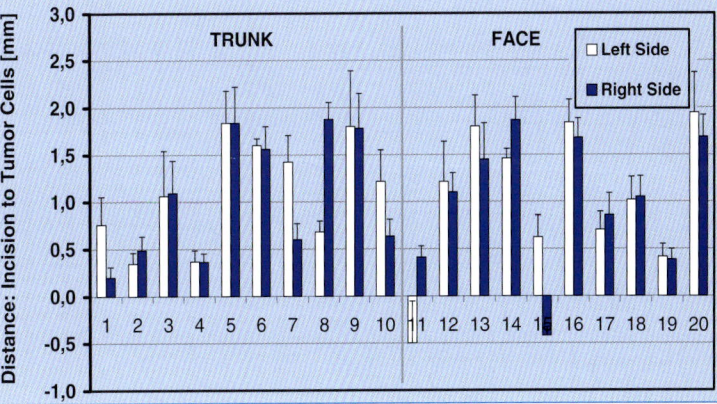

**Fig. 87.** Distance of the clinically visible borders to the tumor edges as measured by histopathology. For each lesion mean ± SD is given for all histopathological sections (varying from 5–11)

appearance (left: −0.6 ± 0.43 to −0.13 ± 0.26 mm; right: −0.83 ± 0.37 to 0.02 ± 0.4 mm).

In FDAP, 3 h after application of ALA-ME, 5 lesions showed false negative results (4 on the left side, 5 on the right side) (Fig. 85). In FDAP 5 h and 24 h after ALA-ME treatment, all lesions on the trunk revealed correct fluorescence (Figs. 86 and 87), except for two lesions on the face, which showed false negative fluorescence (one on the left, the other on the right side). Values of the distance fluorescence / real tumor border increased with the application time of ALA-ME.

### Chapter Discussion

This study showed that the application time of 5 hours is recommendable in the case ALA methylester is used as the photosensitizing prodrug. Upon the analysis of 20 tumors is was clearly shown that FDAP is a suitable method to mark tumorous tissue, which was confirmed by histopathological methods. Although the results concerning complete tumor removal were comparable for 5 and 24 h (90% *vs.* 75% for 3 h), an application time of 5 h should be chosen. For 24 h (1.1 ± 0.3 mm), the number of false positive fluorescence was more pronounced as compared to 5 h (0.7 ± 0.21 mm). In some lesions, the outer borders of FDAP were distant from the outer tumor tissue with maximum distance of 1.2 mm (false negative). In most sections of the lesions, the fluorescence borders were larger than the histopathological extension of the tumor cells (false positive), ranging from 0.05–3.2 mm. The reason for this false positive fluorescence might be a leakage of porphyrins from the tumor tissue into the close tumor-adjacent tissue. This pilot study suggests that tumor surgery would lead to 100% complete excision if the lesions were excised according to the FDAP results adding 2 mm.

## G.7 FDAP: Course of FDAP in Relation to the Number of PDT Sessions

### Material and Methods

Fifty SK, 7 BD and 35 histopathologically proven BCC (14 superficial BCC, 14 nodular BCC, 7 sclerodermiform BCC) were treated by PDT using 10% ALA for SK and 20% ALA for BCC. Incubation time was 4 hours. After FDAP, PDT was performed using 75 J/cm$^2$ red light (125 mW/cm$^2$; Curelight®, PhotoCure ASA, Oslo, Norway) for BCC and 30 J/cm$^2$ green light (25 mW/cm$^2$; PDT Greenlight®, Saalmann, Herford, Germany) for SK. PDT was repeated biweekly until there was no more fluorescence detectable within the treated area. Maximum number of treatments was 4 times. Clinical picture was compared with the results of FDAP.

*Fluorescence measurements.* Fluorescence intensity was given in % of relative grey values according to a fluorescence standard (= 100 %). Fluorescence area was measured to determine the individual homogeneity in any lesion and was given as % of the clinical tumor area. Fluorescence demarcation was measured digitally by image analysis Power Point (Microsoft) and Image Access (Imagic, Germany) and given as % of total fluorescent area. The quality of fluorescence delineation of the total fluorescing area was analyzed by measuring the total length of the lesion's border.

### Results

*FDAP in guiding PDT of SK, BD and BCC.* Prior to PDT, all SK, BD (Figs. 88–97) and BCC, except the sclerodermiform type, showed a bright red fluorescence in FDAP (Table 8)

Table 8. FDAP-guided PDT: Lesions with positive fluorescence

| FDAP | PDT | BCC superficial | BCC nodular | BCC scleroder. | Bowen's disease | Solar keratoses |
|---|---|---|---|---|---|---|
| | | n = 14 | n = 14 | n = 7 | n = 7 | n = 14 |
| | | Fluorescence | | | | |
| | After no. of sessions | Present in n [%] lesions | Present in n [%] lesions | Present in n [%] lesions | Present in n [%] lesions | Present in n [%] lesions |
| Baseline | | 100 | 100 | 43 | 100 | 100 |
| 2 weeks | 1 | 100 | 100 | 57 | 100 | 43 |
| 4 weeks | 2 | 14 | 93 | 43 | 57 | 7 |
| 6 weeks | 3 | 7 | 64 | 57 | 29 | 0 |
| 8 weeks | 4 | 0 | 21 | 29 | 0 | 0 |

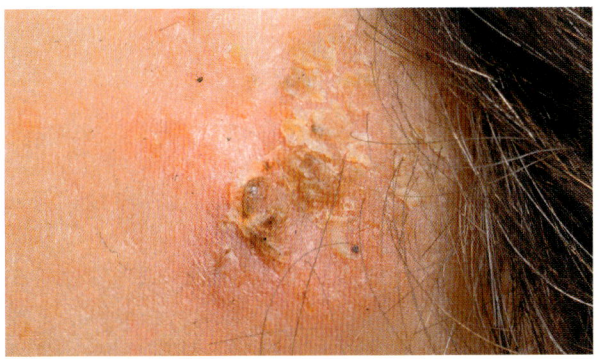

**Fig. 88.** BD on the forehead left. The lesion is ill-defined

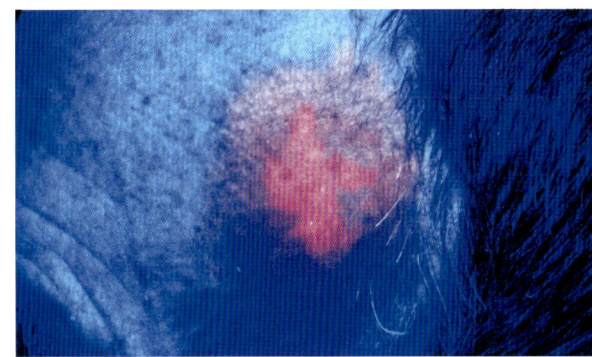

**Fig. 89.** FDAP 1:20% Metvix®. Fluorescence of the tumor tissue

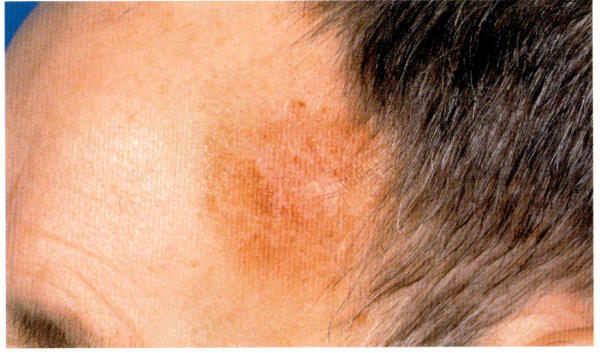

**Fig. 90.** 2 weeks after 1st PDT. Partial response, hyperpigmentation

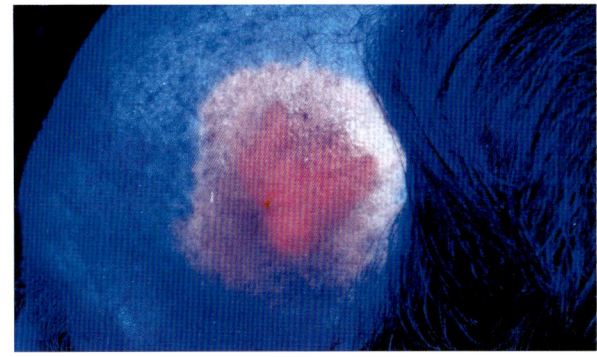

**Fig. 91.** FDAP 2: Increased fluorescence

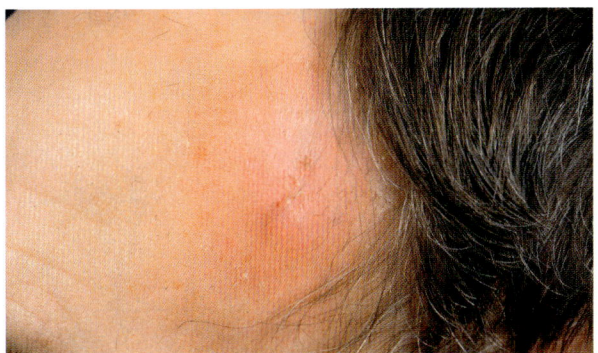

**Fig. 92.** 2 weeks after 2nd PDT. Clinically almost cured lesion

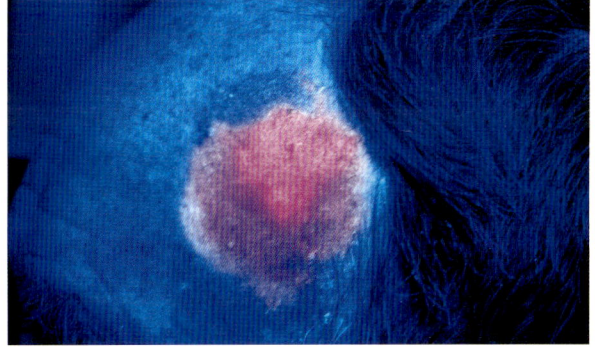

**Fig. 93.** FDAP 3: Decreasing fluorescence intensity

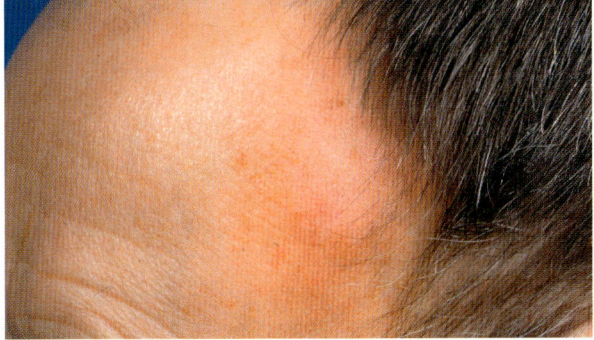

**Fig. 94.** 2 weeks after 3rd PDT. Slight hyperpigmentation

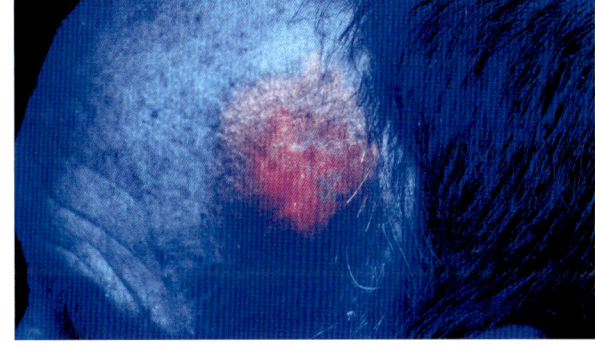

**Fig. 95.** FDAP 4: Decreasing fluorescence intensity

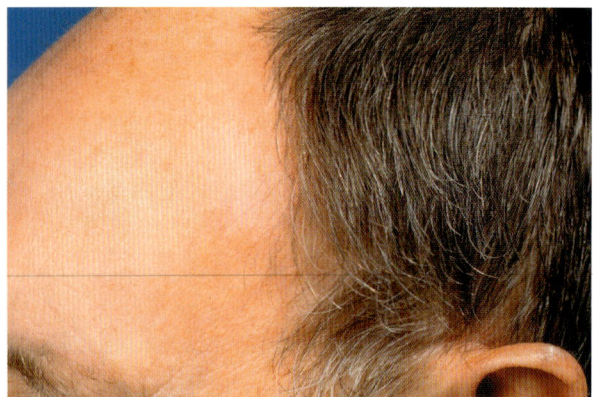
Fig. 96. 2 weeks after 4th PDT (8 weeks after 1st PDT). Complete response

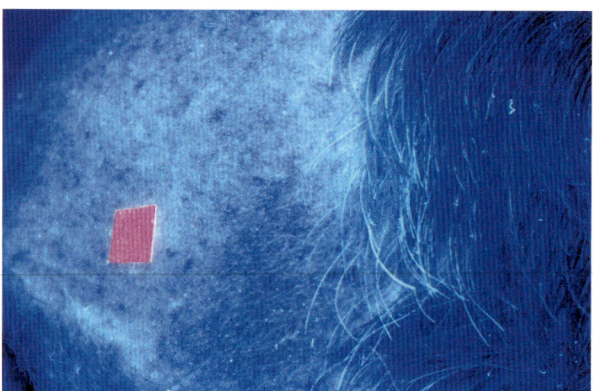
Fig. 97. FDAP 4: Absent fluorescence

The fluorescence was sharply demarcated even in skin areas that clinically seemed to be uninvolved (Figs. 89 and 91). However, sclerodermiform BCC revealed only weak fluorescence intensities with partly ill-defined fluorescence areas. In most BCC, BD and SK cases, beside the tumor-specific intensive red fluorescence a weak pink fluorescence was also demonstrated in normal tumor-surrounding skin in several cases. Fluorescence intensity of SK and BCC decreased with the number of performed PDT sessions (Figs. 91, 93, 95, 97, 98). In BCC, the complete response rates were dependent on the histopathological type (Table 8).

The fluorescing area was dependent on the number of PDT sessions (Fig. 99). It showed an increase during the second FDAP (after the first PDT session) in superficial and nodular BCC as well as in BD. Thereafter, the fluorescing area was continuously decreasing dependent on the number of PDT sessions.

Figure 100 shows if fluorescing areas could be clearly delineated or not – independent on the present size of fluorescent area.

## Chapter Discussion

The increase of fluorescence intensity and also of fluorescence area, as measured in BCC, BD and SK after the first PDT session (Figs. 89 and 91), could be due to the fact that the central (deeper localized) part of the tumor is coming to the surface after removing the superficial part through the first PDT cycle. Additionally, an inflammation reaction in the area adjacent to skin tumors after PDT may enable tumor-surrounding skin to accumulate more porphyrins.

### Fluorescence Intensity of Skin Tumors during PDT Sessions

Fig. 98. Fluorescence intensity in BCC (superficial type: n = 14; nodular type: n = 14; sclerodermiform type: n = 7), BD (n = 7) and SK (n = 50) after topical application of 20 % (SK: 10 %) ALA dependent on the number of PDT cycles. Maximum fluorescence was measured independent of the size of fluorescing area (given as % of a fluorescence standard; mean ± SD). In nodular and superficial BCC and BD, fluorescence intensity increased 2 weeks after the first PDT, followed by a steady decrease after the following PDT sessions. For sclerodermiform BCC only a weak intensity was measured

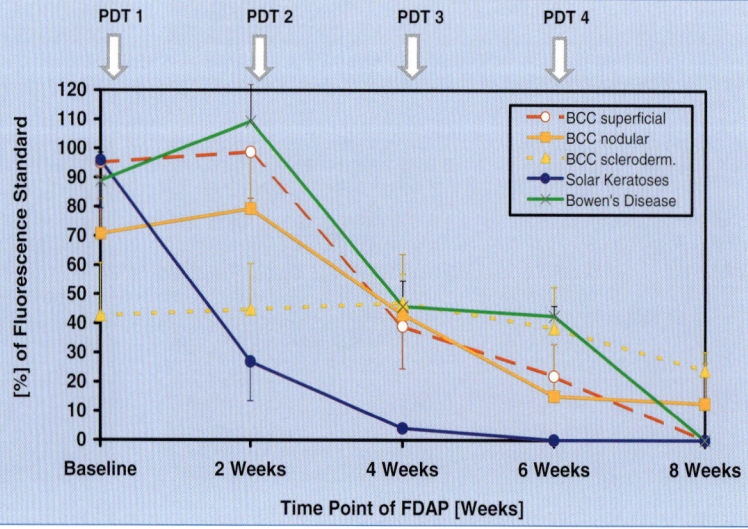

## Fluorescence Area of Skin Tumors during PDT Sessions

**Fig. 99.** Fluorescence area in BCC (superficial type: n=14; nodular type: n=14; sclerodermiform type: n=7), BD (n=7) and SK (n=50) after topical application of 20% (SK: 10%) ALA dependent on the number of PDT cycles. Prior to first PDT, best correlation between tumor extension and fluorescence area was measured for superficial BCC, BD and SK (given as % of the clinical visible tumor area; mean ± SD). Fluorescent area decreased parallel to the number of PDT sessions. For sclerodermiform BCC, the fluorescent area was only partially correlating with the clinical tumor area and was not changing during the time period measured

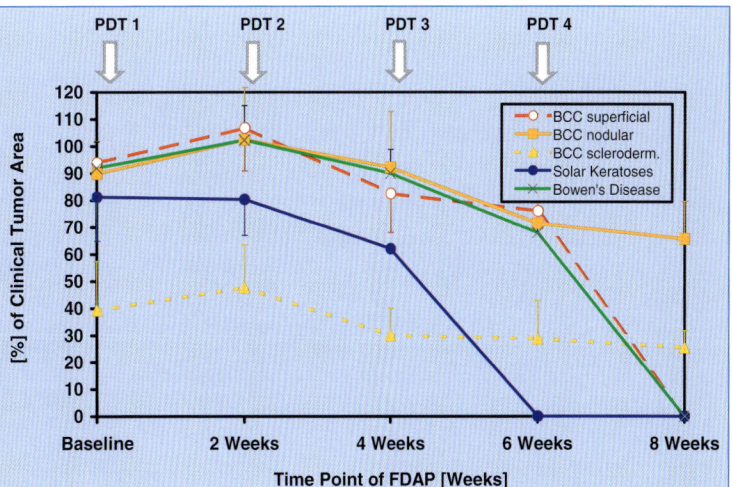

## Fluorescence Area of Skin Tumors during PDT Sessions

**Fig. 100.** Amount of fluorescing area which can be sharply delineated in BCC (superficial type: n=14; nodular type: n=14; sclerodermiform type: n=7) and SK (n=50) after topical application of 20% (SK: 10%) ALA, dependent on the number of PDT cycles. Except for the sclerodermiform type of BCC, the fluorescing areas could be clearly delineated in all lesions (given as % of a total fluorescing area; mean ± SD)

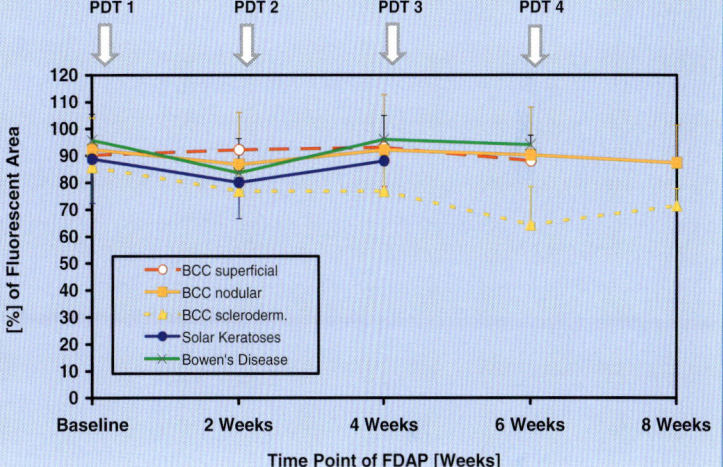

# H  The Clinical Use of FDAP

One of the major promising potentials of FDAP is the detection and delineation of clinically ill-defined neoplastic skin areas. It is a fascinating phenomenon that the topical application of a certain substance (ALA) leads to the specific accumulation of fluorescing molecules in skin tumors. This selectivity of fluorescence takes place although the ALA-containing ointment is applied also to the normal skin within a certain safety margin. Making use of this phenomenon, the total tumor area including the surrounding borders of superficial and nodular BCC, SCC and SK can be visualized prior to excision.

## H.1 FDAP in Clinically Well-defined Tumors

The following figures give some examples for the selective porphyrin accumulation in epithelial skin cancers. The chapter comprises cases that show clinically well-defined lesions.

These 3 cases clearly demonstrate that ALA-induced porphyrins selectively accumulate in the neoplastic tissue (Figs. 101–106) although the tumor-surrounding skin was also treated. Thus, fluorescence in FDAP correlates well with the clinical size of the tumor. Supposing that the histopathological expansion of the tumor corre-

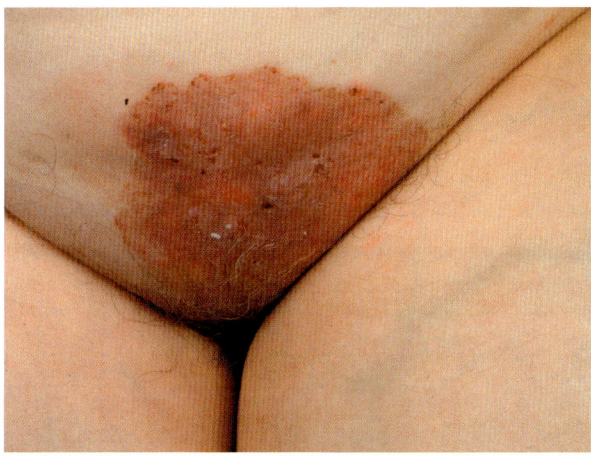

Fig. 101. Large superficial BCC on the suprapubic area. Sharply delineated erythemato-squamous plaque

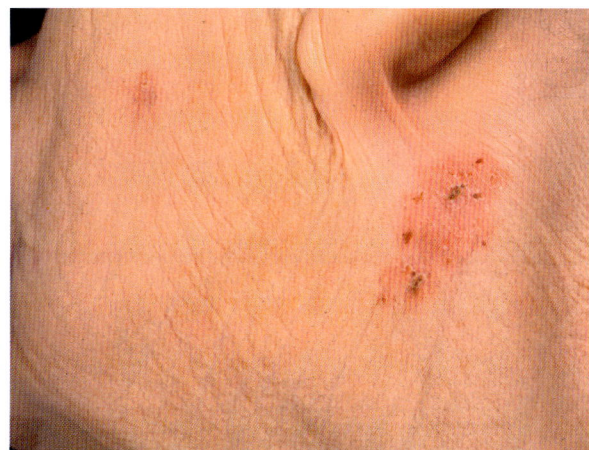

Fig. 103. Superficial BCC in the left retroauricular region. The lesion is well defined

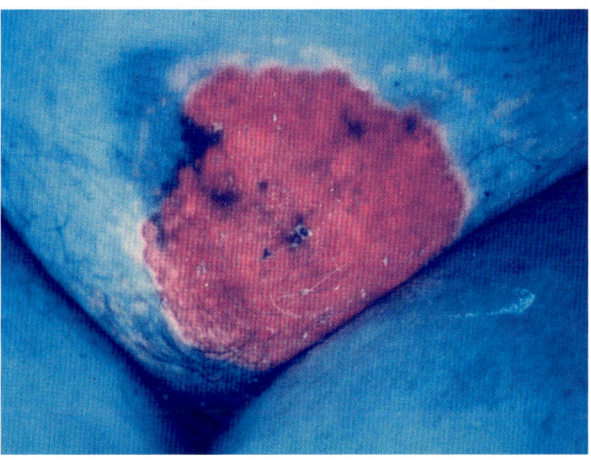

Fig. 102. FDAP: Bright fluorescence, correlating with the clinical extension of the lesion

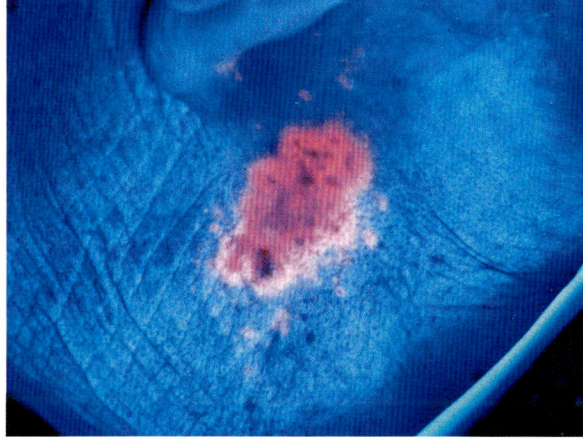

Fig. 104. FDAP: Bright fluorescence, which correlates with the clinical size of the lesion

# H  The Clinical Use of FDAP

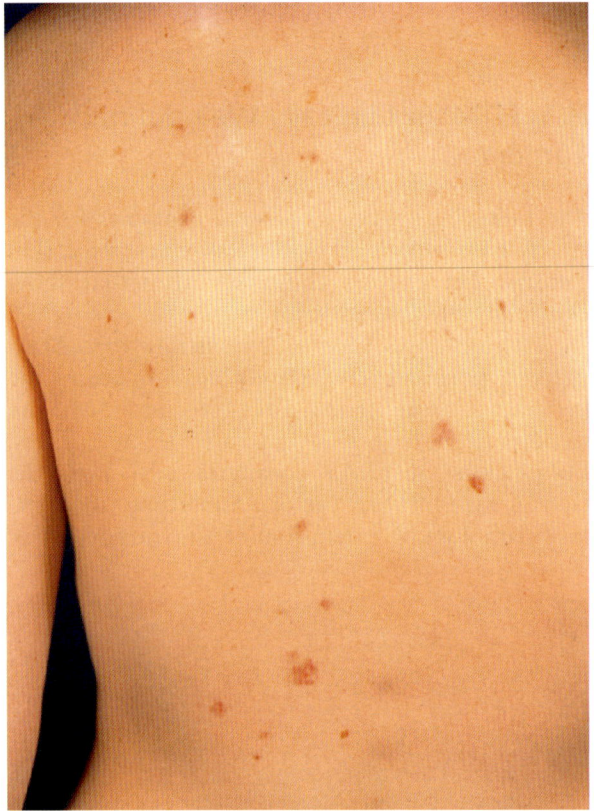

**Fig. 105.** Multiple superficial BCC on the back presenting as erythematous macules or plaques

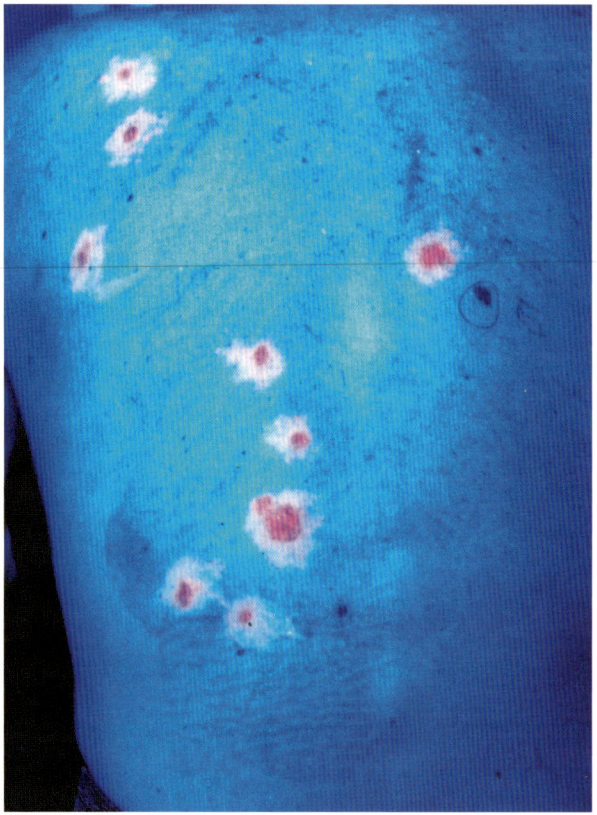

**Fig. 106.** FDAP demonstrates the area of diseased skin. There are 9 brightly fluorescing islands detectable, indicating neoplastic tissues

lates with the clinically visible tumor area (if it is completely visible), FDAP is suitable to detect skin tumors. The case of the patient with several BCC on her back (Figs. 105 and 106) impressively demonstrates the high selectivity of this technique. Normal skin shows different fluorescence kinetics depending on the body site. Lesions on the trunk are generally easier to handle by FDAP than facial ones.

## H.2  FDAP in Clinically Ill-defined Lesions

Most of the epithelial skin tumors present ill-defined lesion borders. Therefore, the clinically visible area of the tumor tissue is frequently not corresponding to the real size of the tumor tissue. Therefore the use of an adjuvant diagnostic tool such as FDAP to detect all neoplastic tissue is of great value.

These cases impressively demonstrate that FDAP is also very effective in detecting neoplastic skin in the case of clinically ill-defined lesions. The lesion-bound fluorescence is partly surrounded by a whitish-pink fluorescence in the skin adjacent to the tumor tisue (Figs. 116 and 120). In some cases, this undesired fluorescence may interfere with that over the tumor-associated tissue and may therefore complicate an exact delineation of the tumor area.

This relatively intensive fluorescence can be demonstrated on the head, the groin and axillae and may be due to the colonization by porphyrin producing bacteria (e.g., propionibacteria). After an application time of 24 h, we detected up to a medium intensive fluorescence in these locations. Here, the contrast between neoplastic and healthy skin can be improved by reducing the application time of the ALA to 2–4 h and also by the use of ALA methylester (Fig. 75) instead of free ALA. Corynebacterium minutissimum, the causative factor in erythrasma, can also form large amounts of protoporphyrin. Therefore, in untreated erythrasma lesions, one can demonstrate red fluorescence, which is similar to the red fluorescence generated in FDAP.

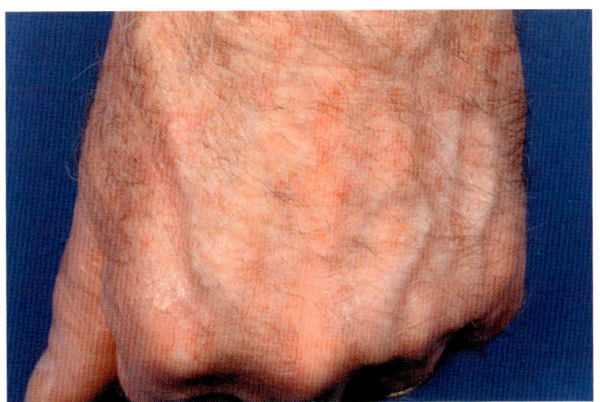

**Fig. 107.** Multiple scales and crusts on the back of the hand. It is impossible to detect and delineate all lesions

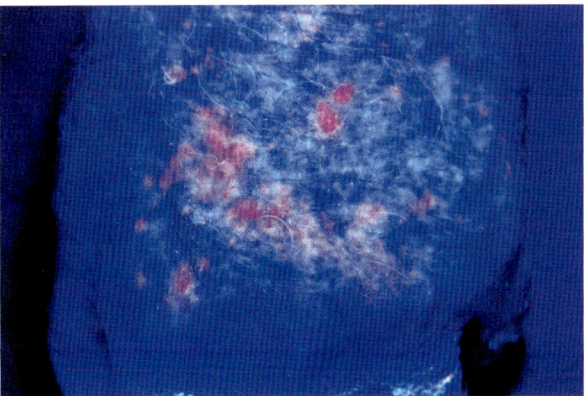

**Fig. 108.** FDAP: All neoplastic tissue reveals bright red fluorescence. FDAP improves the visualization of all lesions

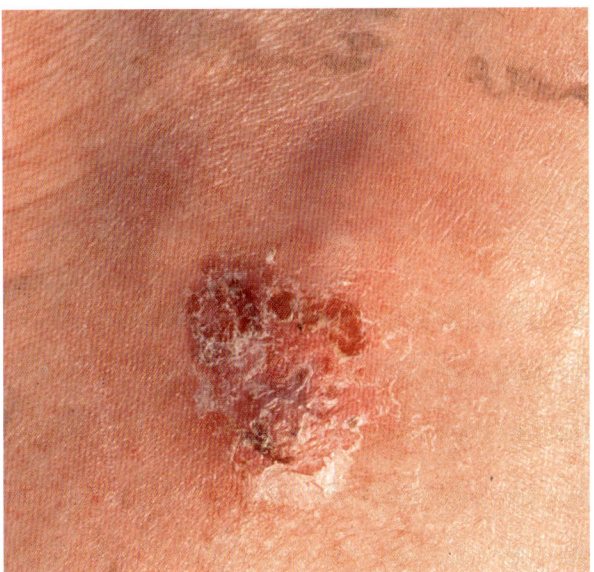

**Fig. 109.** BD on the ankle joint of the lower leg. The borders of the lesion are ill-defined

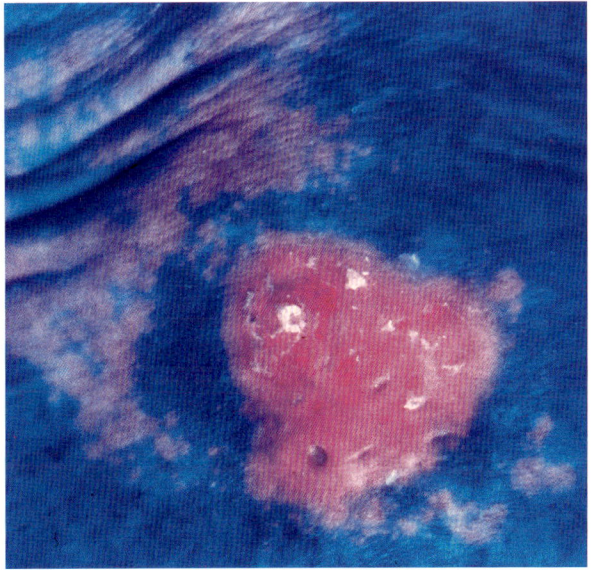

**Fig. 110.** FDAP: Sharp demarcation of the neoplastic skin. Normal skin surrounding the lesions also presents a weak fluorescence

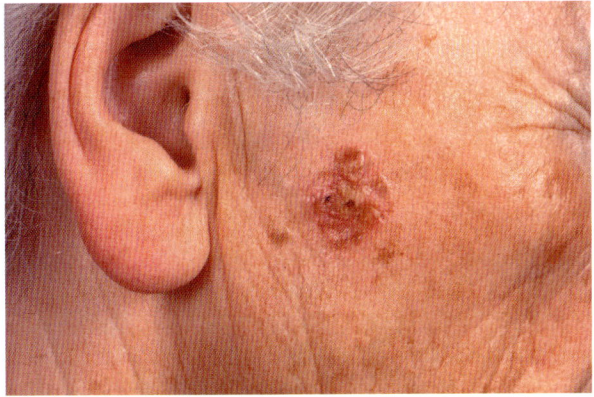

**Fig. 111.** BD on the right cheek. Ill-defined lesion

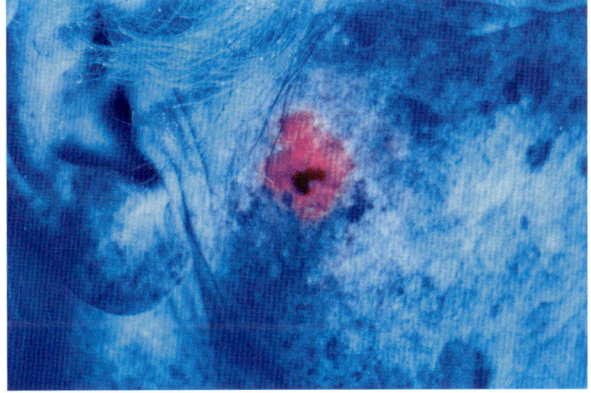

**Fig. 112.** FDAP allows a clear delineation of the BD

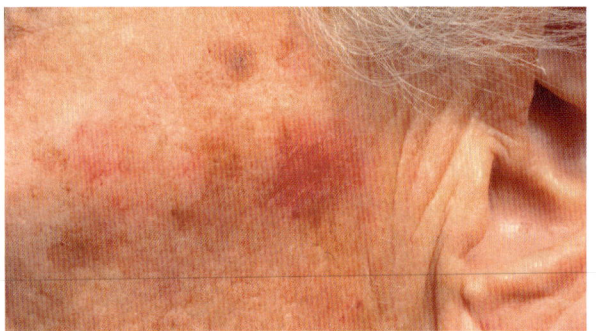

Fig. 113. BD on the left cheek. Erythematous macule, in part ill-defined

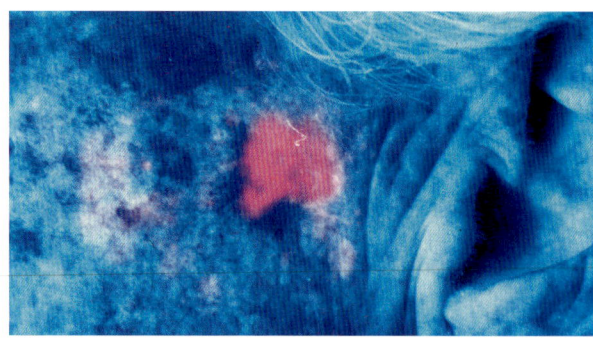

Fig. 114. FDAP allows a clear delineation of the BD

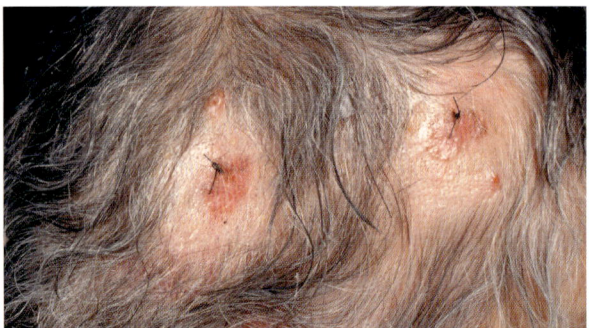

Fig. 115. Two BCC on the capillitium

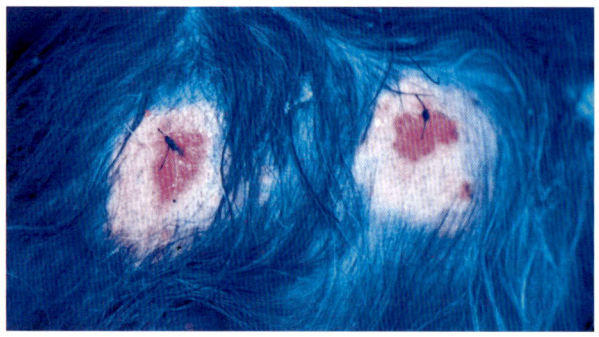

Fig. 116. FDAP allows a clear delination of the BCC and reveals a 3rd lesion

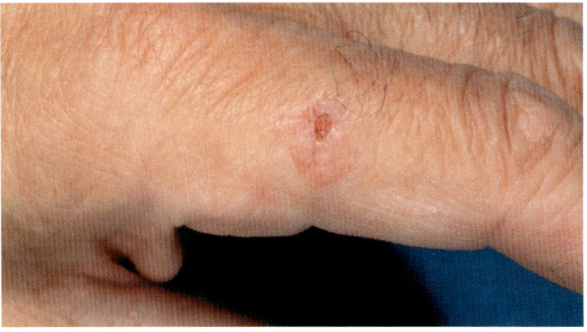

Fig. 117. BD on the index finger of the left hand. The borders of the lesion are not defined

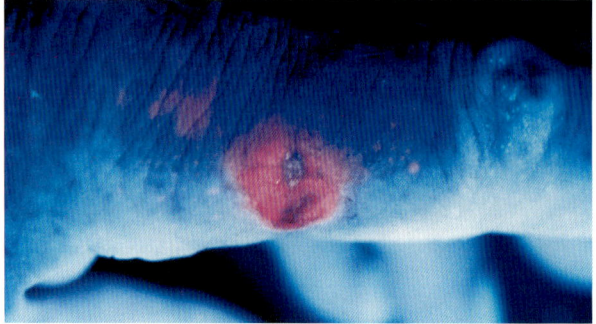

Fig. 118. FDAP presents the entire neoplastic skin. In the upper left corner there is nonspecific fluorescence of normal skin

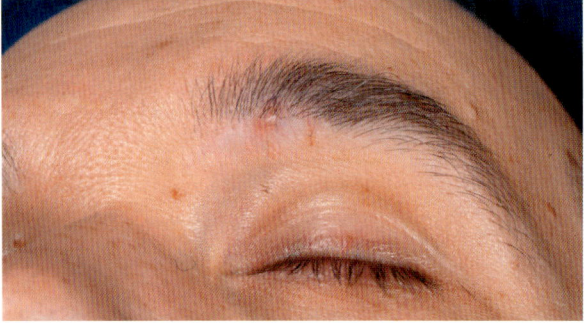

Fig. 119. Histologically verified BCC in the area of the left eyebrow

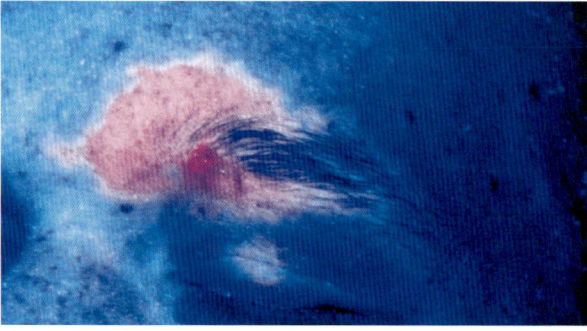

Fig. 120. Although normal skin shows a whitish fluorescence, the tumor tissue can be nicely delineated by means of FDAP

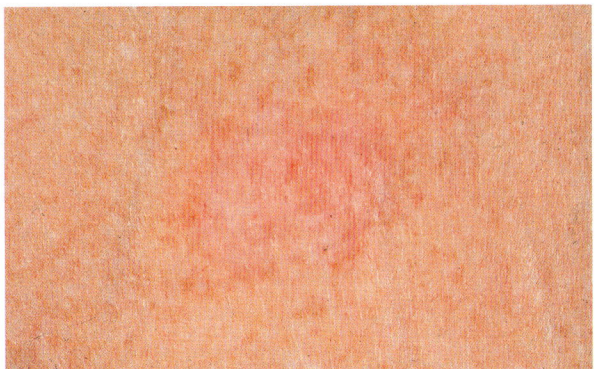

Fig. 121. This whitish red macule was histologically proven to be a BCC. It is not possible to detect the borders of the tumor

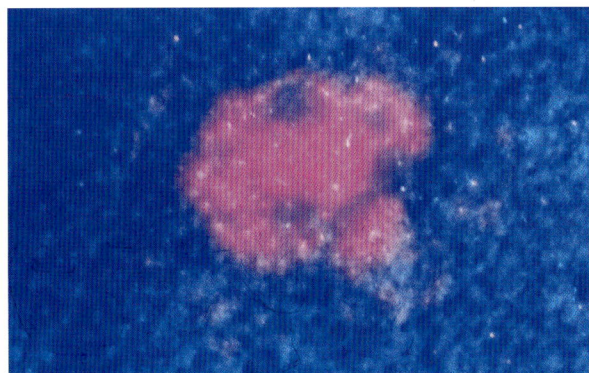

Fig. 122. In FDAP, an excellent delineation of the entire lesion is demonstrated

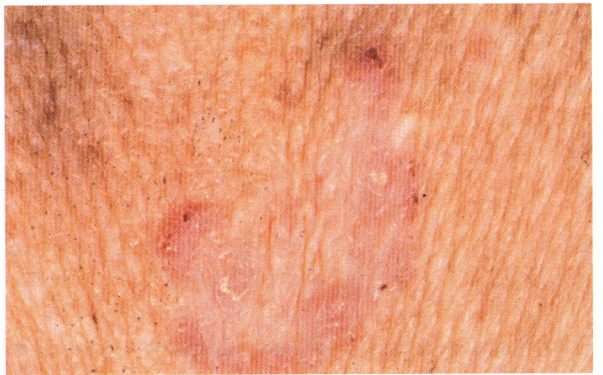

Fig. 123. BCC on the back. Most of the tumor tissue does not show clearly defined borders

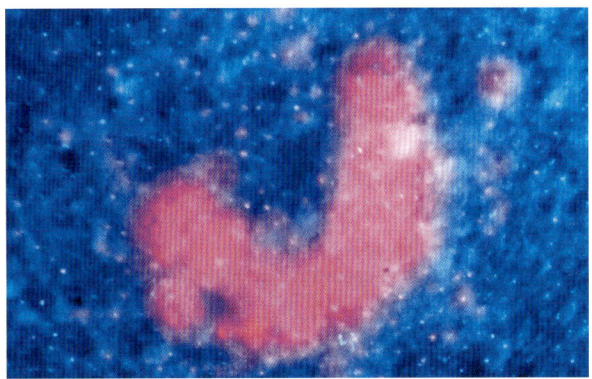

Fig. 124. In FDAP, the demarcation of the exact tumor size is possible

## H.3 FDAP in Pretreated or Damaged Skin

Most epithelial skin cancers develop in actinically damaged skin, in particular on the face. Solar damage and multiple pre-treatments by cryosurgery, surgery, or topical chemotherapy make a clear detection of the tumor tissue difficult.

FDAP offers an easy technique to demarcate neoplastic skin even in actinically damaged skin (Figs. 125 and 126) and in skin areas pre-treated by cryosurgery (Figs. 127 and 128) or surgery (Figs. 129–132). By means of FDAP, surgical procedure is optimized and remaining or regrowing tumor tissue can be detected in time.

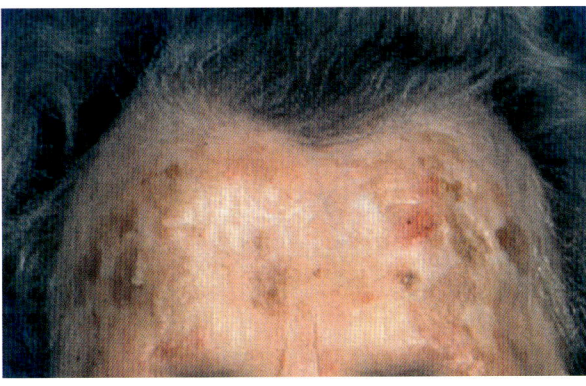

Fig. 125. Multiple SK in actinically damaged skin on the front

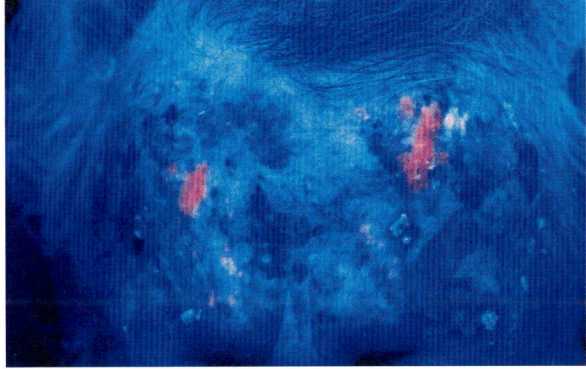

Fig. 126. FDAP demarcates the neoplastic areas

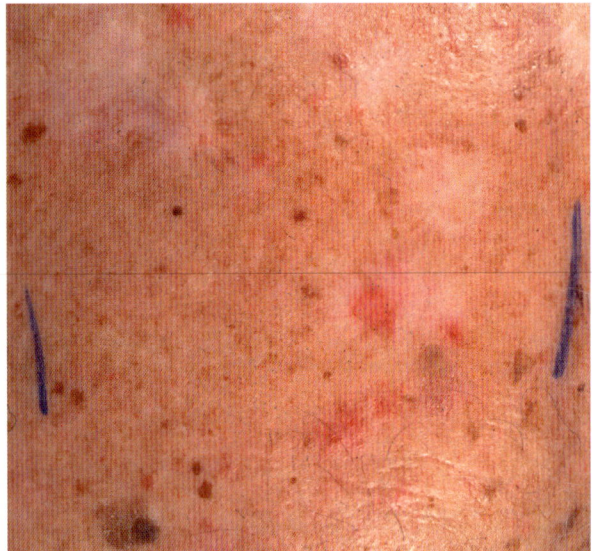

Fig. 127. Multiple BCC on the back pre-treated by cryosurgery (white scars). There are red macules, partly within the cicatrized skin. It is difficult to detect and to delineate newly developing or regressing tumor tissue

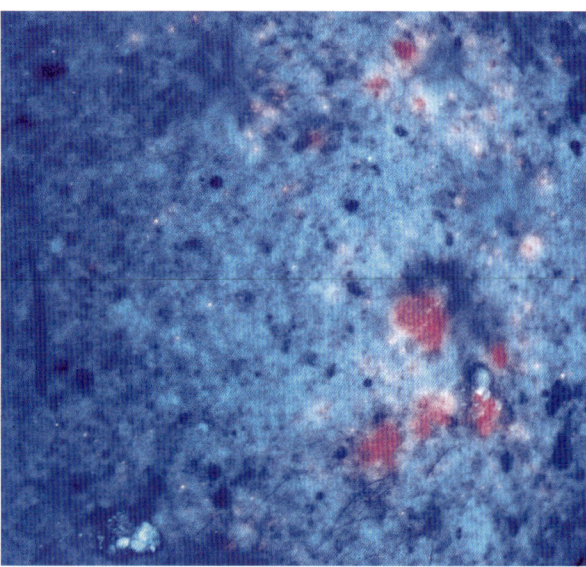

Fig. 128. The red fluorescence in FDAP allows to detect all tumor areas, to mark and to treat them effectively by cryosurgery, surgery or PDT

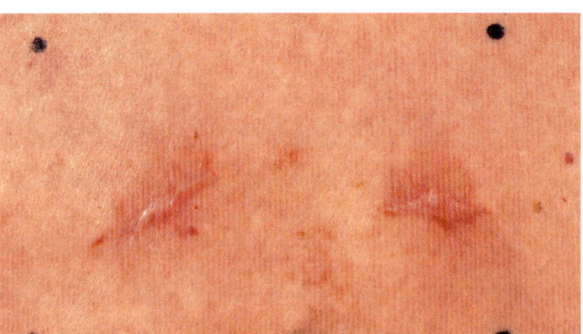

Fig. 129. Multiple scars on the back of a patient whose BCC were treated by surgery 2 years before this consultation. Some reddish areas within the scars are visible

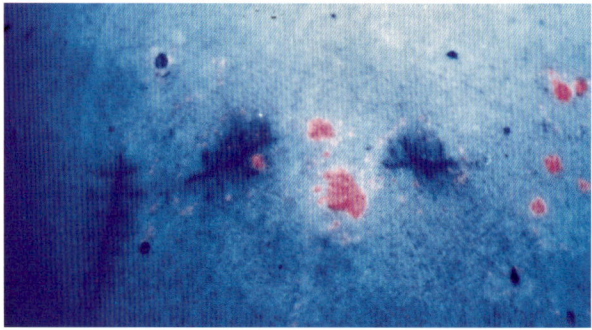

Fig. 130. In FDAP, all BCC can be easily demarcated. One of them is localized within a scar indicating tumor relapse. There, a BCC was formerly excised

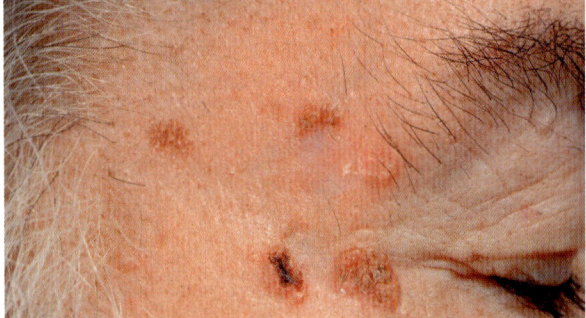

Fig. 131. Multicentric BCC. 2 years before this presentation, a BCC was surgically excised and the tissue defect was covered by a skin flap. Now, there is tumor relapse on all four edges of the former skin flap

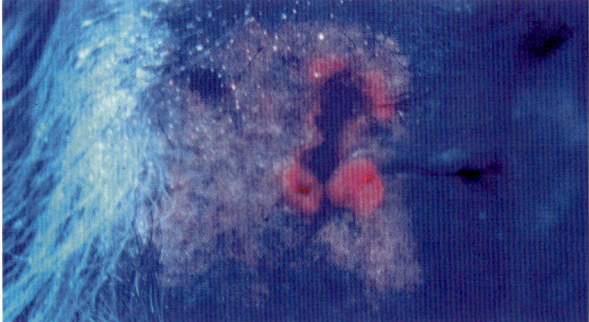

Fig. 132. FDAP describes the total dimension of the tumor area. In addition to the four tumor nodules, there is also fluorescence along the vertical sutures of the skin flap. The lesion in the left upper part of the picture is a seborrhoic wart and does not reveal any fluorescence

## H.4 Limitations of FDAP

In certain cases, the efficacy of FDAP is limited due to partly unkown reasons. Sometimes the fluorescent area in FDAP is smaller than the clinical size of the tumor (Figs. 133 and 134). In the cases of sclerodermiform BCC, the technique is of minor benefit (Figs. 135–138).

Most probable explanations for the limited correlation of the macroscopic fluorescence pattern with the tumor extension in selected cases might be: (a) an ineffective debulking of the exophytic tumor part, (b) relatively deep localization of the tumor cells, or (c) a high amount of sclerodermiform tissue limiting an optimum penetration of the ALA mixture.

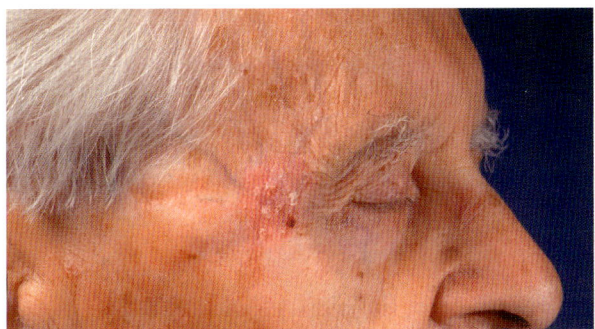

Fig. 133. This BCC is clinically ill-defined

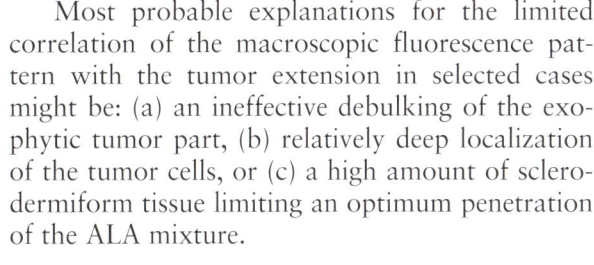
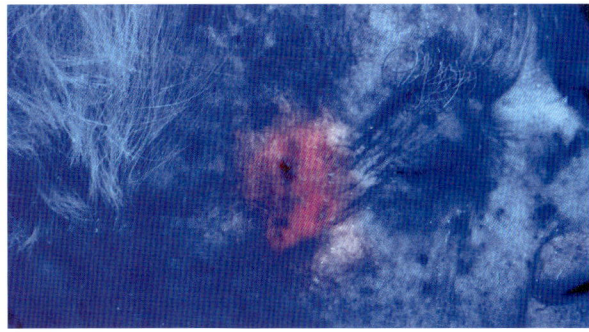

Fig. 134. FDAP improves the delineation of the tumor borders. However, in this case, the efficacy of FDAP is limited. Here, the borders of the fluorescence are not sharply demarcated, particularly at the auricular side of the tumor

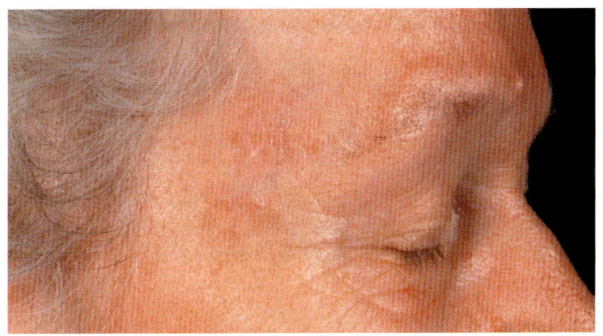

Fig. 135. Sclerodermiform BCC. The tumor tissue is invisible. The skin is indurated

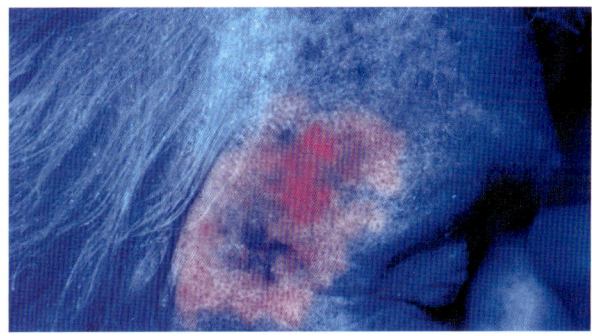

Fig. 136. FDAP clearly visualizes the tumor tissue. However, the fluorescence cannot be sharply delineated along all borders

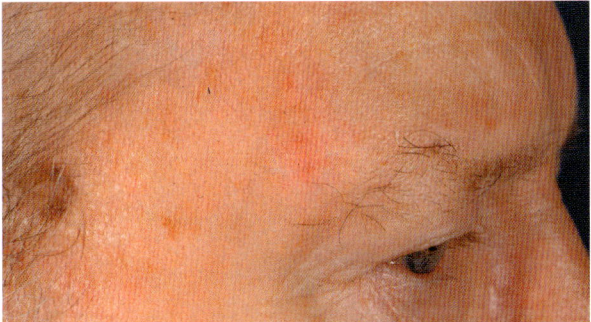

Fig. 137. Sclerodermiform type of BCC, presenting as a reddish macule. The tissue is indurated on palpation

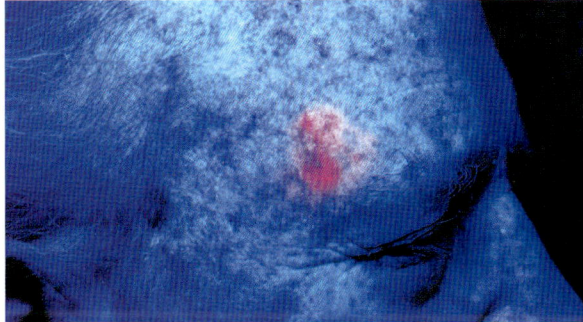

Fig. 138. In FDAP, the tumor can be well delineated. However, it is not possible to define exactly the borders of the fluorescence und thus the extension of the tumor tissue

## H.5 Usefulness of FDAP in Guiding Tumor Therapies

### Material and Methods

FDAP was used to control the efficacy of PDT, cryosurgery or surgery. 12 patients with a total number of 21 superficial BCC (trunk) were treated by **FDAP-guided cryosurgery**. Prior to each cryosurgery session (monthly), FDAP was performed (20% ALA, 4 hours). All fluorescing areas were treated by cryosurgery (Fritsch et al, 1994).

Three patients with extramammary Paget's disease (EDP) were treated by **FDAP-guided $CO_2$-laser therapy**. 20% ALA was topically applied for 6 hours. In the dark, under Wood's light visualization, all fluorescing areas were marked and subjected to $CO_2$-laser treatment (Limmer, Appen, Germany, 15–20 Watt, cw-modus, 3 to 5 layers). The resulting charred surface was removed by lightly scrubbing the surface with 3% hydrogen peroxide to avoid thermal build-up. This process was repeated layer by layer using the same parameters until all remaining abnormal fluorescent tissue had been removed. Vaporization was performed to a depth of approximately 2 mm and horizontally 1 cm beyond the fluorescent area (Becker-Wegerich et al, 1998).

Since 1995 we performed **FDAP-guided surgery** in 856 patients. All patients with lesions clinically suspect for an epithelial skin tumor (newly developed, regrowing tumor or ill-defined borders in pretreated areas) were subjected to FDAP (20% ALA, 3–6 hours). Fluorescing areas were marked by a surgical pen. The lesions were excised including the marking.

### Results

**FDAP-guided cryosurgery** was very useful to detect and cure all BCC (Figs. 139–144).

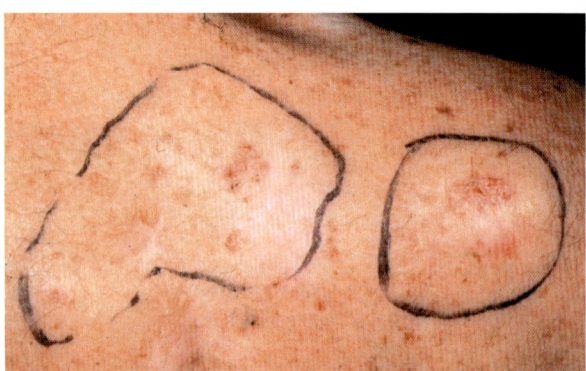

Fig. 139. Multiple BCC pre-treated by cryosurgery. Clinical picture shows a number of scars and ill-defined red macules and plaques

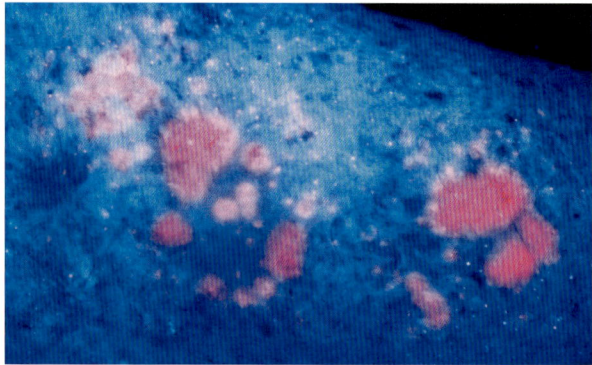

Fig. 140. In FDAP, all tumors can be clearly demonstrated. Fluorescent area was marked and selectively treated by cryosurgery (2 x 20 sec., spray technique)

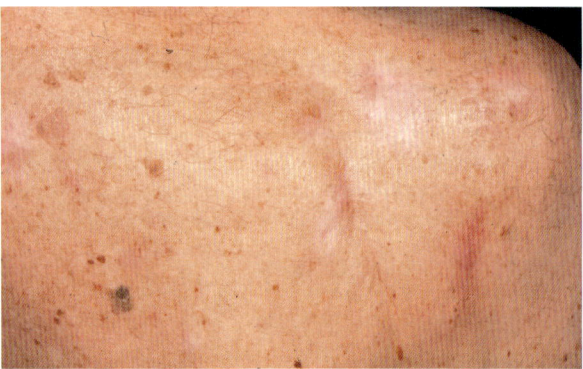

Fig. 141. One month after FDAP guided cryosurgery. A remarkable improvement of the lesions was noted

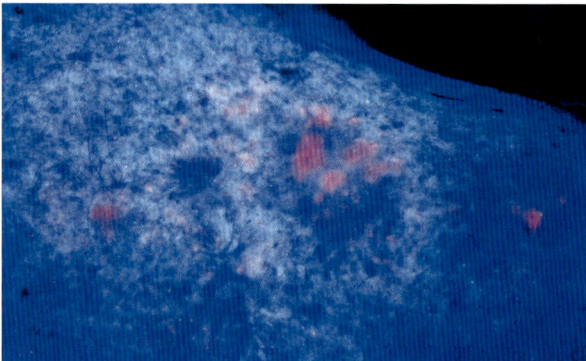

Fig. 142. In FDAP 2, there were still some fluorescing areas remaining. Therefore another session of cryosurgery was performed

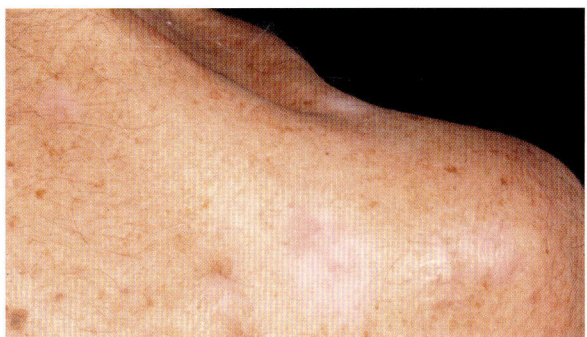

**Fig. 143.** One month after the 2nd FDAP-guided cryosurgery. There was no hint for any remaining or regrowing tumor tissue

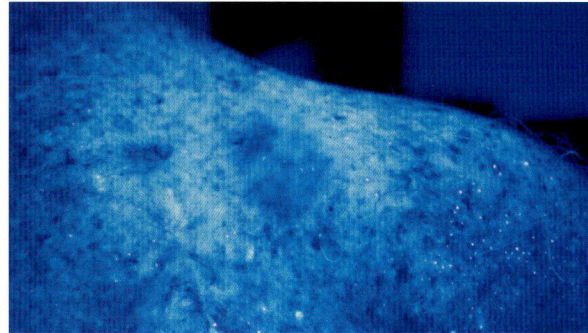

**Fig. 144.** In FDAP 3, the efficacy of crysurgery was underlined. The complete lack of fluorescence indicates absence of neoplastic tissue

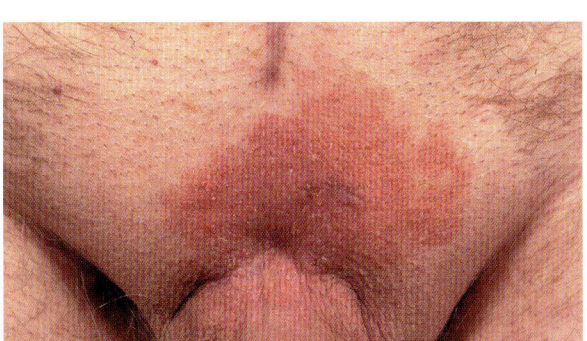

**Fig. 145.** Extramammary Paget's disease, erythematous partly eczematous plaque

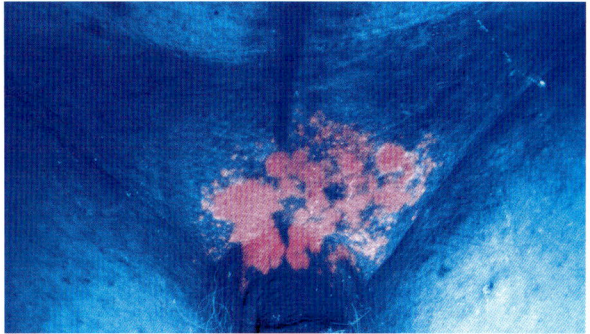

**Fig. 146.** FDAP presents high fluorescence within the clinically detected suspect area. Fluorescent area was marked and treated by $CO_2$-laser under Wood's light irradiation

After the first session, 87% of the BCC lesions were cured (Figs. 141 and 142).

FDAP allowed to detect all remaining BCCs. After another two cryosurgeries all BCCs were cured. In the last FDAP that was performed 1 month after the third cryosurgery, no fluorescing tissue was detected (Figs. 143 and 144) (Fritsch et al, 1994). However, all treated areas healed with scarring.

In the case of **FDAP-guided $CO_2$-laser vaporization** of extramammary Paget's disease, the clinically ill-defined or even undetectable tumor areas (Figs. 145 and 146) were clearly delineated by the typical red porphyrin fluorescence (Fig. 147).

In one patient 18 biopsies from the fluorescing lesions were taken according to a biopsy mapping scheme. In all biopsies extramammary Paget's disease was present. Maximum depth of infiltration was 0.38 mm. After $CO_2$-laser vaporization, a good granulation was evident, and, after 4 weeks, a good cosmetic result was achieved. Three months after therapy, FDAP revealed no fluorescence in the treated area except for a 4 mm spot (Fig. 147). This showed Paget's disease on histopathological examination, and $CO_2$-laser therapy under FDAP was performed again. FDAP control 3 months later displayed no fluorescence, indicating absence of tumor tissue.

The **FDAP-guided surgery** was performed in 815 skin tumor patients: 703 BCC (484 superficial

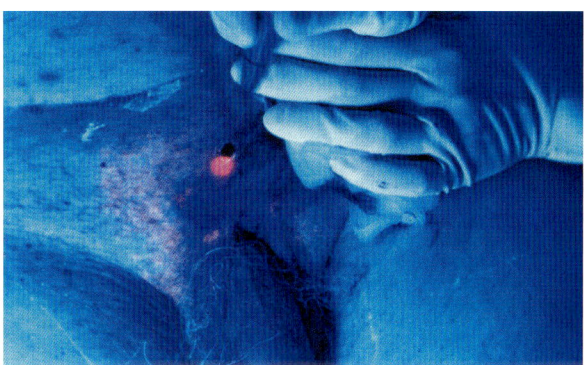

**Fig. 147.** 2nd FDAP one month after the first laser surgery. There is still one remaining tumor area detectable. FDAP-guided $CO_2$-laser surgery was repeated

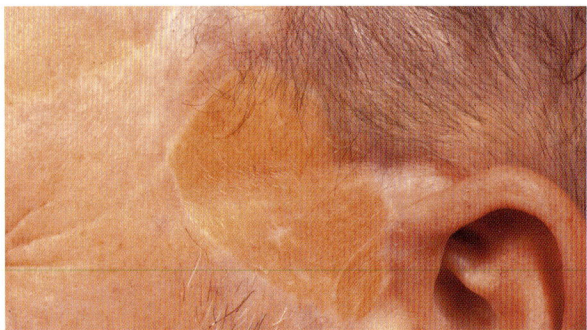

**Fig. 148.** Patient with a history of more than 200 BCC during the last 10 years. Multiple surgical interventions became necessary. Relapse of BCC was suspected surrounding the graft area

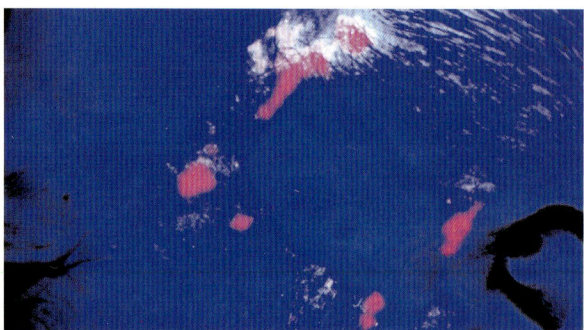

**Fig. 149.** Six brightly fluorescing spots were detected by FDAP. After marking and surgical excision, all fluorescing tissue was shown to be BCC by histopathology. None of these lesions, except that close to the helix of the ear were evident clinically

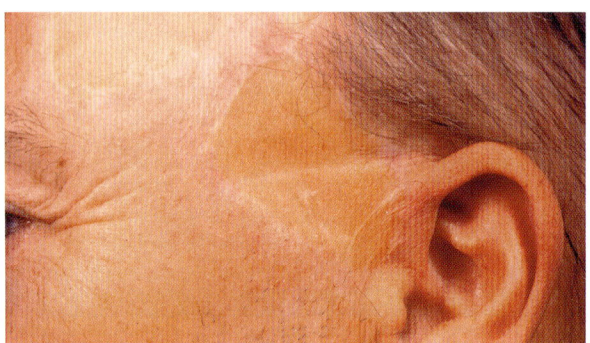

**Fig. 150.** Three months after FDAP-guided surgery of the six lesions. The remaining graft area is now diminished because parts of it were resected during surgical procedure. Clinically, there is no indication for residual tumor tissue

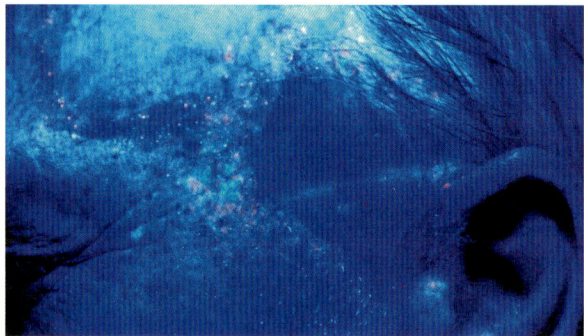

**Fig. 151.** In the corresponding 2nd FDAP, there is also no tumor-specific fluorescence. Therefore, FDAP-guided surgery can be postulated as a pre-surgical technique supporting to treat problematic cases, preferentially in anatomically difficult areas such as the face

type, 36 multicentric type, 154 solid type, 29 sclerodermiform type), 58 SCC and 34 Bowen's disease, 12 SK, 11 lesions of dermatitis and 49 normal skin or scars. In 810 / 856 (94.6%) of the lesions high fluorescence was present. In 3 lesions FDAP was false positive (0.3%). In eight BCC the fluorescence was not present – false negative (0.9%). In summary, FDAP was very useful to detect and delineate neoplastic tissues (99.1%) (Figs. 148–151).

## Chapter Discussion

This study demonstrates the effective treatment of BCC or EPD with cryosurgery or $CO_2$ laser guided by FDAP. EPD usually occurs in the genital, axillary or perianal areas, where the apocrine glands predominate (Potter, 1967). Occurrence in other sites is very rare. Approximately 50% of EPD have been associated with an underlying adenocarcinoma of urinary, genital or intestinal tract. Conventional surgical excision or Mohs' micrographic surgery is the treatment of choice in such tumors. However, in some cases it is difficult to excise the lesion completely, especially if it is widespread or located in a critical anatomical site. Other therapeutic modalities include the application of topical cytotoxic substances (5-fluorouracil and bleomycin), radiation and chemoradiotherapy. These are either ineffective or do not eradicate the tumor cells completely. The recurrence rate in EPD is high, indicating the lack of a sensitive method to visualize the clinically indistinct margin of the lesion as well as the tumor areas not responding to the treatment. Long-term follow up, using FDAP and screening procedures to detect internal malignancies, is mandatory in order to detect local recurrence at an early stage and to exclude tumor invasion.

The data concerning the correlation of the skin tumors with the fluorescence in FDAP clearly demonstrate the high specificity of this technique for neoplastic skin.

# Photodynamic Therapy in Cutaneous Diseases

In general, most published reports on the efficacy of ALA in PDT are case reports or summaries of individual experiences without using a standardized treatment schedule. Most of these studies comprised different treatment parameters (concerning choice of vehicle, concentration and application times of ALA, use of light sources and varying irradiation energies). All these experimental or pilot studies will be summarized in the Phase I-section. There is only a small number of placebo- or alternative-therapy-controlled ALA-PDT studies. They will be mentioned in the Phase II- and Phase III-section, respectively.

Generally, the results have been described as complete response (CR, no clinical and/or histopathologic evidence for the treated disease at the site of drug and light application) and partial response (PR, reduction of >50% in lesion number or size).

Due to sun exposure, most precanceroses and tumors of the skin occur mainly on the face, and therefore therapies with best cosmetic results are desirable. On the other hand, total removal of skin tumors is an aim which up to now has been achieved best with surgery and subsequent histological evaluation. Precancerous lesions are often treated by various nonsurgical methods and, depending on the age and the patient's general health condition, even cancers can be treated by methods other than surgery (Braun-Falco et al, 2000).

## I.1 PDT: Evaluation of the Efficacy in Solar Keratoses

SK and BD, the most frequent precanceroses of the skin, are mainly treated by cryotherapy, topical chemotherapy (5-fluorouracil), carbon dioxide laser vaporization or surgery depending on the size and thickness of the lesion. Except surgery, all these methods lack histological control. Some of these treatment procedures lead to hypopigmentation or hyperpigmentation and scarring. Imiquimod, a promising novel immunomodulatory compound, provokes an inflammation reaction.

### Material and Methods

A total number of 1263 SK on the scalp (n = 1134) and extremities (n = 129) were treated by topical PDT from August 1995 until July 2001.

In 165 lesions, the dependence of the response rate on the *lesion size* and total *light energy* was investigated. ALA (Merck, Darmstadt, Germany, 10% in Neribas® ointment, Schering, Berlin, Germany) was applied for 4 hours. Irradiation was performed using red light with intensities from 50 to 120 $mW/cm^2$ and total energies from 60 to 144 $J/cm^2$ (PDT 1200®, Waldmann, Villingen-Schwenningen, Germany, 570–670 nm). PDT was repeated biweekly (maximum: 3 PDT sessions).

In 250 lesions (n = 129 on the backs of the hands, n = 121 on the scalp), the response rate depending on the *localization* was measured. ALA (Merck, Darmstadt, Germany, 10% in Neribas® ointment, Schering, Berlin, Germany) was applied for 4 hours. Irradiation was performed using green light with an intensity of 20 $mW/cm^2$ and a total energy of 30 $J/cm^2$ (PDT Greenlight®, Saalmann, Herford, Germany, 543–548 nm). PDT was repeated biweekly (total maximum number: 3 PDT sessions).

In 6 SK (capillitium), the response rate depending on the *light source (wavelength)* was measured (see Sect. I.8.).

In 20 lesions (capillitium), the efficacy of *ALA methylester* (20%, Metvix®, PhotoCure ASA, Oslo, Norway) was evaluated. Application time was 3 hours. Red light was applied using 75 $J/cm^2$ of CureLight (PhotoCure ASA, Oslo, Norway). PDT was repeated once (total maximum number: 2 PDT sessions).

The remaining 822 lesions were treated routinely using 10% ALA (Merck, Darmstadt, Germany or medac, Wedel, Germany) and green light with an intensity of 20 $mW/cm^2$ and a total energy of 30 $J/cm^2$ (PDT Greenlight®, Saalmann, Herford, Germany, 543–548 nm). PDT was repeated biweekly until complete response of the lesions (total maximum number: 3 PDT sessions).

### Results

Dependence on *lesion size* and on the total *light energy* (ALA, red light): SK were effectively treated by 10% ALA and red light PDT (Table 9). Smaller lesions responded better to PDT than larger ones. Best results for all lesion sizes were achieved using light energy of 144 $J/cm^2$ and two treatment sessions (100%).

**Table 9.** PDT in SK: Influence of lesion size and light energy

| Size [cm] | Lesions [n] | Irradiation [broad band, red, 570–650] | | Complete response | | |
|---|---|---|---|---|---|---|
| | | [mW/cm²] | [J/cm²] | 1 | 2 | 3 |
| Dependence on the Size | | | | | | |
| <0.5 | 20 | 50 | 60 | 60 | **100** | – |
| | 20 | 80 | 96 | 80 | **100** | – |
| | 20 | 100 | 144 | 95 | **100** | – |
| 0.5 – 1 | 30 | 50 | 60 | 57 | 83 | **100** |
| | 30 | 80 | 96 | 67 | 93 | **100** |
| | 25 | 100 | 144 | 92 | **100** | – |
| >1 | 10 | 50 | 60 | 50 | 90 | **100** |
| | 7 | 80 | 96 | 86 | **100** | – |
| | 7 | 100 | 144 | 86 | **100** | – |
| Dependence on the energy | | | | | | |
| All sizes | 60 | 50 | 60 | 56 | 91 | **100** |
| All sizes | 57 | 80 | 96 | 78 | **100** | **100** |
| All sizes | 52 | 120 | 144 | 91 | **100** | – |
| Best choice | | | | | | |
| All sizes | 52 | **120** | **144** | 91 | **100** | – |

SK of different sizes treated by 20% ALA for 4 h. Irradiation was performed by red light with energies varying from 60 to 144 J/cm². Best results for any size of lesion were achieved using 120 mW/cm² red light irradiation for 20 min (= 144 J/cm²).

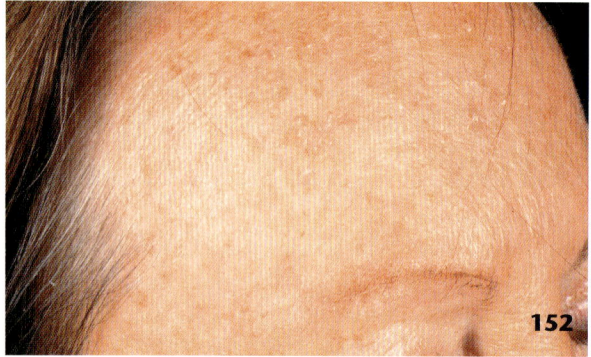

**Fig. 152.** Multiple SK on the front. Lesions are better gropable than visible. PDT was performed using 10% ALA and red light (570 – 750 nm; 96 J/cm²)

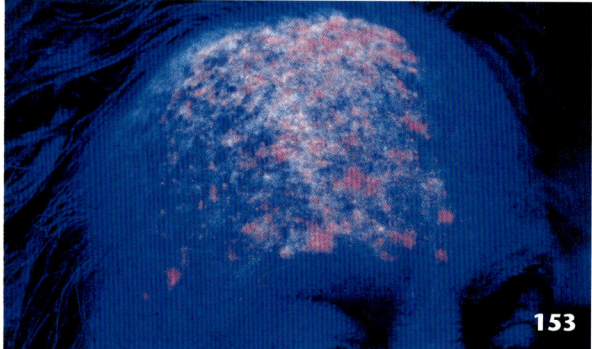

**Fig. 153.** FDAP (10% ALA): There is a large area of fluorescent tissue, indicating SK. The number of SK could not be estimated in the clinical picture alone

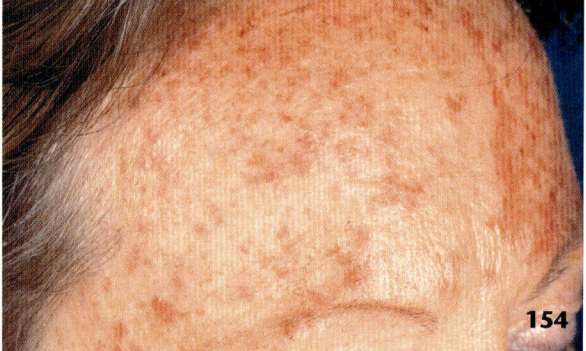

**Fig. 154.** One day after PDT session. Inflammation reaction with demarcation of all skin areas which accumulated high porphyrin levels

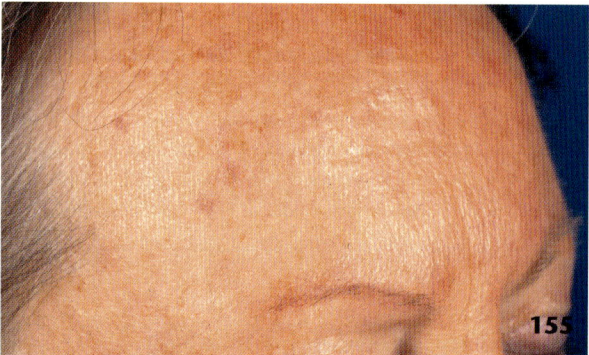

**Fig. 155.** Two weeks after PDT. Besides a slight hyperpigmentation, there is a complete response of all SK

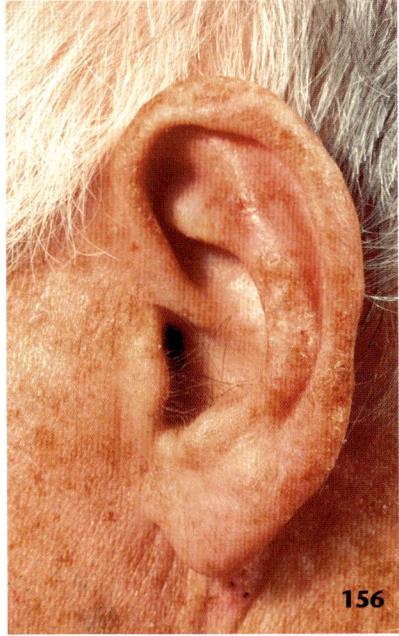
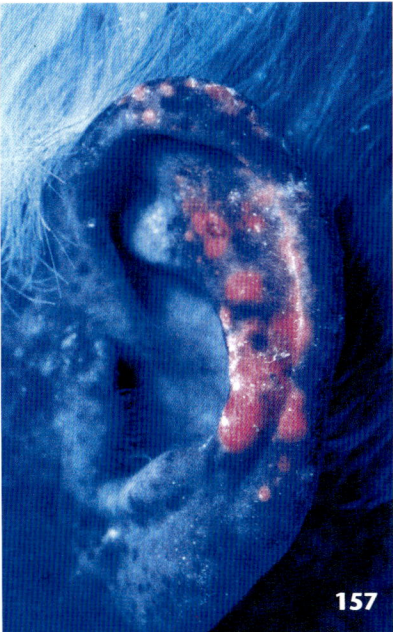
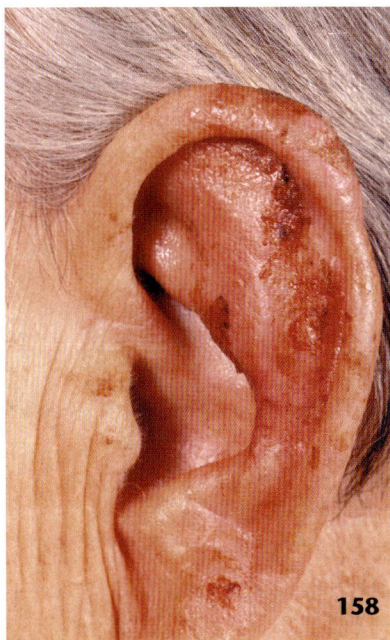

**Fig. 156.** Multiple SK on the helix of the left ear presenting as crusts and hyperkeratotic areas. Detailed detection of all lesions is not possible

**Fig. 157.** FDAP: Specific marking of all neoplastic areas. The ear was treated by 10% ALA and 60 J/cm² red light

**Fig. 158.** One day after PDT. Red crusty tissue, inflammation reaction

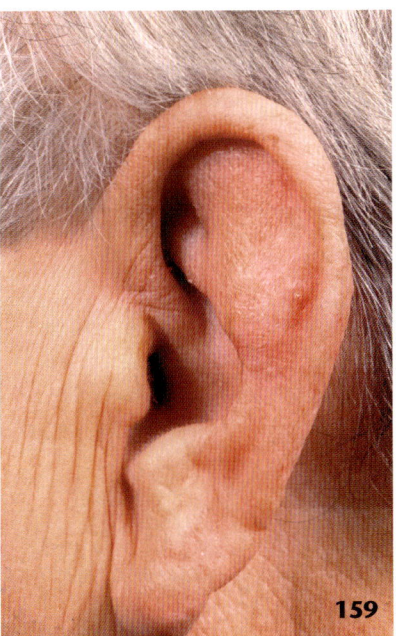
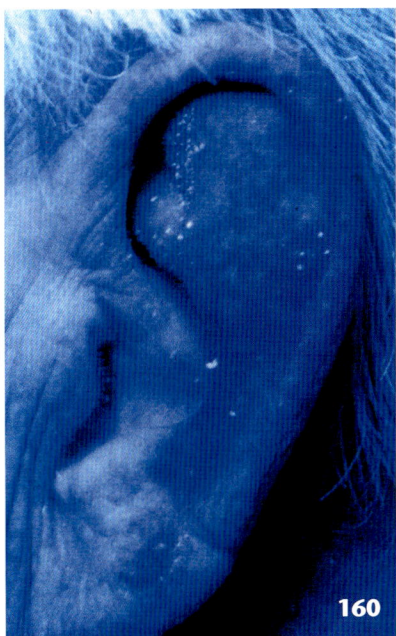

**Fig. 159.** One month after PDT. Ear free of tumor tissue with an excellent cosmetic result

**Fig. 160.** FDAP 2: One month after PDT. No tumor-specific fluorescence detectable

Dependence on the *localization*: The SK on the backs of the hands responded much worse than those on face or scalp. After the first PDT session, 89.3% of the SK on the scalp were cured in contrast to only 40.3% of those localized on the backs of the hands. After the second and third PDT session, all lesions on the scalp were cured (2nd 98.3%, 3rd 100%) (Figs. 152–160). The lesions on the hands showed complete response rates of 52.7% (2nd) and 61.2% (3rd).

The efficacy of *ALA methylester* (20%, Metvix®, PhotoCure ASA, Oslo, Norway) in topi-

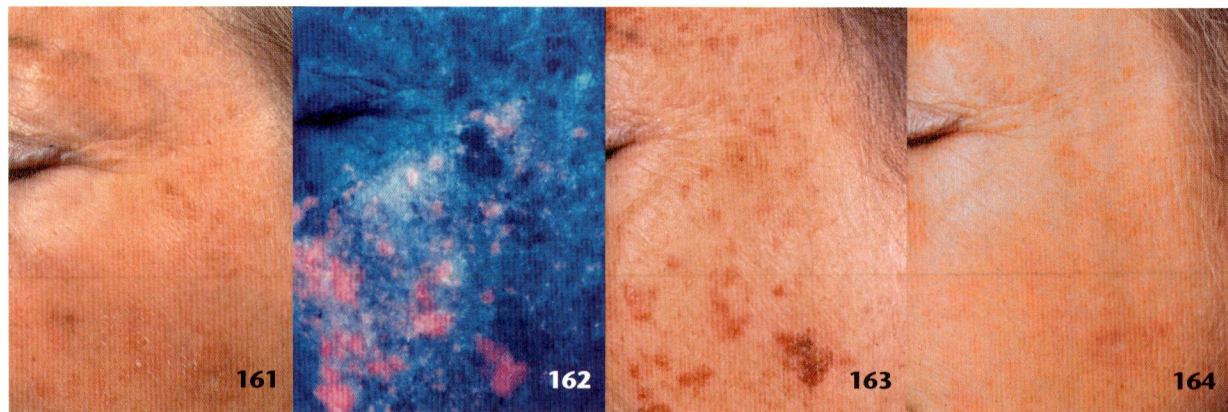

**Fig. 161.** Multiple SK on the cheek; **Fig. 162.** FDAP (20% ALA-ME): Detection of all neoplastic skin areas; **Fig. 163.** One day after PDT with red light (75 J/cm²). Inflammation with crusts; **Fig. 164.** One month after PDT. Facial skin is clear and smooth without any scals or keratosis

cal PDT was found to be very good. All SK were cured after the 2nd PDT (Figs. 161–164).

The remaining 822 lesions in 364 patients were treated with routine regimen (Figs. 165–168) and showed complete response rates as shown in Table 10.

**Table 10.** PDT in SK: Routinely treated lesions

| Localisation | Patients [n] | Lesions [n] | Irradiation [543 – 548] | | Complete response | | |
|---|---|---|---|---|---|---|---|
| | | | [mW/cm²] | [J/cm²] | 1 | 2 | 3 |
| Front | 286 | 498 | 20 | 30 | 84.3 | 98.4 | **100** |
| Temporal | 22 | 60 | 20 | 30 | 86.7 | **100** | – |
| Parietal | 86 | 144 | 20 | 30 | 88.9 | 97.2 | **98.6** |
| Occipital | 41 | 57 | 20 | 30 | 84.2 | 87.7 | **96.5** |
| Face | 39 | 63 | 20 | 30 | 95.2 | **100** | – |
| Total | 364 | 822 | 20 | 30 | 87.9 | 96.7 | **99.0** |

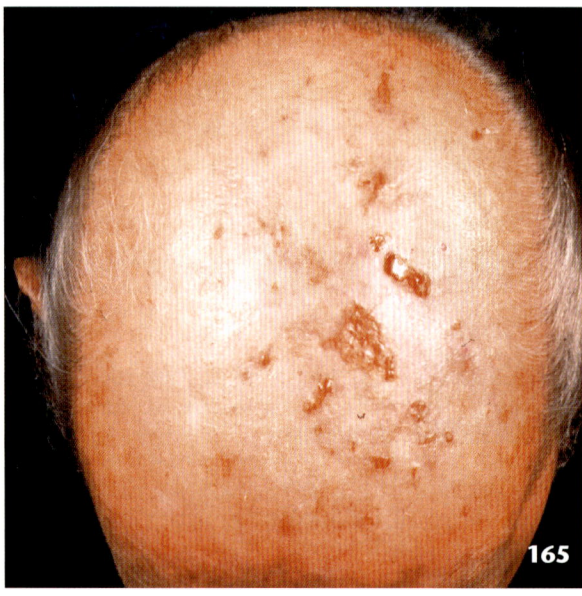
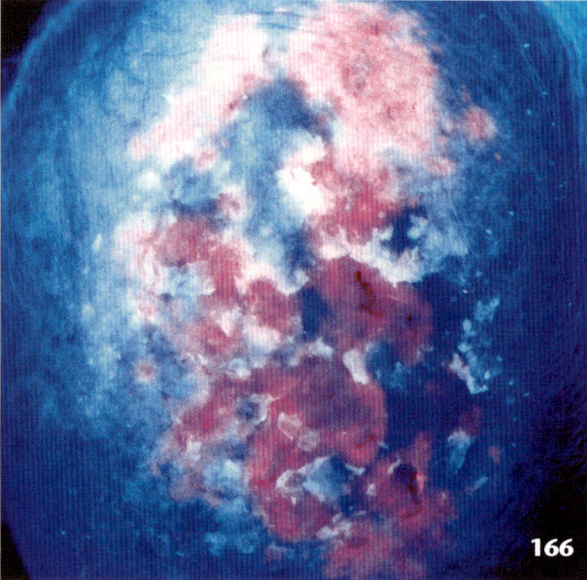

**Fig. 165.** Multiple SK, partly with transition into SCC. The skin was cleansed by isopropanol-soaked gauze. In addition, all exophytic parts of the lesions were removed by curettage using a curette; **Fig. 166.** FDAP (10% ALA): A large number of SK was detected by the porphyrin fluorescence technique. PDT was performed using green light (543 – 548 nm, 30 J/cm²).

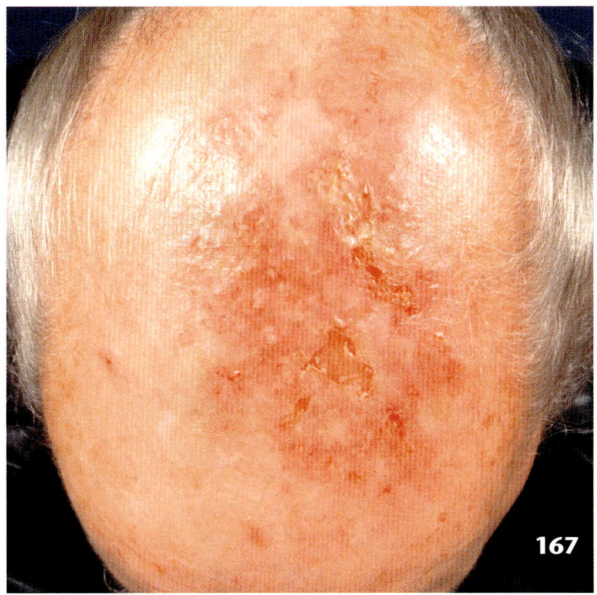 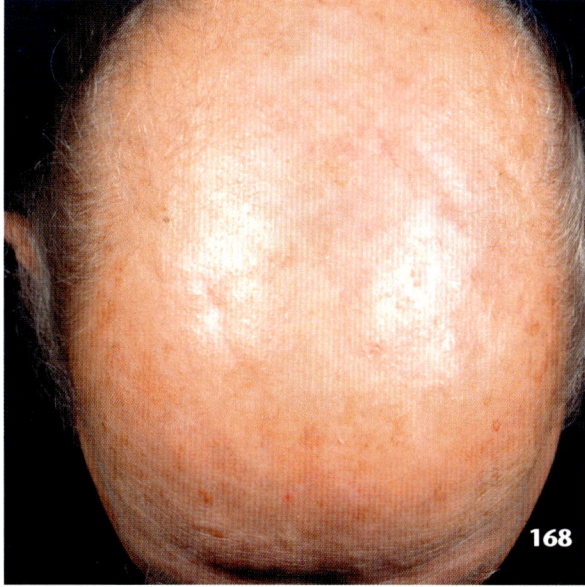

Fig. 167. Two days after PDT. Inflammation reaction. Serous crusts are overlying the treated lesions. Anti-inflammatory and antimicrobial treatment was performed with polyvidone iodine containing solutions and triamcinolone (0.1%) containing creams; Fig. 168. 20 days after PDT. Healthy clear skin free of any tumor tissue presenting an excellent cosmetic result

## Chapter Discussion

*Clinical trials and Phase I-studies.* In 1990, the topical application of 20% ALA to SK, followed by a single exposure to light of a filtered slide projector, resulted in a CR of 90% (Kennedy et al, 1990). Other investigators, using more professional incoherent light sources, obtained a CR in 80 to 100% of all treated SKs (Wolf et al, 1993; Fijan et al, 1995; Calzavara-Pinton, 1995). Using ALA concentrations from 10 to 30%, the CR rate of SKs located on the face and scalp was significantly higher (91%) in comparison with keratoses on the trunk and the extremities (45%) (Jeffes et al, 1997). The poor clinical response (<30%) of the thick hyperkeratotic lesions may be due to ineffective penetration of ALA and consecutive insufficient production of porphyrin molecules. The results in SK in Japanese patients were approximately the same as those reported for SK in Caucasian patients. However, a larger number of treatment sessions was required (Itoh et al, 2000). ALA-PDT using red, green or blue light may already be postulated as the treatment of choice for non-hyperkeratotic SKs of the face or scalp. A standardized protocol for the treatment of SK has been developed by the company DUSA (Valhalla, New York, USA) using Levulan® (ALA-hydrochloride). The product Kerastick™ has been approved for clinical use: 20% wt/vol ALA-solution (48% ethanol) is applied to individual lesions and re-applied once after the initial application has dried. To ensure accurate application of topical ALA solution an applicator is used. The applicator tip is attached to a flexible plastic tube containing 2 glass vials: 1 containing ALA in powder form and the other an ethanol based solvent. The vials are broken by pressing the tube: the contents are mixed by shaking and then applied by gently dabbing the lesion. 14 to 18 hours after application the company recommends to expose the treated lesions to blue light (417 nm; 10 J/cm$^2$). However, PDT with ALA applied for even shorter intervals (3–6 h) and using red or green light is also highly effective in the treatment of SK (Fritsch et al, 1998; Fritsch et al, 1997). Schering AG, Berlin applied for registration of Levulan® Kerastick™ for the treatment of SK in Austria in 2001. Austria acts as a reference member state for the European registration.

*ALA methylester* (20%) was shown to induce a more selective porphyrin accumulation in SK as compared to free ALA (Fig. 75) (Fritsch et al, 1998) and was proven to effectively cure SK on the face and the scalp using red light irradiation 3 h after application (Braathen et al, 2000).

*Phase II-studies.* *ALA hydrochloride*: In a randomized, multicenter, vehicle-controlled, investigator-blinded, light-dose ranging study, maximum therapeutic effects were obtained in ALA-treated SK irradiated with blue light (417 nm) at a dose of

10 J/cm² (10 mW/cm²) (Jeffes et al, 1997; Omrod and Jarvis, 2000). 20% ALA solution or the vehicle was applied to 2 lesions each on the face and scalp in 36 patients. 14 to 18 h after application, lesions were exposed to 2, 5 or 10 J/cm² of blue light (417 nm) delivered at 3, 5 or 10 mW/cm². Eight weeks after treatment a CR was obtained in 66% of ALA-treated lesions versus 17% of those treated with vehicle and light (p < 0.001). The maximum response (80%) was seen in patients treated with the highest dose of light (10 J/cm²). Nonresponding lesions were re-treated at 8 weeks, and by 16 weeks the CR was 85% in ALA-treated lesions.

The efficacy of the higher light dose was confirmed in a second phase II study conducted with the same protocol in 64 patients (Omrod and Jarvis, 2000). 20% ALA or vehicle was applied to 25 cm² of skin containing 3 to 7 lesions. CR were defined as patients who had > 75% of their lesions cleared. Using this criterion up to 100% of patients responded to a single treatment with ALA. Again maximum response was obtained with 10 J/cm² at 10 mW/cm². 14% of patients terminated treatment early or required reduction of the power density of light irradiation because of stinging and burning.

To establish the optimum concentration of the ALA solution, a randomized, vehicle-controlled, investigator-blinded, multicenter study was carried out using ALA 2.5, 5, 10, 20, or 30% wt/vol and blue light at 10 J/cm² (10 mW/cm²) (Omrod and Jarvis, 2000). ALA was applied to lesions (site not specified) in 124 patients. There were significantly more CR (defined as clearance of 75% of lesions) in the groups treated with 10, 20 or 30% ALA than in the groups treated with 2.5 or 5%. A dose-response trend was evident with a plateau emerging at the 10, 20 and 30% concentration levels. The researchers concluded that an ALA concentration of 20% produced the best response.

An earlier dose-ranging study used a red light regimen and was conducted in 40 patients (Jeffes et al, 1997). Topical ALA solution 10, 20 or 30% or vehicle was applied under an opaque occlusive tape to 6 lesions on the head, trunk or extremities which were irradiated 3 h later with red light (630 nm, 150 mW/cm²). The best responses were obtained in lesions on the head (p < 0.05 for lesions on head vs lesions on trunk and extremities treated with ALA 20 or 30%). Moreover, typical SKs (grade 1 or 2, easily seen with palpable hyperkeratosis), but not thick hypertrophic or hyperkeratotic lesions (grade 3), responded well to ALA-PDT. In grade 1 and 2 lesions, CR of lesions occurred in 42, 50 and 61% of patients treated with ALA 10, 20 and 30%, respectively (vs 3% with vehicle) at 16 weeks. Light fluence, which ranged from 10 to 150 J/cm², had no effect on efficacy in this study (Jeffes et al, 1997).

*ALA methylester*: Using 20% ALA methylester in an oil in water formulation (Metvix®, Photocure, Oslo, Norway) and red light irradiation (Curelight®, Photocure, Oslo, Norway), 160 mg ALA methylester/g cream was found to lead to optimum response rates (Braathen et al, 2000; Bjerring et al, 2001).

*ALA hydrochloride vs. 5-fluorouracil*: The purpose of another study was to assess the efficacy and tolerability of ALA-PDT versus topical 5-fluorouracil (FU) in 14 patients with SK on the backs of the hands (Kurwa et al, 1999). Each patient's right and left hands were randomized to receive either a 3-week course of topical 5-FU applied twice per day or PDT using topical ALA and then, after 4 hours, irradiation (incoherent light; 580 to 740 nm; 53–100 mW/cm²; 150 J/cm²). All patients were reviewed at 1, 4, and 24 weeks after starting treatment. The mean lesional area treated with topical FU decreased from 1390 to 297 mm² (mean lesion reduction: 70%). The mean lesional area treated with topical PDT decreased from 1322 to 291 mm² (mean lesion reduction: 73%). There was no statistically significant difference between the treatment methods in overall symptom scores for pain and redness. One treatment with PDT using topical ALA appears to be as effective and well tolerated as 3 weeks of twice-daily topical FU, a cheap and widely available alternative.

***Phase III-studies.*** In phase III trials topical ALA 20% was effective in eradicating SKs of the face and scalp in the majority of patients. A total of 241 patients with 4 to 15 SK were enrolled in 2 randomized, vehicle-controlled, investigator-blinded, multicenter trials (Omrod and Jarvis, 2000). Treatment protocols were identical: a 20% ALA solution was applied to lesions on the face or scalp, 14 to 18 h before exposure to blue light (417 nm; 10 mW/cm²; 10 J/cm²). CR (defined as 75% and 100%) were determined 8 weeks after treatment. Lesions which had not cleared were re-treated (with ALA or vehicle and PDT as appropriate). All patients were re-evaluated 12 weeks after the initial treatment. Eight weeks after treatment a CR was obtained in 66% of patients (119 of 180) treated with ALA whereas only 13% of patients (8 of 61) treated with vehicle showed a CR. A 75% CR was reported in 77 and 23% of patients randomized to ALA and vehicle, respectively. Among patients who required a second treatment, 43% (24 of 56) of ALA recipients were clear of lesions after 12 weeks (versus 4% (2 of 49) among placebo recipients). The CR among ALA-treated patients increased from 66% at week 8 to 72% at week 12, and the >75% CR increased from 77 to 88%. At 12 weeks the 100 and 75% CR for vehicle-treated patients were 20 and 11%, respectively. It should be noted that, among patients treated with ALA whose lesions had CR at 8 weeks, recurrences were detected in 12% (14 patients) at 12 weeks. For vehicle-treated patients the 8 to 12 week recurrence rate was 37.5% (3 of 8 patients). There were 1403 lesions at baseline in the ALA treatment group and by 8 weeks 1161 of these had cleared, representing a 82.8% CR. At week 12, 1103 lesions were clear (78.6% CR) and 58 had recurred. Thus, the recurrence rate for total ALA-treated lesions between 8 and 12 weeks was 5%. For vehicle-treated patients the CR for total lesion numbers (506 at baseline) were 34.4 and 27.9% at 8 and 12 weeks, respectively. Between weeks 8 and 12, 33 of 174 lesions which were clear at 8 weeks recurred; a 27.9% recurrence rate.

The clearance rate was higher for lesions on the face than on the scalp. At 12 weeks CR of 78% and 50%, respectively, were obtained in facial and scalp lesions treated with ALA (*vs* <13 in placebo recipients). At the same time-point the 75% clearance rate among ALA-treated patients was 82% and 56% for face and scalp, respectively (*vs* 20% among placebo recipients).

*ALA methylester*: Multicenter clinical trials using 20% ALA methylester in an oil in water formulation (Metvix®, Photocure, Oslo, Norway) and red light irradiation (Curelight®, Photocure, Oslo, Norway) proved a CR of 80% (*vs.* 20% placebo; single PDT) with comparable CR to those achieved by cryosurgery (Foley et al, 2001).

## I.2 PDT: Evaluation of the Efficacy in Bowen's Disease

### Material and Methods

A total number of 132 BD patients was treated by topical PDT from September 1995 until July 2001.

In 8 lesions, the dependence of the complete response rate on the *lesion size* was investigated. ALA (Merck, Darmstadt, Germany, 20% in Neribas® ointment, Schering, Berlin, Germany) was applied for 4 hours. Irradiation was performed using red light with intensities from 150 mW/cm$^2$ and total energies 180 J/cm$^2$ (PDT 1200®, Waldmann). PDT was repeated biweekly (maximum total number: 3 PDT sessions).

In 124 lesions, the response rate depending on the *light source (wavelength)* was measured (see Sect. I.8.).

### Results

Dependence on the *lesion size* (ALA, red light): Diameters of the eight lesions varied from 1.8 to 15.8 cm. The complete response rates were 50% after the 1st PDT, 75% after the 2nd PDT and 75% after the 3rd PDT session (Figs. 169–174). The two lesions, which were not cured were large ones. In addition, there was a regrowth of 3 of the 6 effectively treated lesions after 6 months.

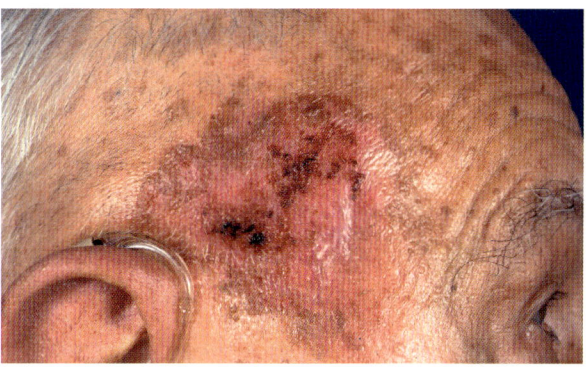

**Fig. 169.** BD with transition into Bowen carcinoma in the central part of the lesion. The carcinomatous skin was surgically excised and the surrounding BD treated by PDT: 20% ALA, 180 J/cm$^2$ red light (570–750 nm). Total of 3 PDT sessions were performed with monthly intervals

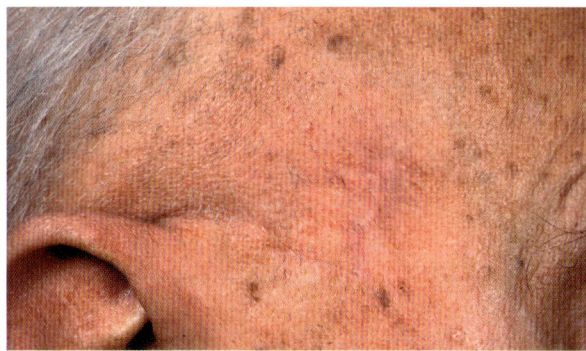

**Fig. 170.** Two months after the 3rd PDT session. The scar represents the area in which the Bowen carcinoma was excised. There is clear skin without evidence of remaining tumor tissue

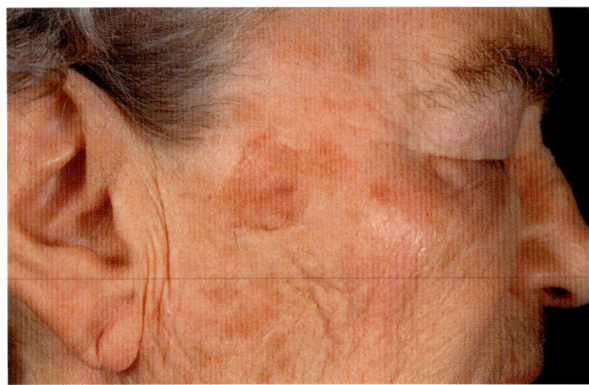

**Fig. 171.** BD within a seborrhoic keratosis, proven by histopathology. It is impossible to distinguish the neoplastic skin from benign changes

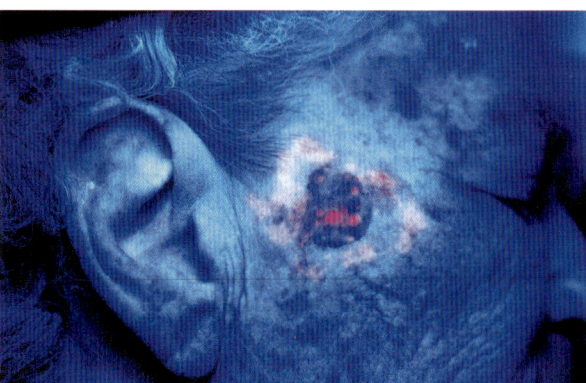

**Fig. 172.** Distinct fluorescence in some areas in the central part of the seborrhoic keratosis

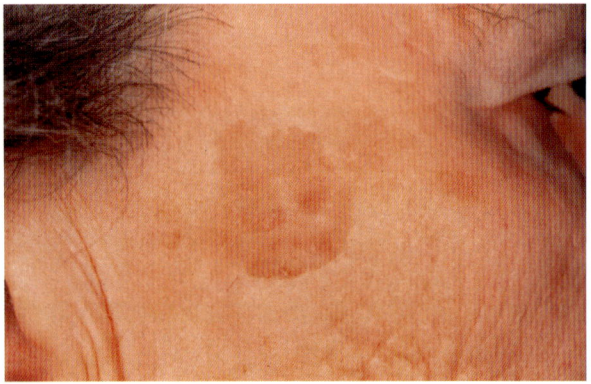

**Fig. 173.** Clinical result after 1 PDT-session using 20% ALA and green light irradiation (543–548 nm, 30 J/cm$^2$ PDT green light, Saalman, Germany)

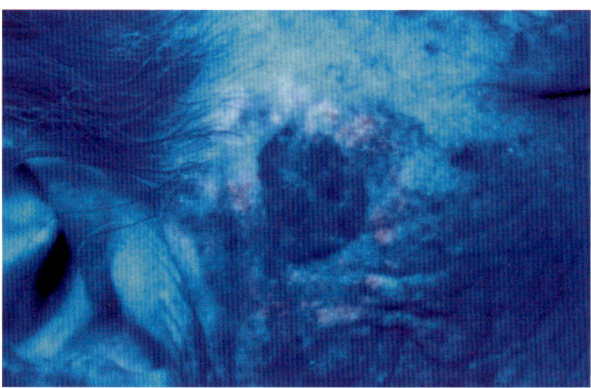

**Fig. 174.** FDAP one month after one PDT-session: there is no fluorescent tissue present

## Chapter Discussion

*Clinical trials and Phase I-studies.* Topical PDT was shown to be effective in BD as demonstrated by a series of studies utilizing the combination of topical 20% ALA and various light sources (Kennedy et al, 1990; Fritsch et al, 1998). Long-term results vary considerably (CR: 30–100%) (Cairnduff et al, 1994; Fijan et al, 1995; Wennberg 1996; Morton et al, 1996). Incomplete response of BD may be due to the thickened epithelial layer with reduced ALA-penetration (Fritsch et al, 1998; Cairnduff et al, 1994, Fijan et al, 1995; Robinson et al, 1988; Pennington et al, 1988, Buchanan et al, 1989; Allen et al, 1992; Wennberg et al, 1996; Morton et al, 1996; Jeffes et al, 1997). Recent clinical trials question the superiority of laser light, demonstrating a 78 to 100% response rate of BD to PDT with conventional lamps (Wennberg et al, 1996). Cryotherapy was shown to be less effective and associated with more complications (ulceration, infection) than ALA-PDT (Morton et al, 1996). Penile BD responded nicely to ALA-PDT (Hart and Hirshovitz, 1998).

## I.3 PDT: Evaluation of the Efficacy in Basal Cell Carcinoma

Basal cell carcinoma (BCC) is the most often occurring semimalignant tumor in humans. Treatment of first choice is surgery but especially in superficial multicentric BCC cryotherapy, 5-fluorouracil or carbon dioxide laser have been proven to be potent alternative strategies. Recently, promising therapeutic results were achieved with imiquimod (5%) containing preparations (Beutner et al, 1999). Radiotherapy might be indicated in the case of large and infiltrating lesions (ulcus rodens, ulcus terebrans) for palliative reasons or for lesions not amenable to any of the methods mentioned above. Side effects are similar to those mentioned in the SK/BD section. Because of the potential risk of tumor progression or recurrence the treated patient needs close follow up.

## Material and Methods

A total number of 452 BCC (superficial BCC: n = 363; nodular BCC: n = 55; sclerodermiform BCC: n = 31) were treated by topical PDT from August 1995 until July 2001.

In 117 lesions (104 superficial, 13 sclerodermiform), the dependence of the response rate on the *lesion size* and the total *light energy* was investigated. ALA (Merck, Darmstadt, Germany, 20% in Neribas® ointment, Schering, Berlin, Germany) was applied for 4 hours. Irradiation was performed using red light with intensities from 80 to 150 mW/cm$^2$ and total energies from 96 to 180 J/cm$^2$ (PDT 1200®, Waldmann, Villingen-Schwenningen, Germany, 570–670 nm). PDT was repeated biweekly (total maximum number: 3 PDT sessions).

In 42 superficial lesions (n = 37 on the trunk, n = 5 on the face), the complete response rate depending on the type of *light source (wavelength)* was measured (see Sect. I.8.).

In 10 lesions, classified as difficult to treat by conventional strategies, the efficacy of *ALA methylester* (20%, Metvix®, PhotoCure ASA, Oslo, Norway) was evaluated. Application time was 3 hours. Red light was applied using 75 J/cm$^2$ of CureLight (PhotoCure ASA, Oslo, Norway). PDT was repeated once after one week and another 2 times 3 months later (total maximum number: 4 PDT sessions).

The remaining 280 lesions (217 superficial, 45 nodular, 18 sclerodermiform BCC) were treated routinely using 20% ALA (Merck, Darmstadt, Germany or medac, Wedel, Germany) and red light (70 J/cm$^2$, CureLight, PhotoCure ASA, Oslo, Norway). PDT was repeated weekly until complete response of the lesions (total maximum number: 3 PDT sessions) was reached.

## Results

Dependence of the response rate on the *lesion size* and on the total *light energy* (ALA, red light): In the 104 superficial BCC, cure rates were dependent on the light energy applied; best response rates were observed for 180 J/cm$^2$ (Table 11). concerning the lesion size, success of PDT was optimum for BCC smaller than 4 cm in diameter. However, larger lesions could be at least reduced in size, reudening these lesions accessible for surgical treatment. Of the 13 sclerodermiform BCC, 85% were cured after three PDT sessions using 180 J/cm$^2$ (follow up time: 6–24 months) (Figs. 175–177).

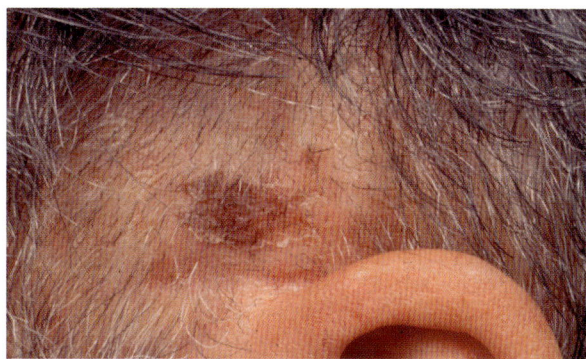

**Fig. 175.** Nodular BCC in the supraauricular area. Crusts and the exophytic tumor mass were removed by gentle curettage

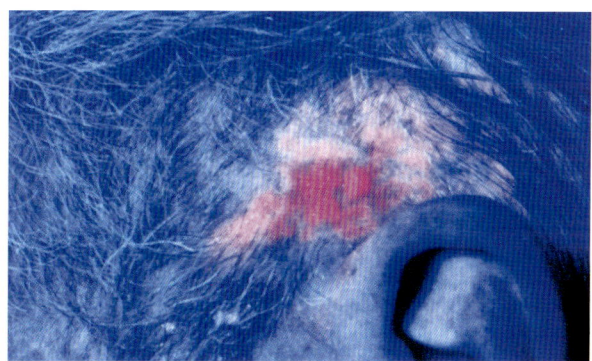

**Fig. 176.** FDAP: Relatively sharp demarcation of the lesion. PDT was performed 3 times with 20% ALA and red light (570–750 nm, 180 J/cm$^2$)

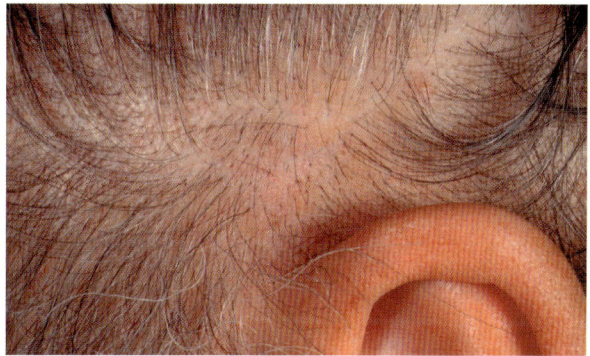

**Fig. 177.** Complete response with excellent cosmetic outcome

**Table 11.** PDT in superficial BCC: Influence of lesion size and light energy

| Size [cm] | Lesions [n] | Irradiation [broad band, red 570–650] | | Complete response | | |
|---|---|---|---|---|---|---|
| | | [mW/cm²] | [J/cm²] | 1 | 2 | 3 |
| Dependence on the size | | | | | | |
| <1 | 5 | 80 | 96 | 60 | 80 | 100 |
| | 5 | 120 | 144 | 80 | 100 | – |
| | 6 | 150 | 180 | 83 | 100 | – |
| 1–2 | 10 | 80 | 96 | 70 | 90 | 90 |
| | 8 | 120 | 144 | 63 | 88 | 100 |
| | 10 | 150 | 180 | 80 | 90 | 100 |
| 2–4 | 8 | 80 | 96 | 60 | 60 | 75 |
| | 5 | 120 | 144 | 80 | 80 | 80 |
| | 12 | 150 | 180 | 67 | 86 | 100 |
| 4–8 | 9 | 80 | 96 | 25 | 50 | 63 |
| | 9 | 120 | 144 | 50 | 50 | 80 |
| | 9 | 150 | 180 | 50 | 75 | 75 |
| 8–12 | 2 | 80 | 96 | 0 | 0 | 50 |
| | 3 | 120 | 144 | 0 | 0 | 33 |
| | 3 | 150 | 180 | 0 | 33 | 33 |
| Dependence on the energy | | | | | | |
| <1–12 | 34 | 80 | 96 | 43 | 56 | 67 |
| <1–12 | 30 | 120 | 144 | 55 | 64 | 79 |
| <1–12 | 40 | 150 | 180 | 56 | 70 | 82 |
| Best choice | | | | | | |
| <1–4 | 69 | **150** | **180** | 77 | 92 | **100** |

Superficial BCC of different sizes treated by 20% ALA for 4 h. Irradiation was performed by red light with light energies varying from 96 to 180 J/cm². Best results were achieved using lesions <4 cm and 150 mW/cm² red light irradiation for 20 min (= 180 J/cm²).

In the 10 BCC, which were difficult to treat by conventional strategies, the PDT with *ALA methylester* and red light (75 J/cm²) (4 sessions, interval one week) led to a complete response rate of 90% (follow up time were 12 months) (Figs. 178–187)

The *BCC treated routinely* by 20% ALA and red light PDT presented cure rates depending on the type of lesion (Table 12).

**Table 12.** PDT: Response of BCC

| Type | Lesion [n] | Irradiation [570 – 650 nm] | | Complete response | | |
|---|---|---|---|---|---|---|
| | | [mW/cm²] | [J/cm²] | 1 | 2 | 3 |
| Superficial BCC | 217 | 60 | 70 | 87 | 97 | 100 |
| Nodular BCC | 45 | 60 | 70 | 78 | 89 | 96 |
| Sclerodermiform BCC | 21 | 60 | 70 | 48 | 61 | 81 |

BCC treated by 20% ALA and red light (75 J/cm², Curelight, PhotoCure ASA, Norway). Best results were achieved for the superficial BCC. Nodular BCC also responded well to PDT. For the sclerodermiform type, 3 PDT sessions were necessary to cure 81% of the lesions.

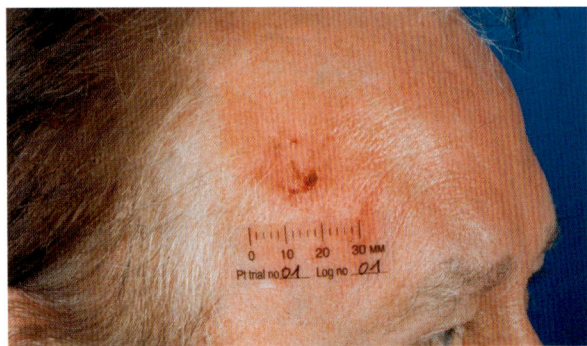

**Fig. 178.** BCC on the front right

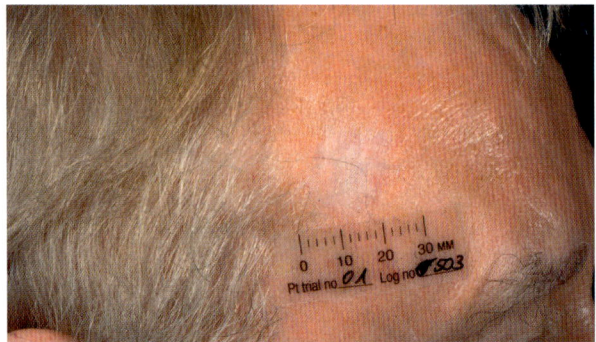

**Fig. 187.** Complete response 3 months after 4 PDT sessions. Slight scarring is present

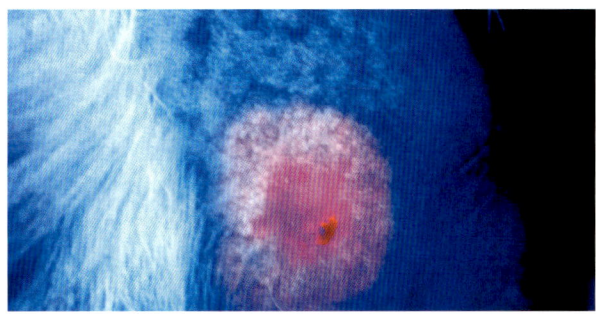

**Fig. 179.** FDAP with 20% ALA: Intensive fluorescence of the tumor. However, the surrounding skin also shows a bright fluorescence

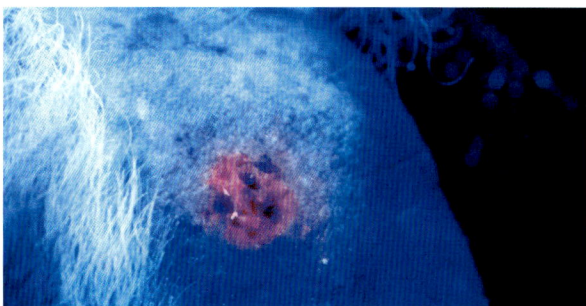

**Fig. 180.** 1st FDAP with 20% ALA methylester: Less intensive but more selective fluorescence than achieved with ALA

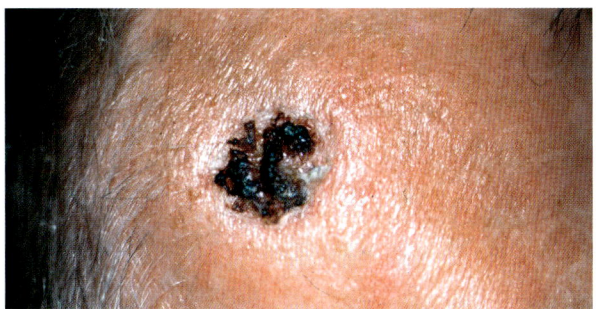

**Fig. 181.** 2 days after PDT with Metvix® and red light (75 J/cm²). Hemorrhagic crusts are formed

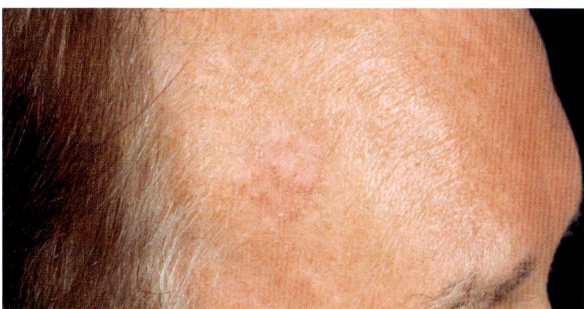

**Fig. 182.** One week after the 1st PDT session. Partial response of the lesion can be seen

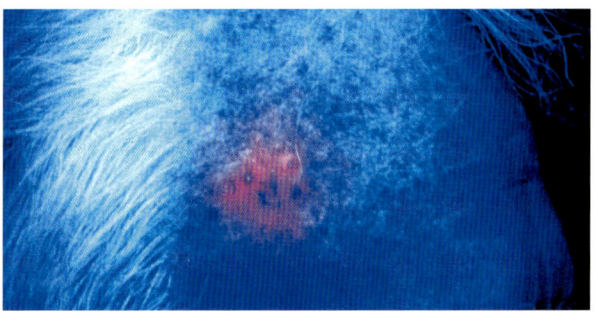

**Fig. 183.** 2nd FDAP with 20% ALA methylester: There is still fluorescence present indicating remaining neoplastic tissue

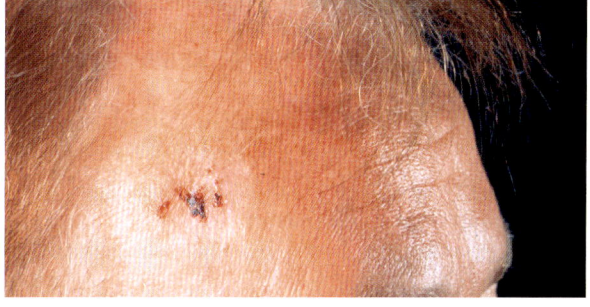

**Fig. 184.** 2 days after the 2nd PDT with Metvix® and red light (75 J/cm²). Hemorrhagic crusts are formed

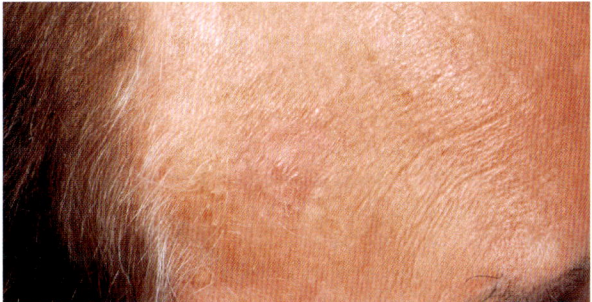

**Fig. 185.** One week after the 4th PDT session the treated area seems to be free of any tumor tissue

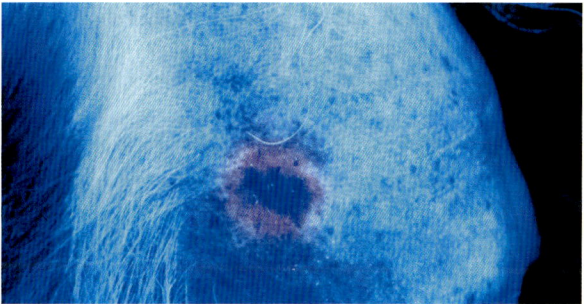

**Fig. 186.** 4th FDAP with 20% ALA methylester: There is no fluorescence present

## Chapter Discussion

*Clinical trials and Phase I-studies.* Superficial BCC showed best response with a remission rate of 99,7% (after the 3rd PDT session). However, also the nodular BCC were responding (3 PDT cycles: 96%). This encouraging result in nodular BCC can be attributed to the debulking procedure which has been routinely performed in all lesions since 1998. Worst response showed the sclerodermiform type of BCC with 81% after 3 PDT sessions. Best results were attained in superficial lesions, with CR rates ranging from 80 to 100% (Wolf et al, 1993; Warloe et al, 1992; Cazavara-Pinton, 1995; Fritsch et al,1998). Nodular and noduloulcerative BCCs showed low CR rates ranging between 10 and 50% in early studies (Wolf et al, 1993; Warloe et al, 1995; Fijan et al, 1995). The limited penetration of ALA into the deeper layers of these tumors contributes at least partly to the lack of sufficient response to PDT (Peng et al, 1995). Distribution of the photosensitizer throughout various BCC types, including nodular and sclerodermiform tumors, was improved after oral or intravenous administration of ALA (Peng et al, 1995; Tope et al, 1998).

It has been demonstrated that a debulking procedure of the exophytic tumor part is essential for a successful PDT in nodular BCC. In addition, best results of topical PDT for nodular BCCs have been obtained with repeated treatment sessions (once per week) using ALA methylester and red light irradiation, leading to a 95–98% CR rate. Sclerodermiform BCCs showed nonhomogeneous or weak fluorescence and responded poorly to topical ALA-PDT (Figs. 98–100) (Fritsch et al, 2000). The porphyrin kinetic studies revealed optimum tumor sensitization 2 to 4 h after topical application of ALA (Fritsch et al, 1999). Large BCC patches were treated successfully by intralesional injection of 10% ALA in a 0.9% sodium chloride solution (Fink-Puches et al, 1997).

FDAP was shown to be highly effective in detecting and delineating BCC affected tissues (Fig. 121–124) (Fritsch et al, 1997; Fritsch et al, 1998).

*Phase II-studies.* In a dose-finding study for the treatment of BCC, 160 mg ALA methylester/g cream (Metvix®, Photocure, Oslo, Norway) was effectively used to cure most of the included lesions (Basset-Seguin et al, 2000). Patients with 'high-risk' BCC (mid-face, large, recurrent) excluding sclerodermiform and highly infiltrating lesions, may be in need of advanced surgery or radiation therapy with the risk of morbidity and/or poor cosmetic outcome (Wolf et al, 2001). Metvix® was also used for PDT in this group of patients to determine CR rate, cosmetic outcome and side effects. Patients (n=85, 108 lesions) received one treatment cycle with Metvix® PDT (two treatments one week apart). After 3 h occlusion, the lesion was illuminated with a dose of 75 J/cm$^2$ red light (Curelight®, Photocure, Norway, 570–670 nm). If an incomplete response was seen after three months (verified by biopsy), the lesion was retreated in the same way. For superficial and nodular lesions CR was 45 and 47%, respectively. Of the patients treated 40% received two treatment cycles. Clinical evaluation showed a 88% CR rate, whereas histopathological results proved only a CR of 74% (Wolff et al, 2001).

## I.4 PDT: Evaluation of the Efficacy in Squamous Cell Carcinoma

Squamous cell carcinomas (SCC) carry the risk of metastases. Surgery with histopathological examination of the tumor is the treatment of choice, particularly in a infiltrating lesion. Alternative procedures mentioned above (Sect. I.3) are also applicable depending on the age and the general health of the patient.

### Material and Methods

A total number of 152 SCC were treated by topical PDT from August 1995 until July 2001.

In 36 lesions, the dependence of the complete response rate on the *lesion size* and the total *light energy* was investigated. ALA (Merck, Darmstadt, Germany, 20% in Neribas® ointment, Schering, Berlin, Germany) was applied for 4 hours. Irradiation was performed using red light with intensities ranging from 80 to 150 mW/cm$^2$ and total energies from 96 to 180 J/cm$^2$ (PDT 1200®, Waldmann, Villingen-Schwenningen, Germany, 570–670 nm). PDT was repeated biweekly (maximum total number: 3 PDT sessions).

In 28 lesions (n=18 on the face, n=10 on the trunk), the complete response rate depending on the *fractionation of the total applied light dose* was measured. ALA (Merck, Darmstadt, Germany, 20% in Neribas® ointment, Schering, Berlin, Germany) was applied for 4 hours. Irradiation was performed using green light with an intensity of 150 mW/cm$^2$ and a total energy of 180 J/cm$^2$ or fractionated in three sessions of 60 J/cm$^2$ each with intervals of 10 min (PDT

CureLight®, PhotoCure ASA, Oslo, Norway). PDT was repeated biweekly (total maximum number: 3 PDT sessions).

The remaining 88 lesions were treated routinely using 20% ALA (Merck, Darmstadt, Germany or medac, Wedel, Germany) and green light (20 mW/cm$^2$; 30 J/cm$^2$; PDT Greenlight®, Saalmann, Herford, Germany, 543–548 nm) or red light (70 J/cm$^2$, CureLight®, PhotoCure ASA, Oslo, Norway). PDT was repeated biweekly until complete response of the lesions (maximum total number: 3 PDT sessions).

## Results

Dependence of the complete response rate on the *lesion size* and the total *light energy* (ALA, red light): SCC were completely cured using 3 PDT sessions and 180 J/cm$^2$ (Figs. 188–200) (Table 13).

Table 13. PDT in SCC: Influence of lesion size and light energy

| Size | Lesion [n] | Irradiation [broad band, red, 570–650 nm] | | Complete response | | |
|---|---|---|---|---|---|---|
| | | [mW/cm$^2$] | [J/cm$^2$] | 1 | 2 | 3 |
| Dependence on the size | | | | | | |
| <1 | 3 | 80 | 96 | 0 | 66 | 66 |
| | 3 | 120 | 144 | 33 | 66 | **100** |
| | 3 | 150 | 180 | 66 | **100** | – |
| 1–2 | 4 | 80 | 96 | 25 | 50 | 75 |
| | 3 | 120 | 144 | 0 | 33 | 66 |
| | 3 | 150 | 180 | 66 | **100** | – |
| 2–4 | 3 | 80 | 96 | 33 | 66 | 66 |
| | 4 | 120 | 144 | 25 | 50 | 75 |
| | 3 | 150 | 180 | 33 | 66 | **100** |
| Dependence on the energy | | | | | | |
| <1–4 | 10 | 80 | 96 | 19 | 61 | 69 |
| <1–4 | 10 | 120 | 144 | 19 | 50 | 80 |
| <1–4 | 9 | 150 | 180 | 55 | 87 | **100** |
| Best choice | | | | | | |
| **<1–4** | 9 | **150** | **180** | 55 | 87 | **100** |

SCC of different sizes were treated by 20% ALA for 4 h. Irradiation was performed by red light with energies varying from 96 to 180 J/cm$^2$. Best results were achieved in lesions <4 cm and using 150 mW/cm$^2$ red light irradiation for 20 min (=180 J/cm$^2$).

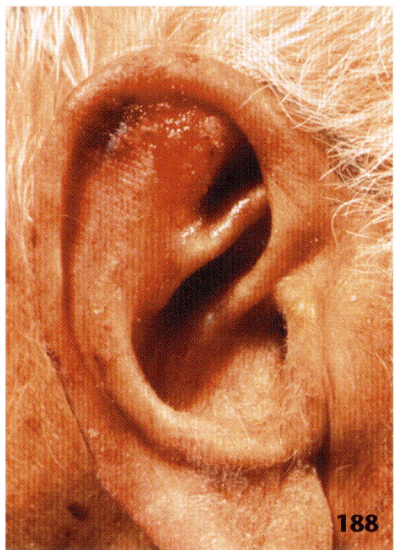 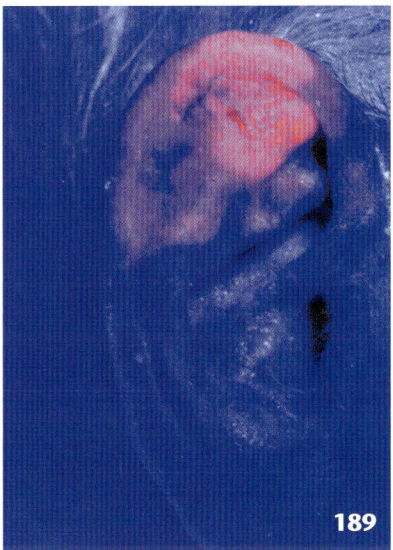 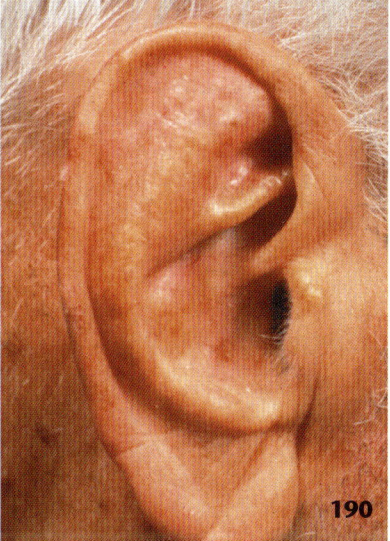

**Fig. 188.** SCC on the upper part of the helix. Inflamed tissue with indistinct borders; **Fig. 189.** FDAP: Fluorescence describes the area of all neoplastic tissue; **Fig. 190.** FDAP: Two months after 3 PDT sessions using 20% ALA and red light (180 J/cm$^2$, 570–750 nm)

Influence of the *fractionation of total applied light* (ALA, red light): 14 SCC were treated by fractionated light application and 14 lesions by continuos light exposure. Complete response rates were (continuous / fractionated): 1st PDT: 64% / 71%, 2nd PDT: 86% / 79%, 3rd PDT: 100% / 93% without statistical difference.

## Chapter Discussion

***Clinical trials and Phase I-studies.*** In situ-SCC and early invasive SCC showed CR rates between 40 and 100%, including data from repeated PDT sessions (Fritsch et al, 1998; Wolff et al, 1993; Calzavara-Pinton, 1995). Topical PDT of advanced SCC resulted only in partial response (PR) (Lui and Anderson, 1993, Kennedy et al, 1990; Cazavara-Pinton, 1995). In a female patient with xeroderma pigmentosum, multiple SCC were effectively treated using a 40% ALA formulation (Wolf et al, 1991).

## I.5 PDT: Evaluation of the Efficacy in Psoriatic Lesions

### Material and Methods

Concerning PDT in psoriatic lesions, there were only some anecdotal reports (Boehnke et al, 1994). Up to now, fundamental studies on the route of photosensitizer administration and the selection of a certain light source are lacking. There are already some very effective therapeutic schedules for psoriasis treatment such as: combined use of topical calcipotriol or corticosteroids with UVB 311 nm irradiation as well as topical or systemic PUVA (psoralen + UVA). In particular, topical PUVA is increasingly performed by applying psoralen as a cream or in a bath. Photosensitization, a side effect in systemic PUVA therapy, is avoided by topical PUVA. In general, using UVB311nm or PUVA, irradiation strategies have to be performed 4 times a week over 3 to 6 weeks or even longer to achieve a benefit of the disease. Therefore, it would be worth while to evaluate if PDT would request fewer sessions and even lead to a longer remission-free interval as compared to UVB 311 nm or PUVA.

A total number of 181 psoriatic lesions in 46 patients was treated by topical PDT from Januar 1999 until July 2001.

In 32 lesions, the dependence of the response rate on the *lesion size* and the total *light energy* was investigated. ALA (medac, Wedel, Germany, 5% in unguentum emulsificans aquosum) was applied for 4 hours. Irradiation was performed using red light with intensities from 20 to 50 mW/cm$^2$ and total energies 30 to 80 J/cm$^2$ (PDT 1200®, Waldmann, Villingen-Schwenningen, Germany, 570–670 nm). PDT was repeated twice per week (total maximum number: 8 PDT sessions = 4 weeks).

In 48 lesions (trunk, extremities), the complete response rate depending on the *ALA concentration* was measured. ALA (medac, Wedel, Germany, 5% in unguentum emulsificans aquosum) was applied for 4 hours. Irradiation was performed using green light with an intensity of 20 mW/cm$^2$ and a total energy of 30 J/cm$^2$ (PDT Greenlight®, Saalmann, Herford, Germany, 543–548 nm). PDT was repeated twice per week (total maximum number: 10 PDT sessions).

In 32 lesions (n = 20 on the trunk, n = 12 on the back of the hands), the complete response rate depending on the *localization* was measured. ALA (Merck, Darmstadt, Germany, 5% in Neribas® ointment, Schering, Berlin, Germany) was applied for 4 hours. Irradiation was performed using green light with an intensity of 20 mW/cm$^2$ and a total energy of 30 J/cm$^2$ (PDT Greenlight®, Saalmann, Herford, Germany, 543–548 nm). PDT was repeated twice per week (total maximum number: 10 PDT sessions).

In 65 psoriatic lesions, the complete response rate depending on the *light source (wavelength)* was measured (see Sect. I.8.).

In 20 lesions (trunk), the efficacy of *ALA methylester* (20%, Metvix®, PhotoCure ASA, Oslo, Norway) was evaluated. Application time was 4 hours. Green light was applied with an intensity of 20 mW/cm$^2$ and a total energy of 30 J/cm$^2$ (PDT Greenlight®, Saalmann, Herford, Germany, 543–548 nm). PDT was repeated twice per week (total maximum number: 10 PDT sessions).

### Results

Dependence of the complete response rate on the *lesion size* and on the total *light energy* (5% ALA, red light) (Table 14):

All light energies chosen here led to comparable complete response rates (maximum 83–92% after 8 PDT sessions). However, treatment resulted in partially intolerable pain.

**Table 14.** PDT in psoriasis lesions: Influence of lesion size and light energy

| Size [cm] | Lesions [n] | Irradiation [broad band, red, 570–650] | | Complete response | | | Pain |
|---|---|---|---|---|---|---|---|
| | | [mW/cm²] | [J/cm²] | 4 | 6 | 8 | |
| *Dependence on the size* | | | | | | | |
| <2 | 4 | 20 | 30 | 50 | 50 | 75 | **2.4** |
| | 3 | 30 | 50 | 33 | 66 | **100** | **2.7** |
| | 4 | 50 | 80 | 50 | 75 | 75 | **2.8** |
| 2–4 | 3 | 20 | 30 | 33 | 66 | **100** | **2.3** |
| | 4 | 30 | 50 | 50 | 50 | 75 | **2.6** |
| | 3 | 50 | 80 | 33 | 100 | – | **2.6** |
| 4–8 | 4 | 20 | 30 | 50 | 75 | **100** | **2.4** |
| | 4 | 30 | 50 | 25 | 50 | 75 | **2.8** |
| | 3 | 50 | 80 | 33 | 66 | **100** | **2.8** |
| *Dependence on the energy* | | | | | | | |
| <8 | 11 | 20 | 30 | 44 | 64 | 92 | **2.4** |
| <8 | 11 | 30 | 50 | 36 | 55 | 83 | **2.4** |
| <8 | 10 | 50 | 80 | 39 | 88 | 92 | **2.7** |
| *Best choice* | | | | | | | |
| <8 | 11 | 20 | **30** | **44** | 64 | 92 | **2.4** |

Psoriatic lesions of different sizes were treated by 5% ALA for 4 h. Irradiation was performed by red light with light energies varying from 30 to 80 J/cm². Comparable results were achieved for all treatment parameters used and all lesion sizes selected. Degree of pain was subjectively ranked and scaled by 1 (moderate), 2 (intermediate) and 3 (severe). Optimum combination of best results and well accepted therapy was achieved using lesions <8 cm and 20 mW/cm² red light irradiation for 25 min (=30 J/cm²).

Therefore, in following studies, we used lower ALA amounts. Furthermore we switched from red light to green light irradiation based on our experience that green light generally causes less pain than red light (Tabs. 20 and 24) (Fritsch et al, 1997).

**Table 15.** PDT in psoriasis lesions: Influence of the ALA concentration

| ALA [%] | Lesions [n] | Irradiation [543–548] | | Complete response | | | | Pain [1–3] |
|---|---|---|---|---|---|---|---|---|
| | | [mW/cm²] | [J/cm²] | 4 | 6 | 8 | 10 | |
| *Dependence on the ALA concentration* | | | | | | | | |
| 0.1 | 10 | 20 | 30 | 10 | 10 | 30 | 40 | 1.4 |
| 1 | 9 | 20 | 30 | 22 | 44 | 78 | **89** | 1.3 |
| 5 | 10 | 20 | 30 | 20 | 40 | 70 | **90** | 2.3 |
| 10 | 10 | 20 | 30 | 30 | 40 | 60 | 80 | 3 |
| 20 | 9 | 20 | 30 | 22 | 55 | 55 | 88 | 2.9 |
| *Best choice* | | | | | | | | |
| **1** | 9 | **20** | **30** | 22 | 44 | 78 | **89** | 1.3 |

Psoriatic lesions treated by different ALA concentrations (0.1 to 20%) for 4 h. Irradiation was performed by green light (20 mW/cm², 25 min). Comparable results were achieved for all ALA concentrations except that of 0.1% ALA. Degree of pain was subjectively ranked and scaled as 1 (moderate), 2 (intermediate) and 3 (severe). Optimum efficacy and tolerability was achieved using 1 and 5% ALA.

Dependent on the *ALA concentration* (0.1, 1, 5, 10 and 20%) the efficacy of PDT and the degree of pain was measured. A total of 10 PDT sessions (twice per week) were performed in 48 lesions (Tab. 15). Results were comparable for ALA doses of 1, 5, 10 and 20%. Only the lowest ALA concentration of 0.1% led to significantly lower response rates. PDT was painful in all cases. For ALA concentrations between 5% and 20%, pain was not tolerable in most cases. ALA concentrations of 0.1 and 1% were generally well tolerated (Figs. 191–198). However, the dose of 0.1% ALA produced insufficient clinical response.

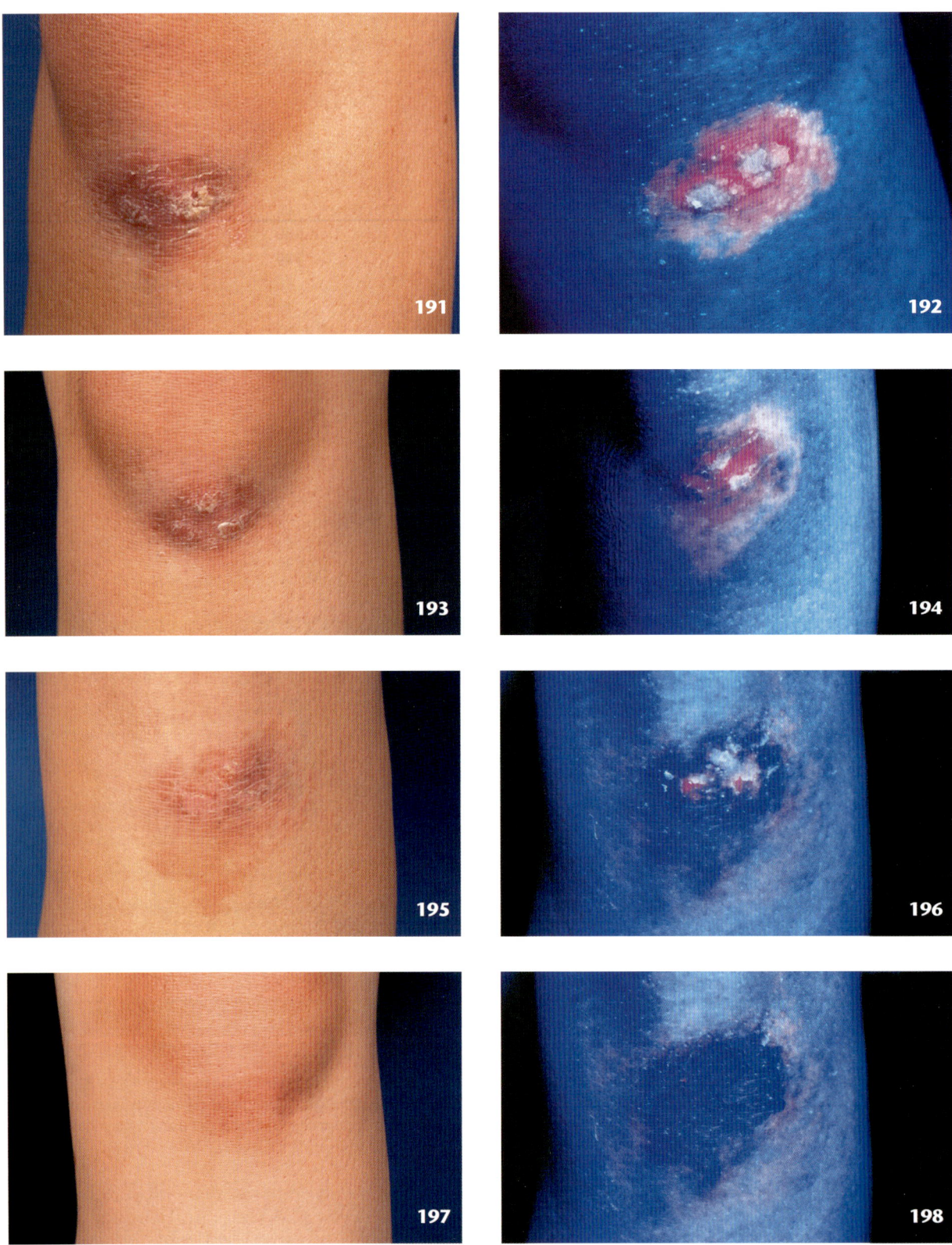

**Figs. 191–198.** Psoriatic lesion on the knee. A total of 10 PDT sessions (once a week) was planned to be performed. 1% ALA and red light irradiation was used. Treatment was stopped if the lesion showed remission and was free of fluorescence in FDAP. In this psoriatic plaque, three PDT cycles (20 days) were sufficient to induce a complete response. The last pair of figures (197, 198) shows the outcome one week after the 3rd PDT session

The influence of the *localization* (trunk: 20, back of the hands: 20 lesions) was evaluated using 1% ALA and green light (Table 16). The lesions localized on the back of the hands showed slower and weaker response compared to lesions on the trunk (Figs. 199–206, 207–214).

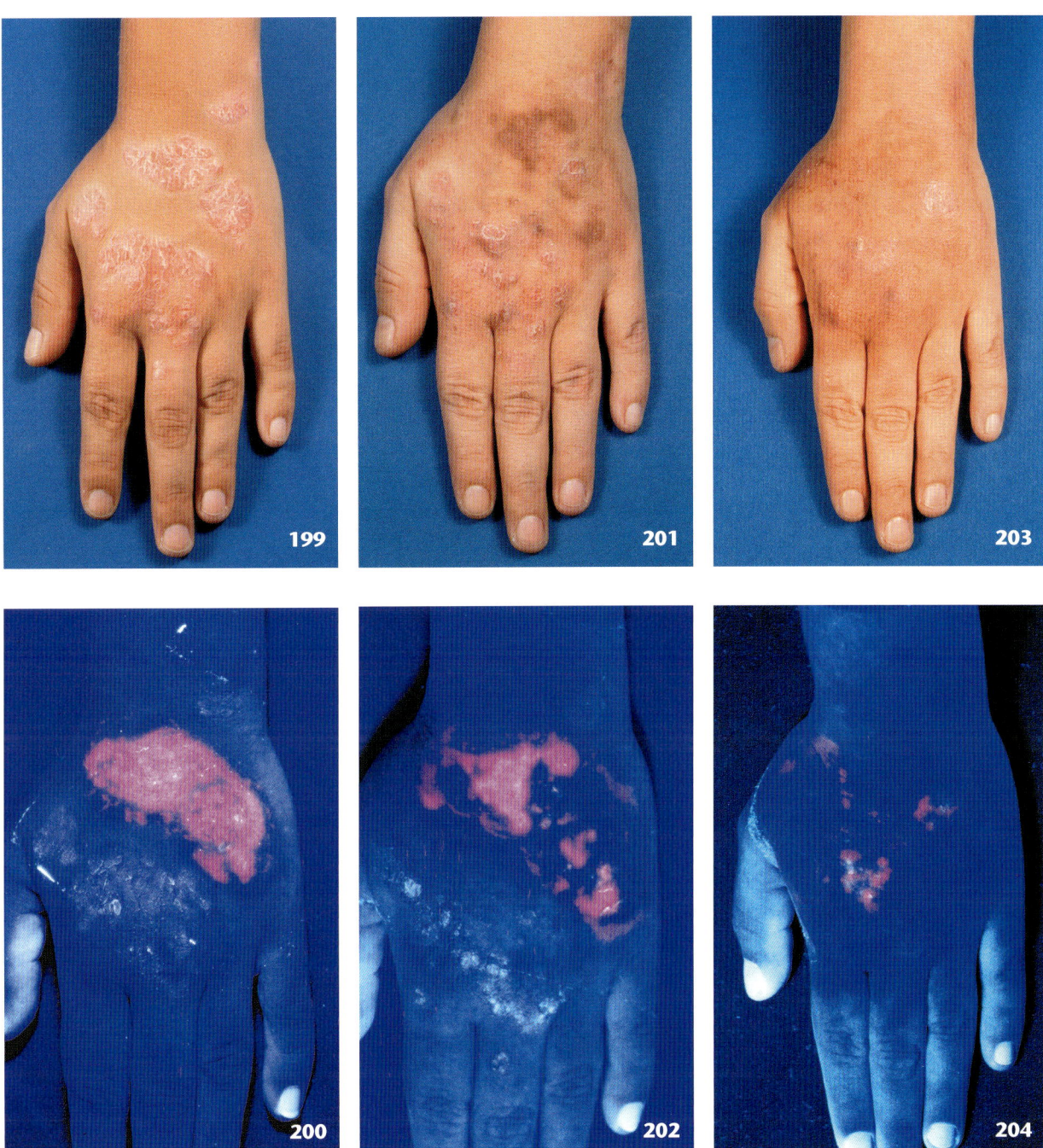

**Figs. 199–204.** Psoriatic plaques on the back of the hand, over years resistant to standard therapy such as topical calcipotriol (also combined with UVB311 nm irradiation), topical corticosteroids, topical PUVA. Initially, the proximal part of the lesion was first treated by topical ALA (5%) and green light. The treated tissue showed a bright fluorescence in FDAP (Fig. 200), whereas the untreated plaques did not fluoresce.
ALA-PDT induced a remarkable improvement of the treated plaque (Figs. 201 and 202). Therefore, the entire back of the hand was treated by PDT twice per week. Figs. 203 and 204 show the clinical and FDAP result after 4 weeks of treatment (= after 8 PDT cycles)

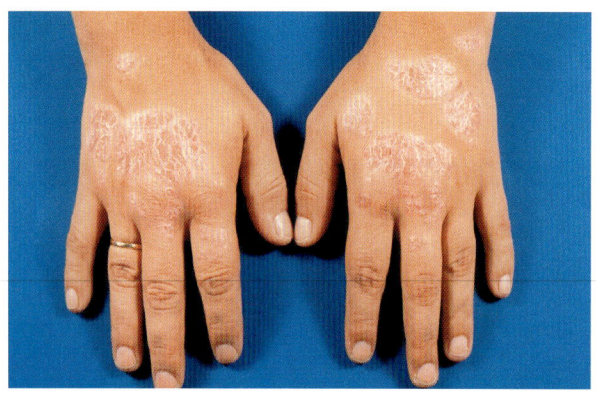

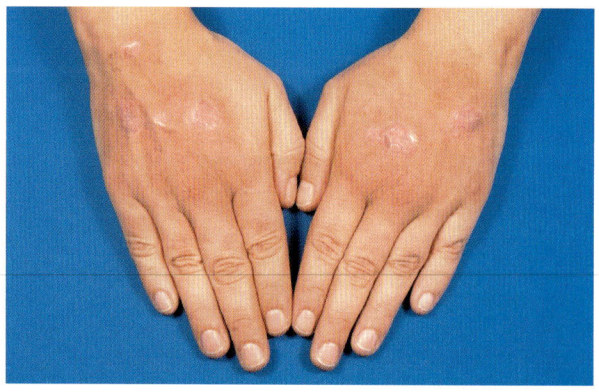

**Fig. 205.** Psoriatic plaques on the back of both hands resistant to multiple therapies. A total number of 20 treatments were performed (twice per week; over 10 weeks) using 5% ALA and green light irradiation (30 J/cm$^2$, 543–548 nm)

**Fig. 206.** Outcome after 20 PDT sessions. There are still some remaining psoriatic islands, but the cure PDT in this case is remarkable due to the lack of efficacy of all other treatments. There is slight hyperpigmentation, which subsided after 2 additional months

**Table 16.** PDT in psoriasis lesions: Influence of the localization

| ALA [%] | Lesions Localization | [n] | Irradiation [543–548] | | Complete response [%] | | | | Pain [1–3] |
|---|---|---|---|---|---|---|---|---|---|
| | | | [mW/cm$^2$] | [J/cm$^2$] | 4. | 6. | 8. | 10. | |
| | | | Dependence on the lesion localization | | | | | | |
| 1 | Trunk | 20 | 20 | 30 | 20 | 45 | 85 | **95** | 1.3 |
| 1 | Hands | 12 | 20 | 30 | 8 | 25 | 58 | **75** | 1.2 |

Psoriatic lesions on the trunk or the hands were treated with 1% ALA for 4 h. Irradiation was performed by green light (30 J/cm$^2$). Lesions on the trunk responded faster and better than those on the back of the hands.

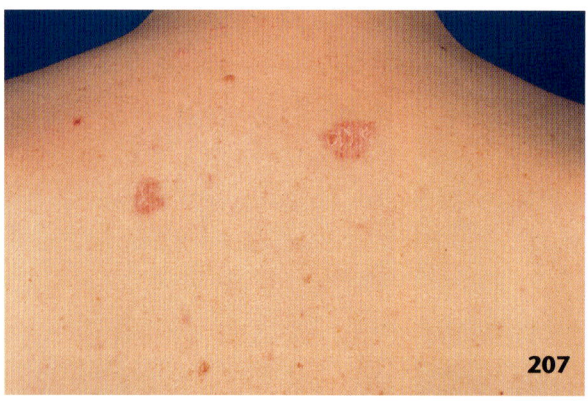

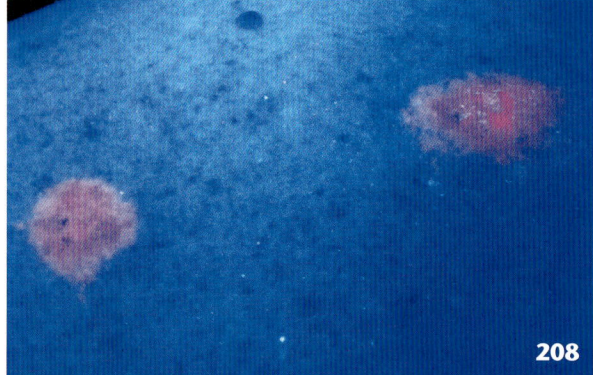

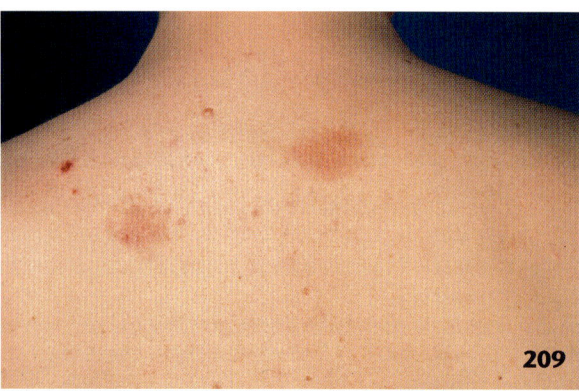

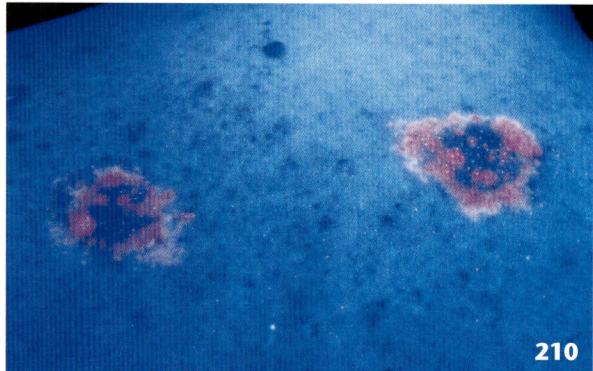

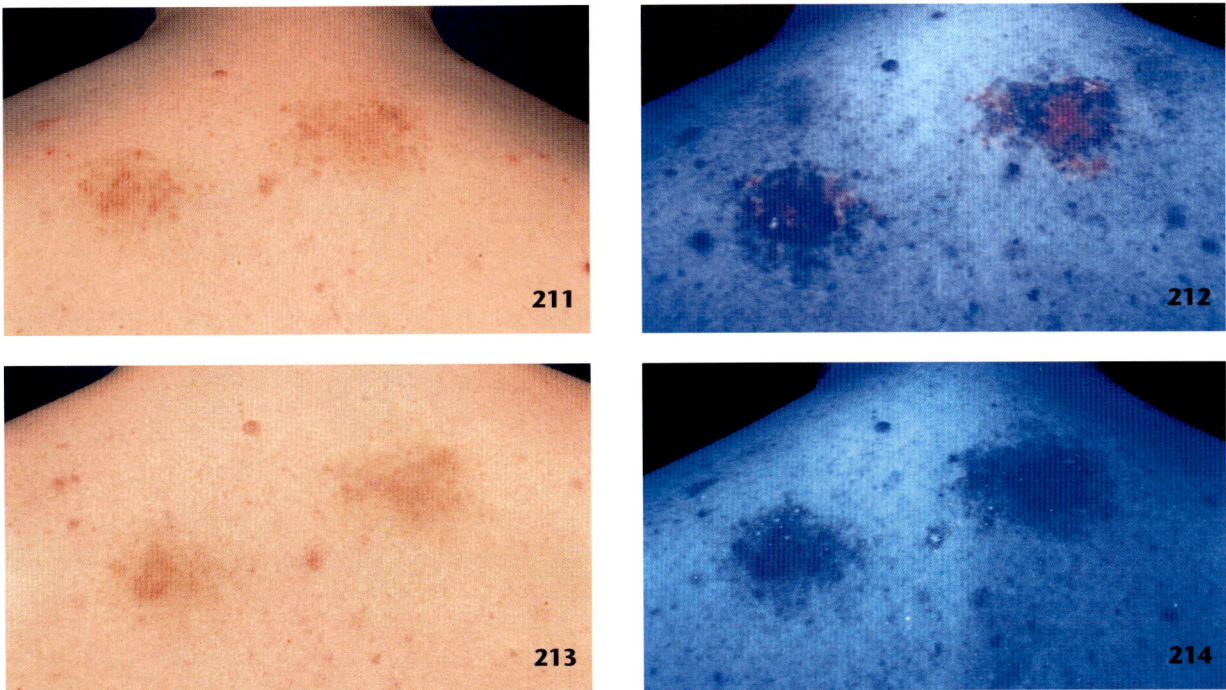

**Figs. 207–214.** Psoriatic plaques on the back. PDT was performed with 1% ALA and green light (543–548 nm, 30 J/cm²) twice per week for 4 weeks. The plaques in this patient responded already after the 3rd PDT session. In the last set of figures (213, 214), there is neither clinically not in FDAP any sign of remaining psoriatic tissue. An occasional side effect of PDT in psoriasis lesions is the long-lasting hyperpigmentation. In this patient, the pigmentation disapeared within 11 weeks

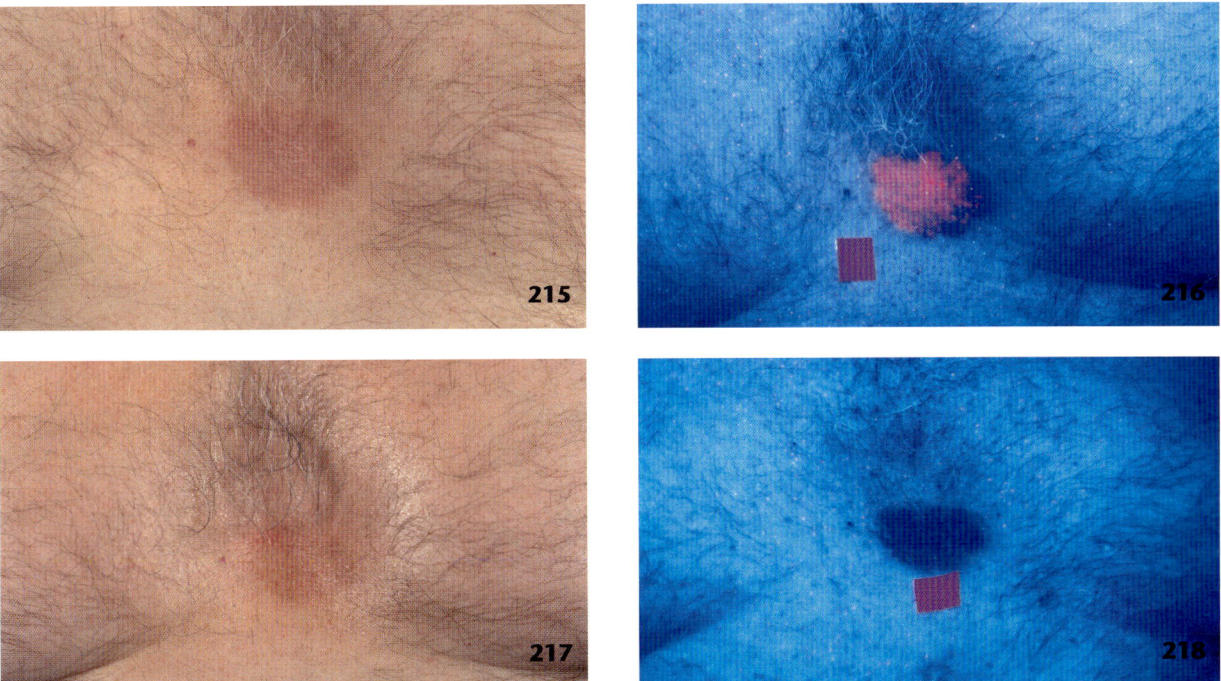

**Figs. 215–218.** Psoriatic plaque in the decollete area. PDT parameters chosen were 1% ALA methylester and green light (543–548 nm, 30 J/cm²). Treatment schedule comprised 10 sessions. This single plaque was cured after the 6th PDT. Although, in FDAP, there is no fluorescence detectable at this time point, the clinical picture still shows a reddish hyperpigmented macule. Therefore, biopsy was performed to control the FDAP result. In histopathology, no specific psoriasiform alterations were found. Therefore, the clinically visible macule represents postinflammatory hyperpigmentation

Using *ALA methylester* (1%) and green light the results were comparable to those achieved by the use of free ALA (Tables 16 and 17). Pain was even less intensive than ALA-PDT (Figs. 215–218).

**Table 17.** PDT in psoriasis lesions: Use of ALA methylester

| ALA ME [%] | Lesions [n] | Irradiation [543–548] | | Complete response | | | | Pain [1–3] |
|---|---|---|---|---|---|---|---|---|
| | | [mW/cm²] | [J/cm²] | 4 | 6 | 8 | 10 | |
| | | | ALA methylester | | | | | |
| 1 | 20 | 20 | 30 | 25 | 45 | 70 | 90 | 1.1 |

Psoriasis lesions on the trunk treated by 1% ALA methylester and green light (30 J/cm²). Degree of pain was subjectively given on a scale as 1 (moderate), 2 (intermediate) and 3 (severe).

## Chapter Discussion

*Clinical trials and Phase I-studies.* Recently, topical ALA-PDT has gained increasing interest in psoriasis therapy. The combination of 10 to 20% ALA with UVA or red light resulted in PR and CR of psoriatic lesions (Boehncke et al, 2000; Robinson et al, 1999). A response similar to therapeutic results achieved by dithranol (Boehncke et al, 1994) has been observed. Direct keratinocyte cytotoxicity and immunomodulatory effects may play an important role for the PDT-induced reduction of psoriatic lesions (Boehncke et al, 1994). We found that ALA concentrations between 1 and 5% are sufficient to induce remission of psoriatic lesions. ALA amounts of 10–20% which are used for treatment of skin tumors lead to a severe burning pain during and after PDT and a strong inflammation reaction lasting for several days after irradiation.

ALA-PDT seems to be a highly interesting therapeutic modality for psoriasis. Treatment frequencies of once to twice per week are sufficient to achieve a response within 2 to 4 weeks, and thus, ALA-PDT might be superior to topical PUVA-therapy. PUVA therapy using the application of psoralen in a cream is generally performed 4 times a week and thus time consuming. Comparative studies of topical ALA-PDT and topical PUVA-therapy have not yet been performed. The length of remission after both treatment modalities needs to be determined. Systemic administration of ALA may offer a convenient therapy to induce a more homogeneous photosensitization of all plaques. Orally administered ALA could even positively influence the psoriatic arthritis (Hendrich et al, 2000). As a cautionary note, it should be mentioned that ALA-PDT can induce a Köbner phenomenon (Figs. 219 and 220) with progression of the disease (Stender and Wulf, 1996).

## I.6 PDT: Evaluation of the Efficacy in Selected Cutaneous Diseases

### Material and Methods

In the treatment of the following diseases, the parameters were: ALA 20% (medac, Wedel, Germany), red light irradiation at 50–100 mW/cm²

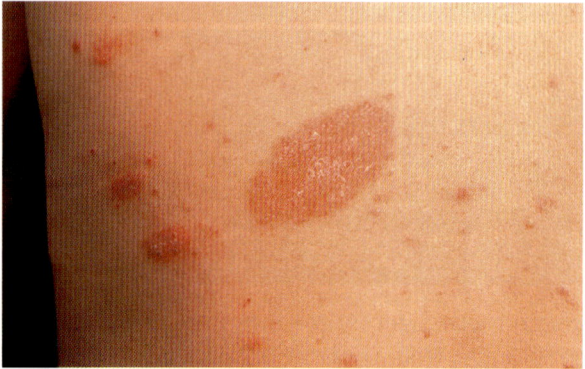

Fig. 219. Psoriatic plaques on the back

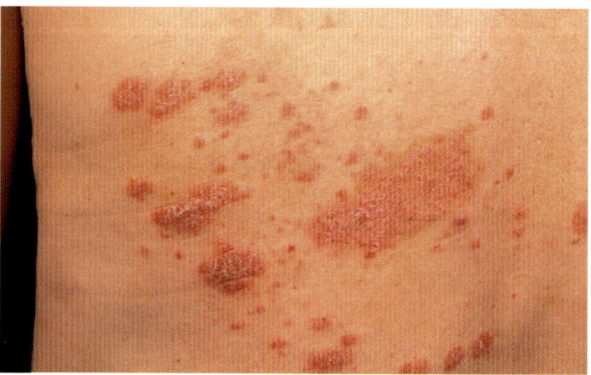

Fig. 220. Provocation of psoriasis upon PDT with 1% ALA and green light (30 J/cm²)

and total energies of 80 to 120 J/cm² (PDT 1200®, Waldmann, Villingen-Schwenningen, Germany, 570–670 nm). PDT was performed biweekly (5 sessions).

Following diseases were treated: 31 lesions of mycosis fungoides (5 patients), 42 lesions of Kaposi's sarcoma (AIDS-related), 6 lesions of lupus erythematosus, 8 patients with acne vulgaris (4 patients with acne vulgaris on the face, 4 with acne conglobata on the back; 30 J/cm²), 8 lesions of leishmaniasis, 3 lesions of lichen sclerosus and atrophicus, 5 keloids, 6 lesions of granuloma anulare, 3 patients with condylomata acuminata (42 lesions), 7 patients with common warts.

Table 18. PDT in various skin diseases

| ALA [%] | Lesions [n] | Patients [n] | Irradiation [nm] [mW/cm²] | [J/cm²] | Complete response Number of PDT sessions 1 | 3 | 5 | Pain¹ [1–3] |
|---|---|---|---|---|---|---|---|---|
| Mycosis fungoides | | | [broad band, red, 570–650] | | | | | |
| 20 | 31 | 5 | 150 | 180 | 0 | 23 | 45 | 1.5 |
| Kaposi's sarcoma | | | [broad band, red, 570–650] | | | | | |
| 20 | 42 | 6 | 150 | 180 | 0 | 0 | 0 | 2.8 |
| Lupus erythematosus | | | [broad band, red, 570–650] | | | | | |
| 20 | 6 | 6 | 150 | 180 | 0 | 33 | 50² | 2.3 |
| Acne vulgaris | | | [543–548] | | | | | |
| 5 | 42 | 4 | 20 | 30 | 0 | 50 | 75³ | 1.8 |
| Acne conglobata | | | [543–548] | | | | | |
| 20 | 31 | 2 | 20 | 30 | 0 | 0 | 50 | 2 |
| Keloid | | | [broad band, red, 570–650] | | | | | |
| 20 | 5 | 2 | 150 | 180 | 0 | 0 | 0 | 1.6 |
| Acne scleroticans nuchae | | | [broad band, red, 570–650] | | | | | |
| 20 | 2 | 2 | 150 | 180 | 0 | 0 | 0 | 1.5 |
| Lichen sclerosus et atrophic. | | | [broad band, red, 570–650] | | | | | |
| 20 | 3 | 3 | 150 | 180 | 0 | 0 | 0 | 1.7 |
| Granuloma anulare | | | [broad band, red, 570–650] | | | | | |
| 20 | 6 | 2 | 20 | 30 | 0 | 0 | 0 | 1.2 |
| Leishmaniasis | | | [543–548] | | | | | |
| 20 | 8 | 1 | 20 | 30 | 0 | 0 | 75 | 1.8 |
| Condylomata acuminata | | | [543–548] | | | | | |
| 20 | 42 | 3 | 20 | 30 | 0 | 5 | 19⁴ | 2 |
| Verrucae vulgares | | | [543–548] | | | | | |
| 20 | 36 | 5 | 20 | 30 | 0 | 11 | 17 | 2.6 |
| Verrucae plantares | | | [broad band, red, 570–650] | | | | | |
| 20 | 11 | 2 | 150 | 180 | 0 | 9 | 18 | 3 |

¹ Degree of pain was subjectively determined on a scale by 1 (moderate), 2 (intermediate) and 3 (severe).
² 3 Lesions of lupus erythematosus got worse during PDT.
³ Acne vulgaris improved in 3 of 4 patients.
⁴ All completely responding condylomata acuminata were flat lesions. None of the thicker lesions was cured.

## Results

The various tissues showed significant differences in their response to topical ALA-PDT (Table 18). Encouraging data were achieved for acne vulgaris and leishmaniasis. All other diseases showed only a poor improvement upon PDT. In addition, the degree of pain associated with treatment was high in most cases. In patients suffering from verrucae vulgares or condylomata acuminata, pain during PDT was not tolerable.

## Chapter Discussion

### I.6.1 PDT in Skin Cancers and Precanceroses Others than Discussed Above

*Mycosis fungoides (MF)*. Topical ALA was effectively used to treat plaque-stage cutaneous T-cell lymphoma (Wolf et al, 1993, Amman et al, 1995). However, the apparent clinical cure was not confirmed by histopathology.

*Malignant melanoma (MM).* So far, there is little information on the efficacy of ALA-PDT in the treatment of primary and metastatic MM (Wolf et al, 1993). The strong pigmentation of melanoma may be the limiting factor of PDT by inhibiting light penetration (Figs. 44 and 45) (Fritsch et al, 2000).

*Skin metastases.* Attempts to palliate metastatic breast carcinoma with topical PDT based on ALA did not lead to acceptable results, probably because of the limited drug penetration of the normal skin covering the peripheral parts of the tumor (Kennedy et al, 1990; Cairnduff et al, 1994; Calzavara-Pinton, 1995). PDT was also used to treat chest wall progression from breast carcinomas (Allison et al, 2001).

*Paget's disease (PD).* A 74-year-old woman with extensive inoperable vulvar extramammary PD was treated with etoposide 100 mg and 5000 cGy electron beam irradiation, which reduced the lesion by 60% (Henta et al, 1999). Following these interventions, the residual lesion was successfully treated with repeated ALA-PDT, which achieved a nearly CR. FDAP was shown to be very useful in detecting and delineating tissue of PD prior to $CO_2$-laser surgery (Figs. 145–147) (Becker-Wegerich et al, 1998).

*Actinic cheilitis* showed CR rates of 100% upon topical 20% ALA and a slide projector treatment in 3 patients (Stender and Wulf, 1996).

*Neoplastic changes of the vulva or penis* comprise SCC and the in situ carcinomas like Bowen's disease, erythroplasia of Queyrat, bowenoid papulosis and Paget's disease. *Genital precancerous stages such as* **erythroplasia of Queyrat** were treated by topical ALA-PDT with encouraging results (Stables et al, 1995). Other intraepithelial neoplasias such as *cervical intraepithelial neoplasia (CIN)* or *vulvar intraepithelial neoplasia (VIN)* were treated effectively by ALA-PDT (Fehr et al, 2001; Hillemanns et al, 2000). Carcinomas of the cervix are the most common cancers of the genital area and are often associated with human papilloma virus type 16 and 18. Although conisation or hysterectomy is the surgical treatment of choice in small tumors (grade I–II), and higher grades are preferentially treated by radiotherapy (Jakus et al, 2000) topical PDT offers an effective alternative treatment. In VIN, vulvoscopy is the major diagnostic step, and neoplastic lesions can be revealed by the local application of acetic acid. Tumor excision or radical vulvectomy are the treatments of choice. Electrosurgery, carbon dioxide laser vaporization, cryosurgery, topical 5-fluorouracil or interferon-α remain as palliative tools (Kurwa et al, 2000). In VIN, ALA-PDT also proved as an alternative treatment modality, easy to perform with the advantage of minimal tissue destruction, low side effects and excellent cosmetic results. While PDT of VIN III seems to show an efficacy similar to conventional treatment modalities, it offers unique advantages: healing time is short, preservation of normal vulvar appearance is excellent, and PDT may be performed without anesthesia.

### I.6.2 PDT in Tumors of the Oral Mucosa

*Leukoplakia.* The outcome of treatment in oral leukoplakia was effectively controlled by follow-up FDAP (Leunig et al, 2000). Twelve patients, who had been suffering from leukoplakia of the oral mucosa for several years, were treated by ALA-mediated PDT (Kubler et al, 1998) (20% ALA, 2 h; 630 nm light, 100 J/cm$^2$). Five patients showed CR, four patients showed a PR and in three patients treatment was unsuccessful.

*SCC of the oral mucosa.* In 58 patients with a suspected cancer of the oral cavity, FDAP was performed by rinsing with a 0.4% ALA solution for 10 to 20 min and UV irradiation after 1–2.5 hours (Leunig et al, 2000). Higher intensities of red fluorescence were measured in neoplastic tissue as compared to the surrounding normal tissue (maximum contrast after 1.5 hours). In 14% of the patients, additional neoplasms were found by means of FDAP. An evaluation of the biopsy specimens resulted in a specificity of 60% and a sensitivity of 99%. FDAP in the oral cavity by rinsing with a 0.4% ALA solution for 20 min was capable to visualize 96% of the histologically confirmed carcinomas in 56 patients (Zenk et al, 1999). In 3 patients additional tumors were detected by fluorescence that were not visible otherwise. However, many patients showed fluorescent areas with no correlation to the histological findings. Bacteria from the oral cavity can also produce protoporphyrin after ALA incubation, which leads to false-positive findings. Reduction of the false-positive findings was achieved by rinsing the oral cavity with hydrogen peroxide and by mechanical plaque reduction. This improves the reliability of a fluorescence-guided biopsy.

### I.6.3 PDT in Non-neoplastic Skin Diseases

*Acne vulgaris (AV).* The production of porphyrins by lipophilic propionibacteria has been utilized for photodynamic destruction of these microorganisms in the management of acne vulgaris (AV) (Meffert et al, 1990). PDT (550–700 nm light, 150 J/cm$^2$) with topical ALA (20%, 3 h) was tested for the treatment of AV in an open-label prospective human study including 22 patients (Hongcharo et al, 2000). Sebum excretion was reduced for several weeks, and was decreased for 20 weeks after PDT. Bacterial porphyrin fluorescence was also suppressed by PDT. There was clinically and statistically significant improvement of inflammatory acne 10 to 20 weeks after PDT. Transient hyperpigmentation, superficial exfoliation, and crusting were observed, which cleared without scarring. Topical PDT seems to be a promising strategy in the treatment of acne lesions. The optimum dosage of ALA and treatment frequency are yet to be determined. In addition, combined therapeutic procedures, e.g., the use of erythromycin-containing creams, could increase the efficacy of PDT.

*Leishmaniasis.* In a patient with 8 lesions of cutaneous leishmaniasis topical ALA-PDT led to a complete response of all lesions (Figs. 221–223).

*Localized scleroderma.* Five patients with progressive disease, in whom conventional therapies had failed, were successfully treated 12 to 24 times by 3% ALA-gel followed by irradiation with an incoherent lamp (40 mW/cm$^2$, 10 J/cm$^2$) (Karrer et al, 2000). The only side-effect was a transient hyperpigmentation of the treated lesions.

*Verrucae vulgares/plantares.* Multiple verrucae vulgares in an immunosuppressed patient have shown considerable improvement after topical ALA-PDT in combination with DMSO and red light at 120J/cm$^2$ (Smetana et al, 1997). 232 recalcitrant foot and hand warts were successfully treated by six repetitive ALA-PDT interventions combined with standard treatment or by placebo (Stender et al, 2000). These findings are in contrast with the results of an open pilot study involving refractory viral warts; only 1 of 6 patients responded to topical 20% ALA and illumination with visible light (Amman et al, 1995). Own experiences with PDT of warts are also rather disappointing. Irradiation is extremely painful and the efficacy of PDT is limited (Figs. 224–229). A rigorous pretreatment using salicylic acid containing preparations is necessary to remove the hyperkeratotic part of the lesions to allow an effective PDT. Compared to $CO_2$-laser therapy, ALA-PDT seems to be only a second choice therapy for warts.

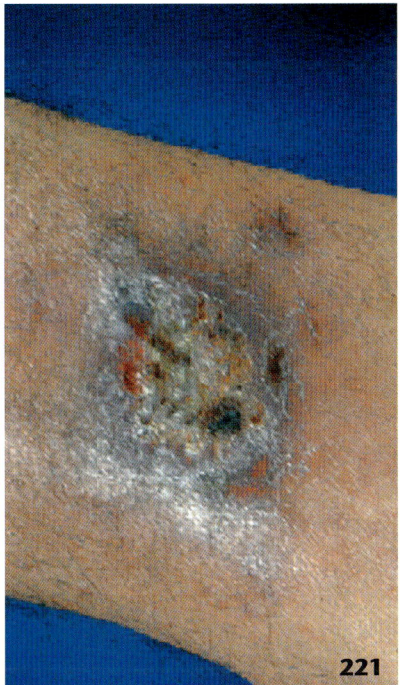
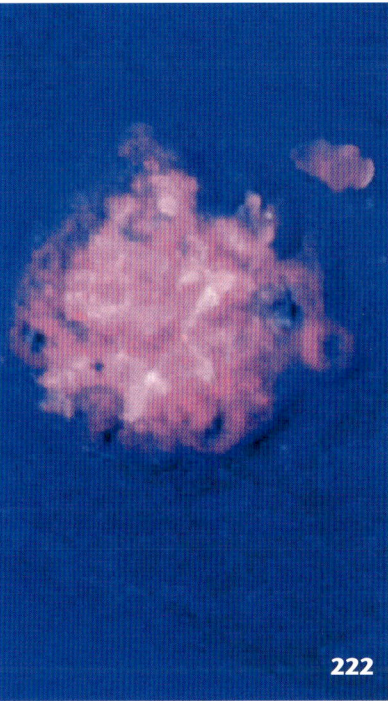
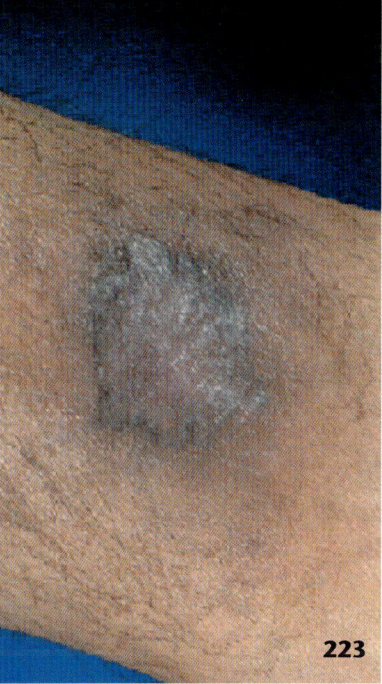

**Fig. 221.** Cutaneous leishmaniasis on the lower leg. Flat exophytic smeary tumor with ulceration and fibrotic areas
**Fig. 222.** FDAP: 6 h after topical application of 20% ALA methylester. Intensive red fluorescence in the entire lesion
**Fig. 223.** After 6 PDT sessions. Neither clinically nor in histopathology there were signs for remaining infectious tissue

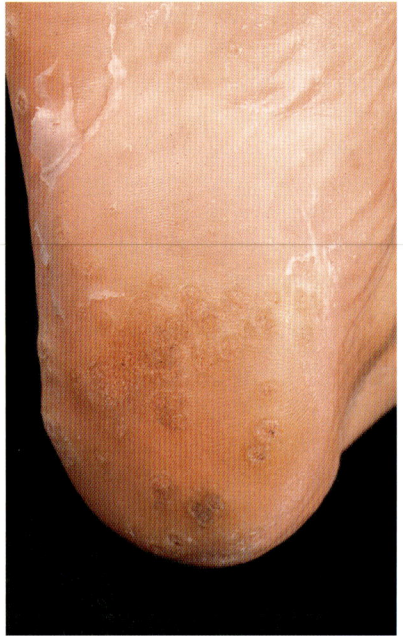

**Fig. 224.** Multiple plantar warts

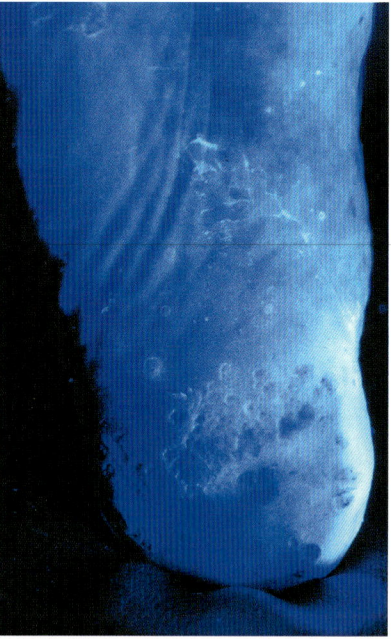

**Fig. 225.** In FDAP, not a single wart shows fluorescence

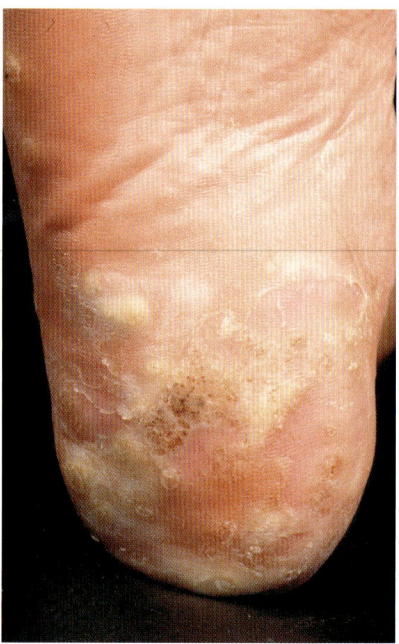

**Fig. 226.** Pre-treatment of the lesions with 5% salicylic acid containing cream for one week. This was done to enhance the permeability of the ALA mixture

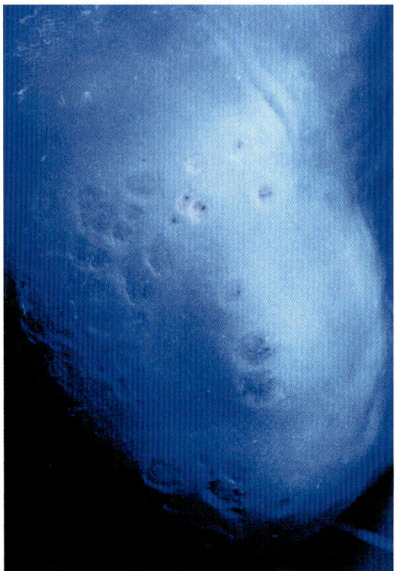

**Fig. 227.** FDAP 2: Although the lesions were pre-treated, the warts did not fluoresce. Nevertheless, PDT was performed using red light (570–750 nm, 180 J/cm²). Interestingly, PDT was extremely painful. It seems that warts accumulate porphyrins upon ALA treatment, however, physical reasons may limit fluorescence

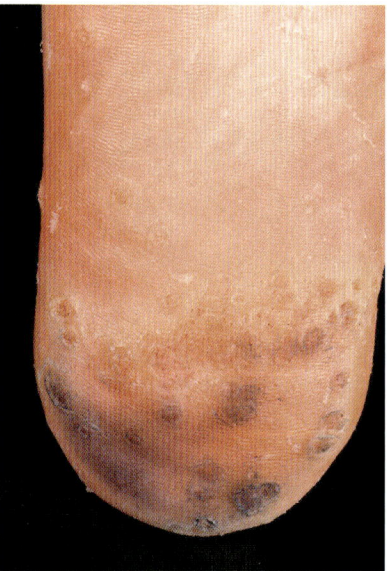

**Fig. 228.** One week after PDT. There is no regression, but profound hyperpigmentation

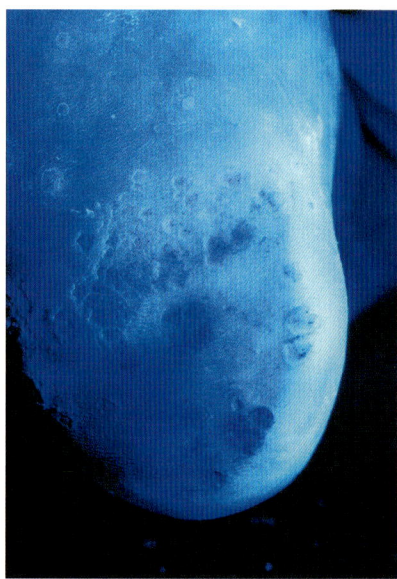

**Fig. 229.** FDAP 3: Again, the warts did not reveal any visible fluorescence

*Condylomata acuminata.* In FDAP, using 2.5% ALA ointment or 20% ALA cream selective fluorescence of condylomata of the labia minora and vestibule was demonstrated. Peak selectivity was reached 90 minutes after drug application and higher levels were achieved using the ointment mixture (Fehr et al, 1996). A 75 to 100% reduction of genital warts was reported in 5 of 7 patients after topical administration of 20% ALA and laser irradiation (Frank and Bos, 1996). Similarly multiple penile condylomata acuminata responded to ALA in combination with a noncoherent light source (Ross et al, 1997). Own data confirm these findings, however, the overall efficacy of PDT in condylomata acuminata is not convincing.

*Epilation.* There are reports that the application of ALA leads to accumulation of porphyrin metabolites in hair follicles and sebaceous glands, suggesting the potential use of PDT for disorders originating from these skin adnexa (Grossman et al, 1995). 20% ALA and 100–200 J/cm$^2$ of light were used for the treatment of hirsutism.

The sites treated with low fluences showed more than 90% hair regrowth versus 50% in areas irradiated with 200 J/cm$^2$, indicating that higher light doses may lead to permanent hair loss. This case report as well as other personal information point to the possible use of PDT in epilation. Further studies should focus on selective PDT of the follicular glands after cleansing the surrounding skin from formed porphyrins to avoid general side effects such as burning pain during and after PDT or pigmentations disorders after PDT.

### I.6.4 PDT in Non-dermatological Indications

*Malignant gliomas.* Although this tumor is not a cutaneous one, latest research activities will be mentioned due to their high relevance for FDAP-guided surgery. To verify the efficacy of FDAP-guided resection of malignant gliomas, a multicentric prospective controlled **Phase III-study** was initiated in autumn 1999. Twelve neurosurgical centers are participating. 270 patients with a primary, not pretreated, uniloculary localized, surgically treatable malignant glioma have been randomized. One part of the tumors is FDAP-guided resected, the other part by conventional surgical technique. The study should provide unique information on the efficacy of presurgical FDAP and on the growth characteristics and prognostic factors of malignant gliomas (Stummer et al, 2000).

*Bladder cancer.* Data concerning this frequent tumor are also included because urologists introduced FDAP-assisted cystoscopy already 10 years ago. Since then urologists have developed this technique to a standard diagnostic tool. In a **Phase III-study**, in 328 cases FDAP-guided (3% ALA solution, intravesically, 3 h) endoscopy was carried out to determine whether neoplastic disease which was missed under white light can be found during transurethral resection of bladder cancer. The fluorescence was excited by a special incoherent light source which provided blue light in addition to white light. In 82 (25%) cases additional neoplastic lesions were found only because of their red porphyrin fluorescence which was induced by ALA. 31% of these neoplastic foci which were found in normal and nonspecific inflamed mucosa had a poorly differentiated histology (Kriegmair et al, 1999; Waidlich et al, 2001). In addition, PDT is effectively used in the destruction of high grade dysplasia and early cancer of the esophagus (Gossner et al, 1999; Tan et al, 1999).

## I.7 PDT: Evaluation of the Optimum Photosensitizing Substance or its Prodrug

### Material and Methods

In the last decade we performed PDT mainly with the porphyrin prodrugs ALA and ALA methylester. As there were early reports on effective PDT of BCC using tetraphenylporphine sulphonate (TPPS$_4$) (Santoro et al, 1990), we evaluated the response of 15 superficial BCC and 15 SK to topically applied porphyrin products such as TPPS$_4$, protoporphyrin IX, and uroporphyrin. The TPPS$_4$ solution was prepared as 2% in isopropylalcohol/water (50:50) according to Santoro et al, (1990). Protoporphyrin IX and uroporphyrin (0.01%) was diluted in isopropylalcohol/water (50:50).

### Results

The topically applied porphyrin products TPPS$_4$, protoporphyrin IX and uroporphyrin induced different response rates of BCC and SK to PDT (Table 19).

Best results were achieved using protoporphyrin IX, which, however, caused the highest

Table 19. PDT in cutaneous neoplasms with porphyrin products

| | Lesion [%] | [n] | Irradiation [543 – 548] [mW/cm²] | [J/cm²] | Complete response 1 | 2 | 3 | Pain [1–3] |
|---|---|---|---|---|---|---|---|---|
| | | | TPPS | | | | | |
| BCC | 2 | 5 | 20 | 30 | 0 | 0 | 20 | 0.6 |
| SK | 2 | 5 | 20 | 30 | 0 | 40 | 60 | 0.4 |
| | | | Protoporphyrin IX | | | | | |
| BCC | 0.01 | 5 | 20 | 30 | 40 | 80 | 100 | 2.6 |
| SK | 0.01 | 5 | 20 | 30 | 60 | 100 | – | 2 |
| | | | Uroporphyrin | | | | | |
| BCC | 0.01 | 5 | 20 | 30 | 60 | 80 | 100 | 1.6 |
| SK | 0.01 | 5 | 20 | 30 | 40 | 60 | 100 | 1.8 |

Treated lesions were solar keratoses (SK) and superficial types of basal cell carcinomas (BCC). Degree of pain was subjectively assessed and graded on a scale as 0 (no), 1 (moderate), 2 (intermediate) and 3 (severe) pain.

degree of pain. Uroporphyrin also led to encouraging results in topical PDT of BCC, but showed weak efficacy in SK. The results of topical TPPS$_4$ therapy were disappointing. Therefore, we could not confirm previous reports (Santoro et al, 1990).

## Chapter Discussion

The data of this particular study do not reproduce the encouraging results of TPPS$_4$ in topical PDT of BCC achieved by other investigators (Santoro et al, 1990). However, we could also verify that the treated skin area was highly photosensitive for several days. This photosensitivity which was much higher than with ALA-PDT was also noticed with protoporphyrin IX and uroporphyrin.

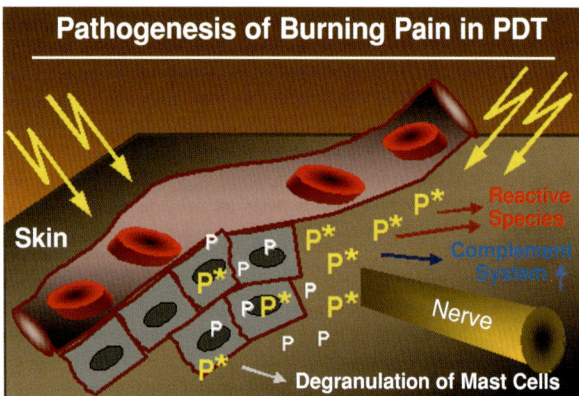

Fig. 230. Schematic illustration of the possible pathogenesis of pain in PDT. Porphyrin molecules (P) are formed in the (neoplastic) skin. Through light irradiation, the energetic niveau of the porphyrins is eleveated (P*). Reactive oxygen species (ROS) are formed, complement factors are activated and mast cells are degranulated. All these factors may react directly or by indirect mechanisms with nerve endings or neurotransmitters

It is an interesting phenomenon that the topical application of protoporphyrin induces a higher degree of pain than uroporphyrin or TPPS$_4$ in PDT. Patients suffering from porphyria diseases report about pain sensations if their skin is exposed to sunlight. Depending on the type of porphyria, a specific porphyrin pattern is accumulating in skin, blood, liver and other organs. Patients with erythropoietic protoporphyria (defect of ferrochelatase) store high amounts of protoporphyrin in their red blood cells. These patients have painful burning in the skin during sunlight exposure. However, patients with porphyria cutanea tarda (reduced activity of the uroporphyrinogen decarboxylase) do not complain of burning discomfort in the sunlight. Patients with porphyria cutanea tarda accumulate preferentially uroporphyrin and heptacarboxylated porphyrin. Thus, the type of porphyrin molecule accumulating in the body and its localization might be responsible for the presence and the degree of pain.

The phenomenon of burning pain during PDT is still not clarified. The ALA-PDT-induced pain is thought to result from a locally induced porphyria and might be comparable to skin symptoms of patients with erythropoietic porphyria (Fig. 230)

Reactive oxygen species lead to an oxidation of membrane lipids, cross linking of several proteins, and oxidative damage of DNA. Activation of the complement factors induces membrane damage, activation of mast cells, chemotaxis of polymorphous leukocytes, vasodilatation and increase of vessel permeability. Degranulation of mast cells may be an additional factor responsible for the burning and tingling in PDT. In order to make topical PDT more attractive for both parties, the patient and the physician, several additional strategies with different degree of success were performed.

Topical application of xylocain-containing creams such as Emla Cream® is ineffective. Local infiltration anesthesia is effective, but, in the case of large or multiple lesions rather invasive and also painful. Recently, there were encouraging reports that the simultaneous application of PDT light and cold air by cooling devices significantly diminishes the pain (Lang et al, 2001). In our own experiences this effect is minimal and does not increase the patient's comfort. Therefore, we tested the influence of different wavelengths on the degree of pain in PDT.

## I.8 PDT: Evaluation of the Optimum Exciting Light Source

### Material and Methods

Six patients with symmetrically spread, extensive **SK** on the forehead and the scalp were included in the study. Skin was cleansed with isopropanol (55%), and ALA (10% in Neribas ointment, Schering Germany) was applied to the whole forehead and the upper temporal area, including the clinically visible lesions, and extended to the surrounding normal skin. Treated skin areas were covered by an occlusive foil (Tegaderm TM, 3M, Canada) to increase penetration and to avoid photobleaching of the compound. After 6 hours, tape and ointment were removed and treated skin was illuminated with Wood's light (370–405 nm). Two identical and symmetrical square-shaped skin areas (<8×8 cm; one side of the forehead respectively) exhibiting deep red fluorescence were marked. Subsequently, one area was irradiated with green light (PDT Greenlight®, Saalmann, 543–548 nm) and the other with red light (Waldmann, PDT 700, 570–750 nm) with comparable light energies (30 J/cm$^2$; 15 mWcm$^2$ for 33.5 min). Patients' forehead was irradiated as a whole (irradiation output field of light sources: red light: 14.5×14.5 cm; green light: 8.5×8.5 cm). Both lamps show a comparable distribution of the emitting intensities with decreasing values of 10% from the center to the peripheral area. Irradiations were performed consecutively; that is, in three patients red light PDT was given first, followed by green light PDT, and in the other three patients the sequence of treatments was reverse. Degree of pain was given subjectively by the patients with values from 1–3. PDT was repeated after 1 month if clinical signs of remaining SK were present.

In 124 cases of **Bowen's diseases** PDT was applied using 20% ALA (Merck, Darmstadt, Germany or medac, Wedel, Germany) and red light with an intensity of 150 mW/cm$^2$ and a total energy of 180 J/cm$^2$ (PDT 1200®, Waldmann, Villingen-Schwenningen, Germany, 570–670 nm) or green light (30 J/cm$^2$; PDT Greenlight®, Saalmann, Herford, Germany, 543–548 nm). PDT was repeated biweekly until complete response of the lesions occured (maximum total number: 3 PDT sessions). The different light energies were used according to data achieved in previous studies on SK and BCC.

In 42 superficial **BCC** (n=37 on the trunk, n=5 on the face), the complete response rate depending on the light source (wavelength) was measured. ALA (Merck, Darmstadt, Germany, 20% in Neribas® ointment, Schering, Berlin, Germany) was applied for 4 hours. Irradiation was performed using green light with an intensity of 20 mW/cm$^2$ and a total energy of 30 J/cm$^2$ (PDT Greenlight®, Saalmann, Herford, Germany, 543–548 nm). PDT was repeated biweekly (maximum: 3 PDT sessions).

88 **SCC** lesions were treated with 20% ALA green light (20 mW/cm$^2$; 30 J/cm$^2$; PDT Greenlight®, Saalmann, Herford, Germany, 543–548 nm) or red light (70 J/cm$^2$, CureLight®, PhotoCure ASA, Oslo, Norway). PDT was repeated biweekly until complete response of the lesions (total maximum number: 3 PDT sessions).

In 65 **psoriatic lesions**, the complete response rate depending on the light source (wavelength) was measured using 1% ALA and red light (30 J/cm$^2$, PDT 1200®, Waldmann, Villingen-Schwenningen, Germany, 570–670 nm), green light (30 J/cm$^2$; PDT Greenlight®, Saalmann, Herford, Germany, 543–548 nm) or blue light (30 J/cm$^2$, UVA700®, Waldmann, Villingen-Schwenningen, Germany, 320–400 nm).

### Results

In all six patients with SK (Figs. 231 and 232), topical ALA application (10%) led to a bright red fluorescence in FDAP, indicating sufficient levels of intralesional porphyrins for PDT (Figs. 233 and 234). During and several hours after irradiation with red light, all patients complained about mild to severe burning pain. In contrast, during irradiation with green light all patients reported sensitivity to heat only, and none of the

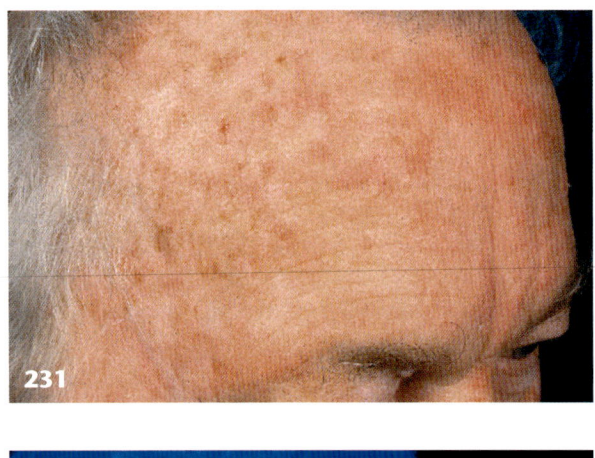
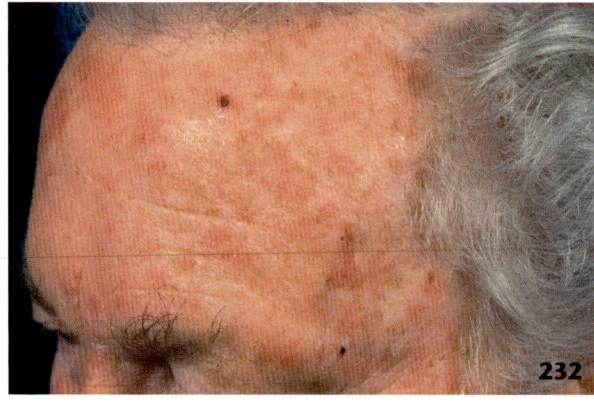
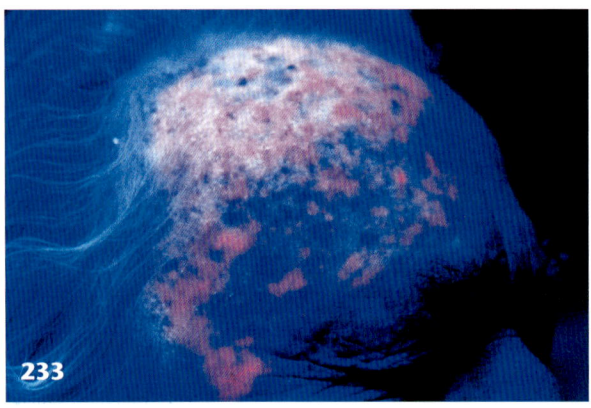
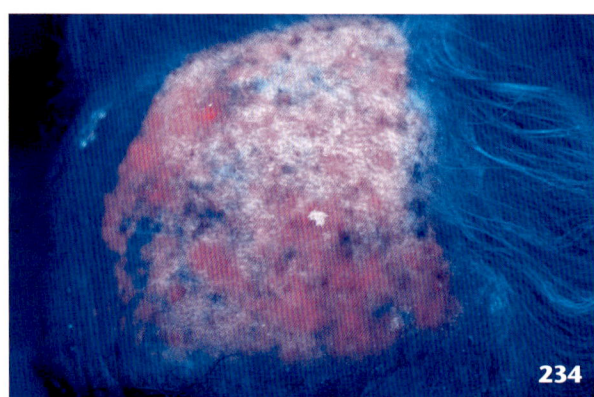
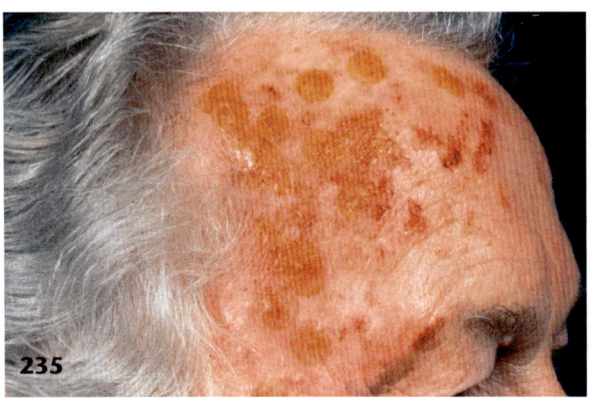
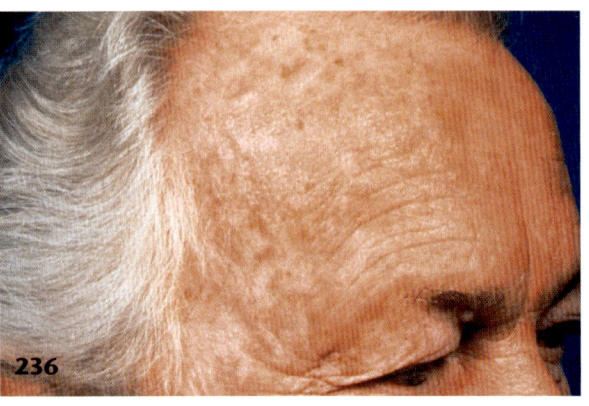

**Figs. 229–236.** Multiple SK on the front right (Fig. 231) and left (Fig. 232). FDAP using 10% ALA and Wood's light irradiation (Fluolight® Saalmann): Note the intralesional bright red fluorescence of the ALA-induced porphyrins (Figs. 233 and 234). Two identical symmetrical square-shaped areas (<8x8 cm; one side of the front, respectively) exhibiting deep red fluorescence were marked. Subsequently, one area was irradiated with green light (Saalmann, PDT Greenlight, 543–548 nm) and the other one with red light (Waldmann, PDT 700, 570–750 nm) with comparable light energies (30 J/cm$^2$; 15 mW/cm$^2$ for 33.5 min). During and several hours after irradiation with red light, the patient complained about severe burning pain. In sharp contrast, during irradiation with green light, sensitivity to heat was reported only. Erythema and crusting developed (Fig. 235) and dissapeared after a few days. Transient hyperpigmentation was noted after one month (Fig. 236.)

patients treated with green light suffered from pain (Table 20).

Erythema and inflammation (Fig. 235) developed in the first hours after both green and red light PDT. Crusting was common in treated areas and disappeared after a few days. Hyperpigmentation lasting for 1 to 3 months was seen in three patients. Therapeutic efficacy did not differ between red and green light PDT. Accordingly, in four patients after one PDT cycle and in two patients (patients 1 and 3) after two PDT cycles, a complete clinical response of the solar keratoses was observed independent of the light source (Fig. 236). After a follow-up period of 15 months, only in one patient (patient 4) signs of recurrence became evident, regardless of whether red light or green light PDT had been performed. This patient was treated again effectively by green light PDT only. For all patients included in the present study, therapeutic efficacy of ALA-PDT was also controlled by FDAP (Fritsch et al, 1997). One month after ALA-PDT, in patients 1 and 3, there were still brightly fluorescing areas indicating remaining neoplastic tissue. One month after the second PDT-session in these patients, and 15 months later in all patients, there was no tumor-specific fluorescence detectable.

The 42 superficial **BCC** using 20% ALA and red or green light showed a comparable response to both light sources (Table 21). Pain was more pronounced in facial lesions compared to those localized on the trunk. Green light PDT was much more comfortable for the patients than red light irradiation (Figs. 237–241).

The 124 routinely treated lesions of **Bowen's disease** using 20% ALA and red or green light showed a better response to red light PDT than to green light irradiation (Table 22). Overall, the effectivness of PDT in Bowen's disease was not as high as in BCC.

Table 20. PDT in SK: Red versus green light

| ALA [%] | Patient [n] | Front | Irradiation [nm] | | CR 1. | Pain | CR 2. | Pain |
|---|---|---|---|---|---|---|---|---|
| | | | [mW/cm²] | [J/cm²] | | | | |
| | | | 25 | 30 | | | | |
| 10 | 1 | left | [570–650] | | N | 3 | Y | 2 |
| 10 | | right | [543–548] | | N | 1 | Y | 1 |
| 10 | 2 | left | [570–650] | | Y | 2 | – | – |
| 10 | | right | [543–548] | | Y | 1 | – | – |
| 10 | 3 | left | [570–650] | | N | 3 | Y | 1 |
| 10 | | right | [543–548] | | N | 1 | Y | 1 |
| 10 | 4 | left | [543–548] | | Y | 1 | – | – |
| 10 | | right | [570–650] | | Y | 3 | – | – |
| 10 | 5 | left | [543–548] | | Y | 1 | – | – |
| 10 | | right | [570–650] | | Y | 3 | – | – |
| 10 | 6 | left | [543–548] | | Y | 1 | – | – |
| 10 | | right | [570–650] | | Y | 2 | – | – |

SK on the forehead were treated by 20 % ALA for 6 h. Irradiation was performed by either red light or green light with an energy of 30 J/cm². Degree of pain was subjectively given and scaled by 1 (moderate), 2 (intermediate) and 3 (severe). Comparable results were achieved for both types of light sources. Green light irradiation, however, led to less pain than red light.

Table 21. PDT in BCC: Red (broad band) versus green light

| ALA [%] | Local. | Lesions [n] | Irradiation [nm] | | Complete response | | | Pain [1–3] |
|---|---|---|---|---|---|---|---|---|
| | | | [mW/cm²] | [J/cm²] | 1. | 3. | 5. | |
| | | | [570–650] | | | | | |
| 20 | Trunk | 16 | 150 | 180 | 38 | 81 | 100 | 2.0 |
| 20 | Face | 5 | 150 | 180 | 40 | 80 | 100 | 2.4 |
| | | | [543–548] | | | | | |
| 20 | Trunk | 16 | 20 | 30 | 43 | 88 | 94 | 1.2 |
| 20 | Face | 5 | 20 | 30 | 60 | 80 | 100 | 1.6 |

Degree of pain was subjectively assessed and graded on a scale as 1 (moderate), 2 (intermediate) and 3 (severe). Green light PDT was less painful than red light irradiation. The complete response rates were comparable for both types of light sources used.

Table 22. PDT in Bowen's disease: Red (broad band) versus green light

| ALA [%] | Lesions [n] | Irradiation [nm] | | Complete response | | | Pain[1] [1–3] |
|---|---|---|---|---|---|---|---|
| | | [mW/cm²] | [J/cm²] | 1 | 3 | 5 | |
| | | [570–650] | | | | | |
| 20 | 66 | 150 | 180 | 38 | 71 | 86 | 1.8 |
| | | [543–548] | | | | | |
| 20 | 58 | 20 | 30 | 31 | 42 | 66 | 1.2 |

[1] Degree of pain was subjectively assessed and graded on a scale as 1 (moderate), 2 (intermediate) and 3 (severe). In Bowen's disease red light PDT was more effective than green light PDT.

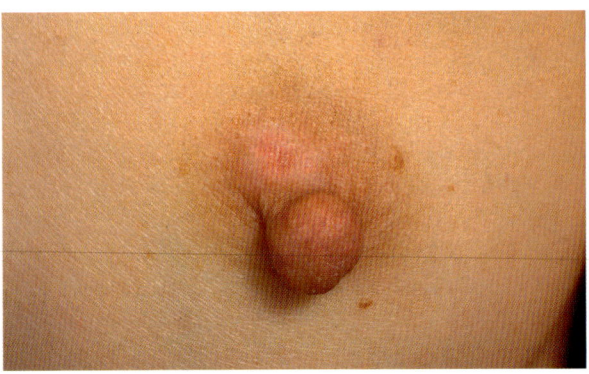

Fig. 237. Superficial BCC within the areola of the left breast. The tumor borders are not visible

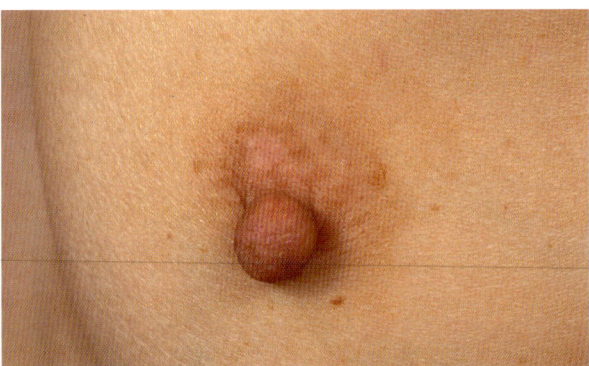

Fig. 240. Two months after three PDT sessions (PDT Saalmann, PDT Green light, 543–548 nm, 30 J/cm$^2$). Excellent cosmetic result without residual lesions

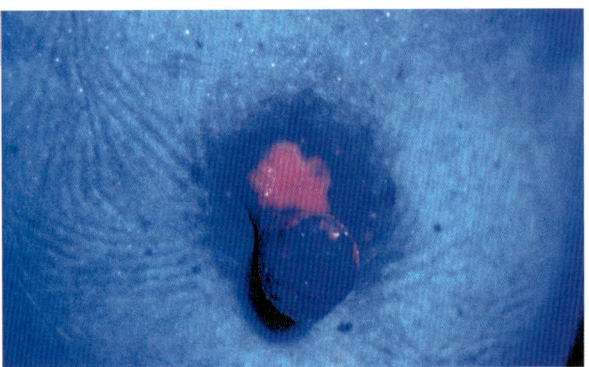

Fig. 238. FDAP with 20% ALA: Bright and sharply delineated fluorescence pattern

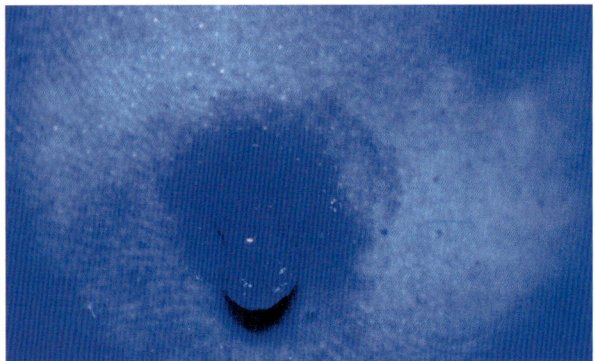

Fig. 241. FDAP 2: Lack of fluorescence indicating absence of tumor tissue

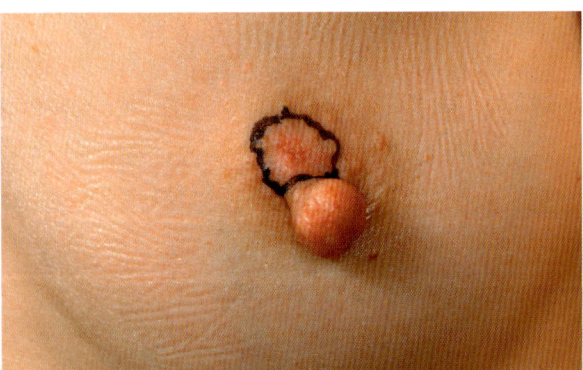

Fig. 239. Marking of the fluorescence pattern. With the help of this marking, one can better decide on surgery, crysurgery, PDT or any other tumor therapy

The 88 **SCC** treated by 20% ALA and green or red light responded nicely to topical PDT (Table 23). Concerning the effects of wavelength, red light PDT showed somewhat higher success rate than green light irradiation. However, the difference was not significant, except the values after the 2nd PDT session. Taking the degree of pain into account, green light irradiation in SCC is much more comfortable than red light PDT.

In 65 **psoriatic lesions**, the complete response rate was not depending on the light source (wavelength) (Table 24). Interestingly, blue light irradiation achieved comparable results to green and red light PDT. Pain was most pronounced after red light PDT.

In these studies comparing different light sources, the energy of green and blue light used was six times lower than red light energy.

## Chapter Discussion

In the present study, it was demonstrated for the first time that green light PDT may be effectively used to treat patients with SK and even SCC or psoriatic lesions. In the case of SK, the therapeutic

**Table 23.** PDT in SCC: Red (broad band) versus green light

| ALA [%] | Lesions [n] | Irradiation [nm] | | Complete response | | | Pain[1] [1–3] |
|---|---|---|---|---|---|---|---|
| | | [mW/cm²] | [J/cm²] | 1 | 3 | 5 | |
| | | [570 – 650] | | | | | |
| 20 | 36 | 150 | 180 | 47 | 81 | 97 | 2.5 |
| | | [543 – 548] | | | | | |
| 20 | 52 | 20 | 30 | 46 | 62 | 92 | 1.5 |

[1] Degree of pain was subjectively assessed and graded on a scale as 1 (moderate), 2 (intermediate) and 3 (severe).

**Table 24.** PDT in psoriatic lesions: Red versus green versus blue light

| ALA [%] | Lesions [n] | Irradiation [nm] | | Complete response | | | Pain[1] [1–3] |
|---|---|---|---|---|---|---|---|
| | | [mW/cm²] | [J/cm²] | 1 | 3 | 5 | |
| | | [570–650] | | | | | |
| 1 | 20 | 150 | 180 | 20 | 55 | 90 | 2.4 |
| | | [543–548] | | | | | |
| 1 | 23 | 20 | 30 | 30 | 52 | 87 | 1.2 |
| | | [320–400] | | | | | |
| 1 | 22 | 20 | 30 | 32 | 63 | 95 | 1.8 |

Degree of pain was subjectively assessed and graded on a scale as 1 (moderate), 2 (intermediate) and 3 (severe).

efficacy of green light PDT was essentially identical to that achieved by standard red light PDT (Wolf et al, 1993, Fritsch et al, 1998, Calcavara-Pinton, 1995). Most remarkably, however, green light PDT, in contrast to red light PDT, did cause less burning and pain during the irradiation process, although identical energies were used. This difference in pain generation might be caused by the deeper penetration of red light into the skin (Lui and Anderson, 1992) and the included infrared part of those lamps. These observations strongly imply that for SK localized on the face or the scalp, green light PDT is superior to red light PDT, because it is equally effective, but at the same time has fewer an desired side effects. Green light PDT led also to excellent results in the treatment of superficial BCC. In the case of BD and marginally also SCC, however, red light PDT was superior to green light PDT. It has to be taken into consideration that red light energy was 6-fold higher than green light. These different light energies were chosen because they were found to lead to optimum therapeutic efficacy in previous studies (Fritsch et al, 1998).

In contrast to surgical procedures, ALA-PDT is particularly suited to treat patients with numerous precancerous lesions or superficial skin tumors. However, the usefulness of ALA-PDT has been substantially limited by the fact that this modality is associated with burning pain. Approximately 90% of all ALA-PDT-treated patients in our department have reported to suffer from burning pain within the treated skin areas, in particular during and several hours after the irradiation process (Fritsch et al, 1998; Fritsch et al, 1998).

The present observation that green light ALA-PDT has caused none or only little burning and pain, but at the same time has exerted photodynamic effects on (pre)malignant skin cells, indicates that the desirable and unwanted effects of ALA-PDT are caused by different wavelengths.

# J General Discussion

FDAP and PDT proved to be highly effective diagnostic and therapeutic tools in skin diseases.

## J.1 FDAP: Indications and Limits

In contrast to PDT, there are only few reports about the application of the ALA-induced porphyrin fluorescence in the detection and delineation of tumors. The present work summarizes the first studies evaluating the efficacy of FDAP in dermatology.

Tumor diagnosis and therapies vary depending on the affected tissue, progression of the tumor and the health condition of the patient. In general, surgery of a cancer with a wide safety margin is the treatment of choice for a curative procedure. An important and difficult step in tumor surgery is the early detection and exact demarcation of neoplastic tissue. Often tumors grow without symptoms and may progress and infiltrate adjacent tissues before they lead to clinical signs. Therefore, efforts have been made to develop procedures such as FDAP which are highly reliable for early tumor diagnosis, noninvasive and easy to perform. The data presented here prove that FDAP is a reliable diagnostic tool in skin cancer detection with the additional possibility of early demarcation of the tumor margins for better preoperative evaluation and a further tool to ensure total excision of the tumor in one session.

Besides dermatological indications, FDAP is used for the detection of gastrointestinal dysplasias improving the endoscopic surveillance of patients with an increased risk for dysplasia. FDAP is currently established as a standard procedure for bladder tumor detection and resection, especially in endoscopically difficult situations (carcinoma in situ, multifocal tumors, multiple prior resections, or previous drug instillation therapy) (Table 25). FDAP facilitates the detection of neoplastic tissues during transurethral resection of bladder cancer and increases the accuracy of diagnosis. It may also be helpful in determining the boundaries of the resected tissue when carrying out conservative kidney-preserving surgery. Therefore, methods that permit intraoperative identification of residual tumor tissue may be of great benefit. In intraepithelial neoplasias of the vulva or the cervix, the application of fluorescence spectroscopy achieved a high degree of detection of lesions and may be a valuable tool for the diagnosis of these lesions.

Indication for FDAP is detection of cutaneous tumor tissue in actinically damaged skin and in pretreated (cryosurgery, surgery) skin areas. Thus, newly arising or regressing tumors can be identified early (Figs. 242–251).

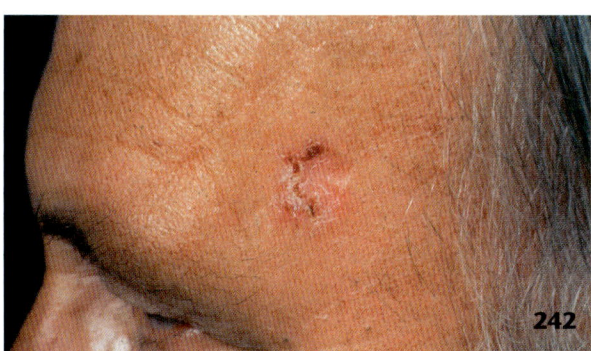

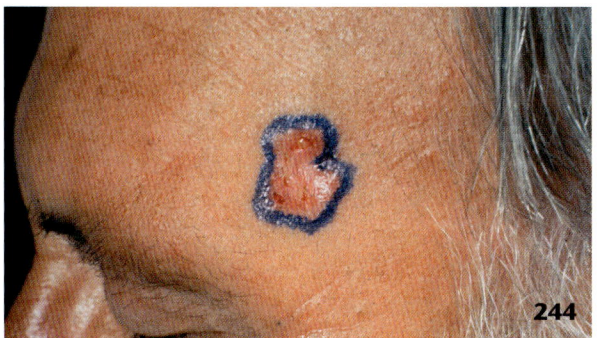

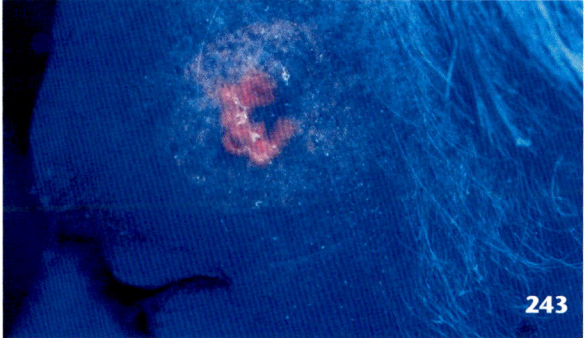

**Figs. 242–244.** Sclerodermiform BCC with ill-defined borders. FDAP (Fig. 243) assisted to delineate the lesion more accurately. According to the marking, surgical excision was performed. Histology confirmed a total excision

**Table 25.** Indications of FDAP

| Speciality | Tumor | ALA application route | Amount | Time | Reference |
|---|---|---|---|---|---|
| Gynaecology | VIN, CIN, Ca | Topical | 10–20% | 2–4 h | (Pahernik et al, 1998) |
| Urology | Bladder Ca | Intravesical | 1.5 g in 50 ml 8.4% $Na_2CO_3$ | 2–3 h | (Kriegmair et al, 1996) |
| Neurosurgery | Malignant Glioma | Oral | 10 mg kg/KG | 3 h | (Stummer et al, 1998) |
| Otorhinology | SCC (Mucosa, Toung) | Mouth rinsing (for 20 min) | 0.4% Solution | 1.5 h | (Leunig et al, 2000) |
| Laryngology | Larynx Ca | Vaporisation (for 20 min) | 0.6 wt% ALA-NaCl | | (Mehlmann et al, 1999) |
| Dermatology | BCC, SCC, SK | Topical | 10–20% ointment | 4 | (Fritsch et al, 2000) |

The route of ALA administration for the diagnosis or treatment of different tumors.

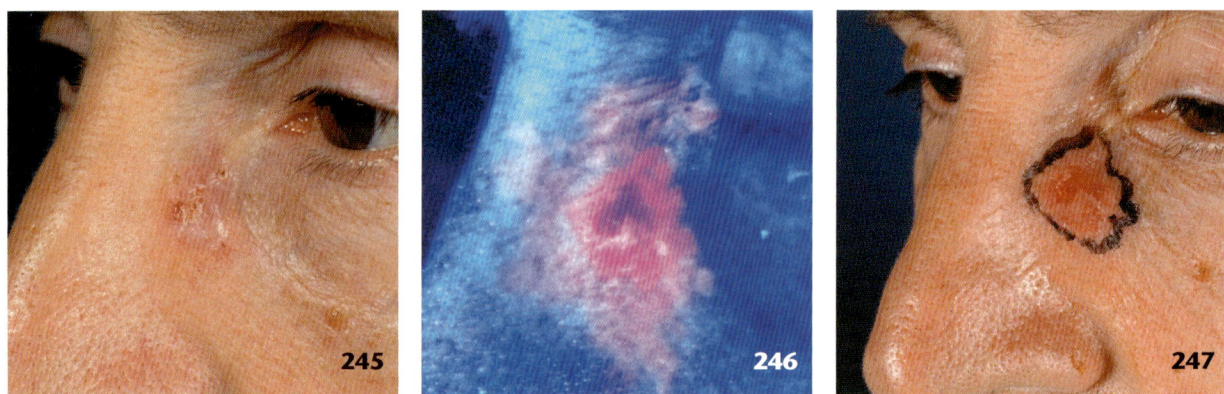

**Fig. 245–247.** BCC with ill-defined borders. FDAP guided surgery was performed and led to a complete excision of the lesion. In this case, the tumor-surrounding skin also showed a bright fluorescence. Tumor fluorescence was more intensive than that of normal skin, thus delineation was still possible

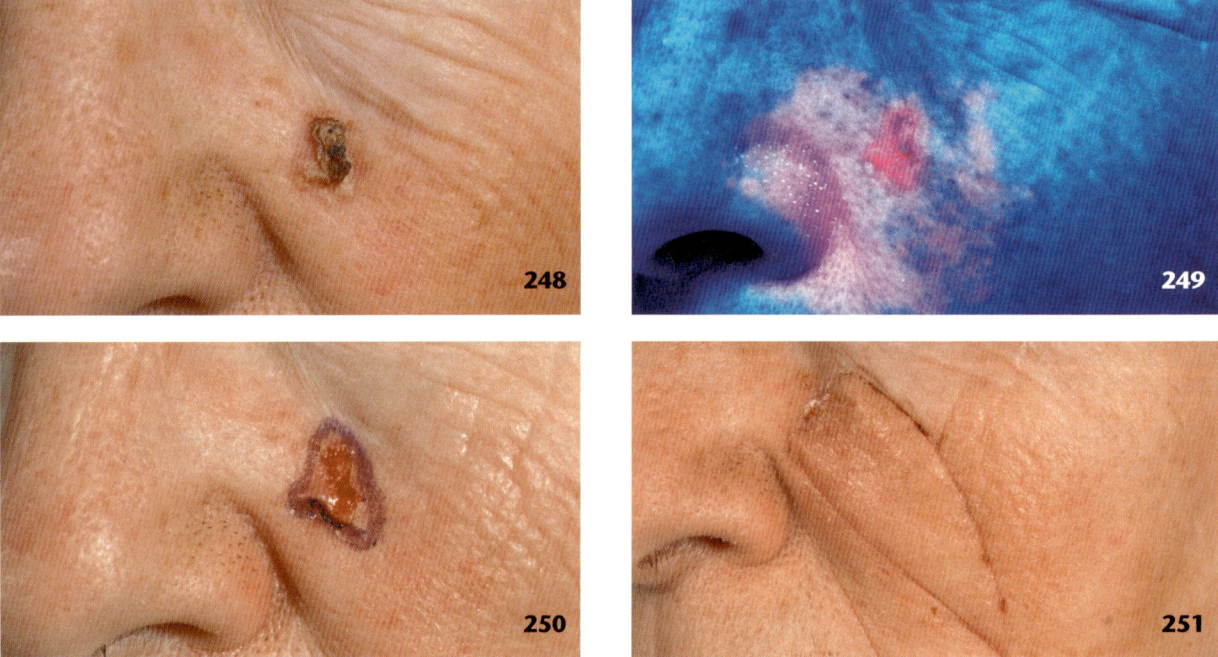

**Figs. 248–251.** SCC presenting with hemorrhagic crusts and ill-defined borders. After debulking the exophytic parts, FDAP enabled clear delineation of the tumor. The lesion was excised according to the fluorescence pattern. Tissue defect was closed by a skin flap

In addition, FDAP is a very effective technique to control the efficacy of any tumor treatment (Figs. 252–265).

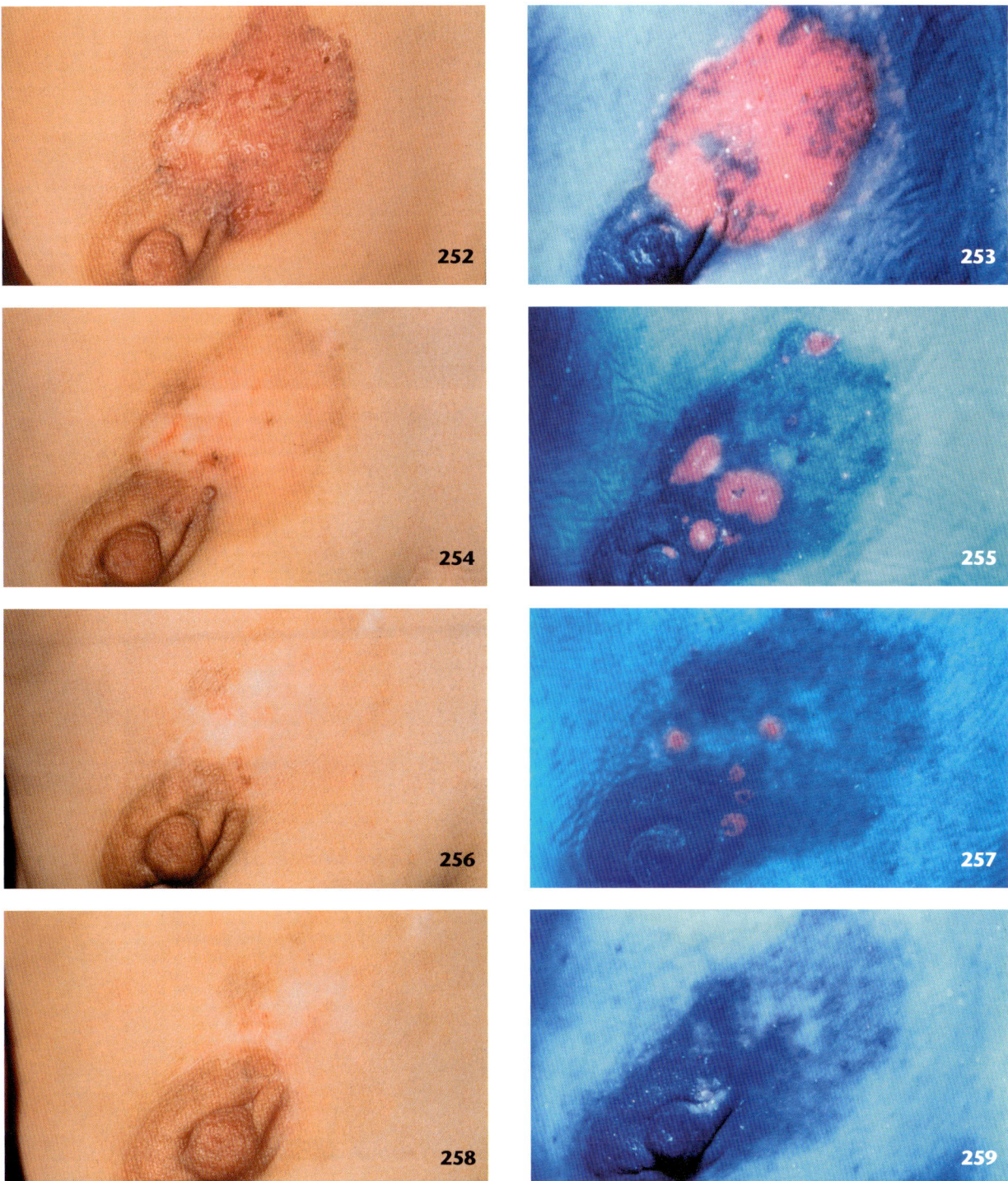

**Figs. 252–259.** BCC on the skin of the right breast. PDT was performed using red light (570–750 nm, 180 J/cm²). A total of four therapeutic sessions were applied, one per month (Figs. 254 and 255 = one month after 1st PDT). FDAP was very effective in detecting and delineating all residual tumor parts. One month after the 4th PDT cycle, there were still some tumor-suspect areas (Figs. 256 and 257). Due to their close proximity to the nipple areola complex, these tumor parts were surgically excised (Figs. 258 and 259 = one month after 4 PDT sessiones and surgical treatment of the nipple area – surrounding residual lesions)

# J General Discussion

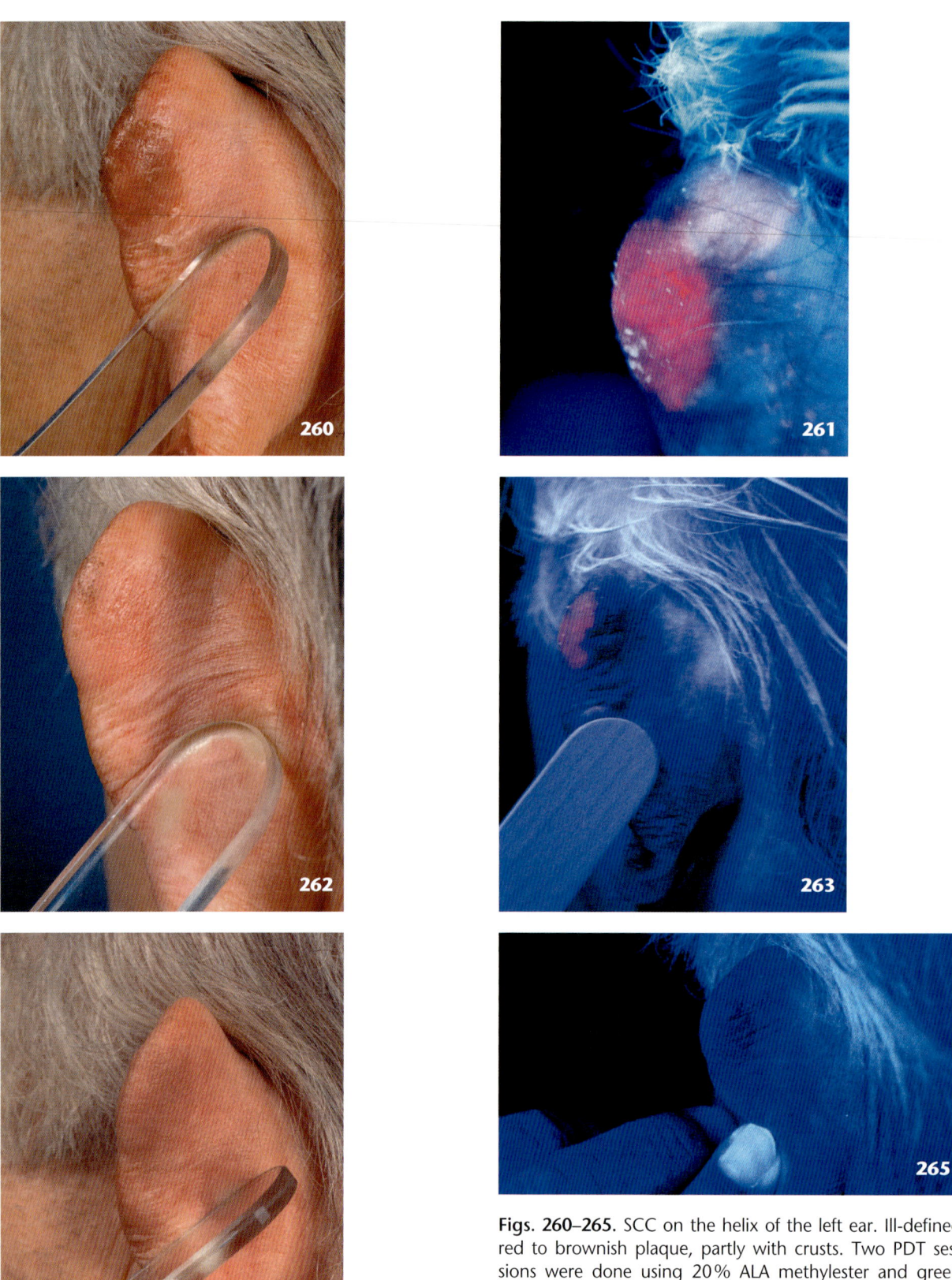

**Figs. 260–265.** SCC on the helix of the left ear. Ill-defined red to brownish plaque, partly with crusts. Two PDT sessions were done using 20% ALA methylester and green light (Saalmann, PDT green light, 543–548 nm, 30 J/cm²). (Figs. 262, 263 – two weeks after the 1st PDT session). Three weeks after the 2nd PDT neither clinically (Fig. 264) nor in the 3rd FDAP (Fig. 265) there were signs of neoplastic tissue

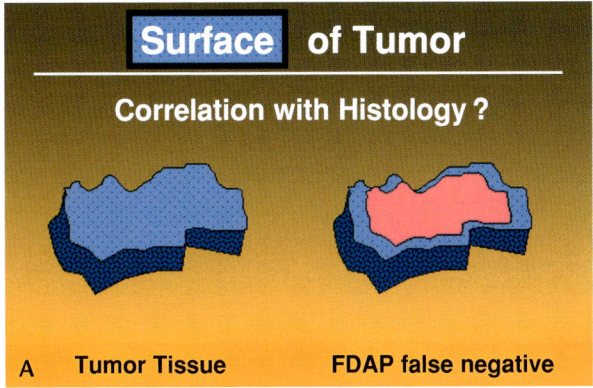
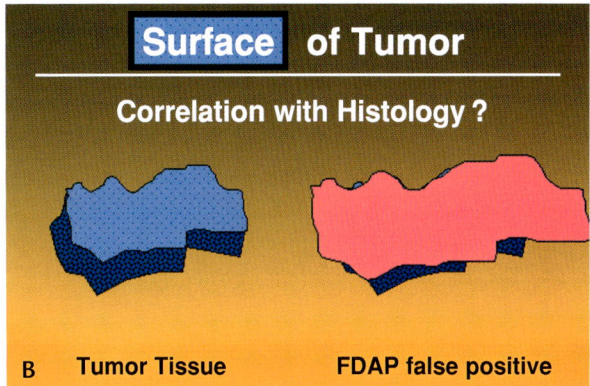

**Fig. 266 A and B:** Schematical illustration of the efficacy of FDAP in skin tumor detection. Concerning the horizontal extension of the tumor tissue, fluorescing area could be smaller or larger than the histological tumor area

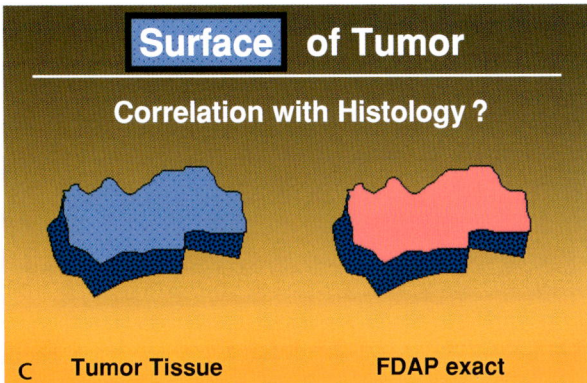
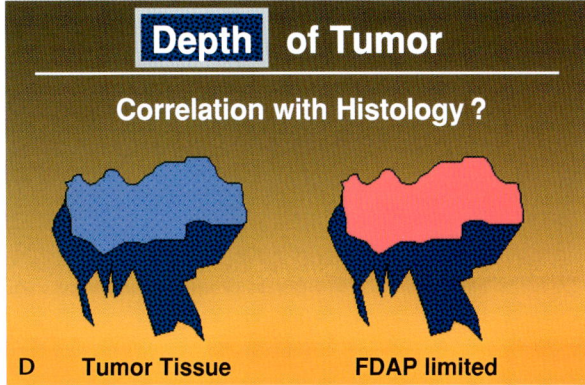

**Fig. 266 C and D:** Optimum use of FDAP is guaranteed if its fluorescence corresponds exactly to the histological tumor area. FDAP will never give any information on the penetration depth of a tumor

FDAP allows determination of only the horizontal extension of a tumor tissue. It provides no information on the infiltration depth of a certain tumor. This can be verified only by histopathological evaluation.

## J.2 PDT: Indications and Limits

As of today, topical ALA-PDT may already be suggested as the treatment of choice in SK. In our opinion, the CR rates of 75–85% as published in the Phase II- or III-studies (Tables 26A–26F) (Omrod and Jarvis, 2000) do not justify the use of the described treatment parameters (14–18 h application time of ALA, irradiation with blue light, 10 J/cm$^2$). We and others showed much higher CR of SK to PDT using only 10% ALA and red (75 J/cm$^2$) (Fritsch et al, 1998; Braathen et al, 2000) or green light (20 mW/cm$^2$, 24 J/cm$^2$) (Fritsch et al, 1997). However, rather than the ALA concentration or the light source used, the ALA application time of 14–18 h does not seem to offer optimum conditions for intralesional porphyrin accumulation. Biochemical studies on porphyrin metabolite kinetics also revealed best lesion/non-lesional skin ratio of porphyrins 2–6 h after ALA application (Fig. 72) (Fritsch et al, 1999; Fritsch et al, 1998). These data do not support an application time of 14–18 h as recommended by DUSA. The use of Metvix® leads to similar results in PDT of SK as compared to free ALA, however, with an improved selectivity. In the treatment of widespread SK, ALA-ME is therefore superior to free ALA, and causes less burning pain.

Regarding epithelial skin tumors, PDT using 20% ALA is strongly recommended for superficial BCC and initial SCC. Nodular tumors should only be treated by experienced physicians. The debulking of the exophytic tumor part is a prerequisite prior to PDT. In general, red and green light is used

**Table 26A.** Clinical Studies on PDT Efficacy in Basal Cell Carcinomas (BCC)

| Treated Lesion | n | Photosensitizer Type | Time [h] | Dose [mg/kg] | Light Source Type | λ [nm] | Intensity [mW/cm²] | Fluence [J/cm²] | CR[1] [%] | Follow up [mo] | Reference |
|---|---|---|---|---|---|---|---|---|---|---|---|
| | | **Intravenous** | | | | | | | | | |
| BCC | 3 | Photofrin | 96 | 5 | Xenon Arc | 600–700 | 100 | 120 | 100 | 7 | (Dougherty, 1981) |
| BCC | 6 | Photofrin | 24/72 | 1–2 | Argon-PDL | 630 | 29–90 | 40–60 | 100 | 3 | (Waldow et al, 1987) |
| BCC | 15 | DHE | 72 | 2 | Cop. Vap-PDL | 628 | n.d. | 50 | 93 | 6 | (Robinson et al, 1988) |
| BCC | 21 | HpD | 72 | 5 | n.d. | 630 | n.d. | 30 | 0 | 6 | (Pennington et al, 1988) |
| BCC | 36 | Photofrin | 48–144 | 2 | Argon-PDL | 630 | 11–110 | 40–144[2] | 31 | 6 | (McCaughan et al, 1989) |
| BCC | 7 | DHE | 72 | 1.5–2 | Argon-PDL | 630 | n.d. | 50–100 | 50 | 6 | (Buchanan et al, 1989) |
| BCC | 3 | NPe6 | 4–8 | 0.5 | Argon-PDL | 664 | 50–400 | 25–200 | 33 | n.d. | (Allen et al, 1992) |
| BCC | 67 | Photosan 3 | 48 | 2 | Argon-PDL | 630 | 100 | 100 | 97 | 54 | (Feyh et al, 1993) |
| BCC | 149 | Photofrin | 48–72 | 1 | Argon-PDL | 630 | 150 | 72–288 | 88[3] | 20–43 | (Wilson et al, 1992) |
| BCC superficial | 5 | mTHPC | 24–96 | 0,1 mg | LED[4] | 652 | 100 | 5–15 | 86 | 12–18 | (Baas et al, 2000) |

[1] Complete response rate is generally based on the results after one treatment. [2] Treatment was given either by surface irradiation or interstitially. [3] CR of lesions was dependent on the body site. [4] LED=Light emitting diodes

**Table 26B.** Clinical Studies on PDT Efficacy in Basal Cell Carcinomas (BCC)

| Treated Lesion | n | Photosensitizer Type | Time [h] | Dose [mg/kg] | Light Source Type | λ [nm] | Intensity [mW/cm²] | Fluence [J/cm²] | CR[1] [%] | Follow up [mo] | Reference |
|---|---|---|---|---|---|---|---|---|---|---|---|
| | | **Topical** | | | | | | | | | |
| BCC | 292 | TPPS | 3+6+24 | 2 | Argon-PDL | 645 | 20–200 | 120/150 | 94 | n.d. | (Santoro et al, 1990) |
| BCC | 98 | ALA | >3 | 20 | Cop. Vap-PDL | 630 | 100–150 | 50–100 | 96 | 3 | (Warloe et al, 1992) |
| BCC | 27 | ALA | 4 | 20 | Xenon Arc | 615–645 | 20–86 | 150 | 59 | 1 | (Morton et al, 1998) |
| BCC superficial | 62 | ALA | 6 | 20 | PDT 1200 | 640 | 105–168 | 105 | 82 | 12 | (Warma et al, 2001) |
| BCC superficial | 26 | ALA | 3 | 20 | Paterson | 615–645 | 50–100 | 120–134 | 96 | 27 | (Haller et al, 2000) |
| BCC superficial | 47 | ALA | 6 | 20 | Argon-PDL | 635 | 60–100 | 60 | 75 | 3 | (Wang et al, 1999) |
| BCC superficial | 55 | ALA | 6 | 10 | Slide-Projector | >600 | 200 | 240 | 85 | 6 | (Hürlimann et al, 1998) |
| BCC superficial | 58 | ALA | 6 | 20 | Xenon | 615–645 | 20–86 | 100–150 | 88 | 12–52 | (Morton et al, 1998) |
| BCC superficial | 95 | ALA | 4 | 20 | Slide-Projector | >600 | 50–100 | 18–131 | 50 | 36 | (Fink-Purches et al, 1998) |
| BCC nodular | 10 | ALA | 4–8 | 20 | Slide-Projector | >570 | 50–100 | 90 | 10 | 3–12 | (Wolf et al, 1993) |
| BCC nodular | 24 | ALA | 4–6 | 20 | Nd: YAG-PDL | 630 | 100 | 150 | 64 | 6–14 | (Svanberg et al, 1994) |
| BCC nodular | 22 | ALA+Desferal | 20 | 20 | PTL-Penta | 570–680 | 150–250 | <300 | 32 | 20 | (Fijan et al, 1995) |
| BCC nodular | 30 | ALA | 6–8 | 20 | Argon-PDL | 630 | 100 | 60–80 | 80 | 29 | (Calzavara-Pinton et al, 1995) |
| BCC nodular | 10 | ALA | 3 | 20 | Xenon Arc | 620–670 | 125, 166 | 75, 100 | 22,0 | 6 | (Wennberg et al, 1996) |
| BCC pigmented | 4 | ALA | 6–8 | 20 | Argon-PDL | 630 | 100 | 60–80 | 0 | 29 | (Calzavara-Pinton et al, 1995) |
| BCC superficial | 80 | ALA | 3–6 | 20 | Slide-Projector | >600 | 150–300 | 54–540 | 90 | 2–3 | (Kennedy et al, 1990) |
| BCC superficial | 30 | ALA | 4–6 | 10–40 | n.d. | 630 | n.d. | 75–200 | 100 | 3 | (Shanler et al, 1993) |
| BCC superficial | 37 | ALA | 4–8 | 20 | Slide-Projector | >570 | 50–100 | 90 | 97 | 3–12 | (Wolf et al, 1993) |
| BCC superficial | 8 | ALA | 3 | 20 | Slide-Projector | red light | 19–44 | 100 | 50 | 1–3 | (Lui, Anderson, 1995) |
| BCC superficial | 55 | ALA | 4–6 | 20 | Nd: YAG-PDL | 630 | 100 | 150 | 100 | 6–14 | (Svanberg et al, 1994) |
| BCC superficial | 34 | ALA+Desferal | 20 | 20 | PTL-Penta | 570–680 | 150–250 | <300 | 88 | 20 | (Fijan et al, 1995) |
| BCC superficial | 23 | ALA | 6–8 | 20 | Argon-PDL | 630 | 100 | 60–80 | 100 | 29 | (Calzavara-Pinton et al, 1995) |
| BCC superficial | 40 | ALA | 6 | 20 | PDT 700 | 570–750 | 150 | 180 | 0–83[2] | 12–24 | (Fritsch et al, 1998) |
| BCC superficial | 157 | ALA | 3 | 20 | Xenon Arc | 620–670 | 125, 166 | 75, 100 | 43,100 | 6 | (Wennberg et al, 1996) |
| BCC pigmented | 16 | ALA | 16 | 20 | Xenon Arc | 650–670 | 120 | 140 | 87 | 12 | (Itoh et al, 2000) |
| BCC nod.+debulk | 24 | ALA | 6 | 20 | Versa® | 630–635 | 100 | 120 | 92 | 3 | (Thissen et al, 2000) |
| BCC | 31 | ALA | 18 | 20 | Versa® | 630–635 | 120 | 140 | 88,9 | 19 | (Haddad et al, 2001) |
| BCC | 245 | ALA+DMSO | 3 | 20 | Halogen | 570–750 | 80 | 75 | 82 | 6 | (Soler et al, 2000) |
| BCC | | ALA+DMSO | 3 | 20 | Laser | 690 | 120–150 | 100–150 | 86 | 6 | (Soler et al, 2000) |
| BCC | 31 | ALA | 12 | 20 | Versa® | 585–720 | 150 | 50 | 84 | 24 | (Hart et al, 1998) |
| BCC | 5 | ALA | 3,5–5 | 20 | ? | ? | ? | ? | 70,6 | 10 | (Stefanidou et al, 2000) |

[1] Complete response rate is generally based on the results after one treatment. [2] CR was dependent on the size of lesions and was improved by repetition of PDT (maximum 3 sessions): superficial BCC 33–100%

**Table 26C.** Clinical Studies on PDT Efficacy in Bowen's Disease (BD)

| Treated Lesion | n | Photosensitizer Type | Time [h] | Dose [mg/kg] | Light Source Type | λ [nm] | Intensity [mW/cm²] | Fluence [J/cm²] | CR[1] [%] | Follow up [mo] | Reference |
|---|---|---|---|---|---|---|---|---|---|---|---|
| | | **Intravenous** | | | | | | | | | |
| BD | 3 | Photofrin | 24 | 2 | Argon-PDL | 630 | 80–194 | 40–60 | 100 | 3 | (Waldow et al, 1987) |
| BD | 87 | DHE | 72 | 2 | Cop. Vap-PDL | 628 | n. d. | 25 | 85 | 4–6 | (Robinson et al, 1988) |
| BD | 3 | Photofrin | 48–144 | 2 | Argon-PDL | 630 | 11–110 | 40–144[2] | 66 | 6 | (McCaughan et al, 1989) |
| BD | 50 | DHE | 72 | 1.5–2 | Argon-PDL | 630 | n.d. | 25 | 50–100 | n.d. | (Buchanan et al, 1989) |
| BD | 8 | Photofrin | 48 | 1 | Argon-PDL | 630 | 150 | 185–250 | 100 | 12–24 | (Jones et al, 1992) |
| BD | 32 | HpD | 72 | 5 | n. d. | 630 | n. d. | 30 | <50 | 6 | (Pennington et al, 1988) |
| | | **Topical** | | % | | | | | | | |
| BD | 36 | ALA | 3–5 | 0.05 | Cop. Vap-PDL | 630 | <150 | 125–250 | 89 | 17 | (Cairnduff et al, 1994) |
| BD | 10 | ALA | 4–6 | 20 | Nd: YAG-PDL | 630 | 100 | 150 | 90 | 16–14 | (Svanberg et al, 1994) |
| BD | 10 | ALA+Desferal | 20 | 20 | PTL-Penta | 570–680 | 150–250 | <300 | 30 | 20 | (Fijan et al, 1995) |
| BD | 6 | ALA | 6–8 | 20 | Argon-PDL | 630 | 100 | 60–80 | 100 | 29 | (Calzavara-Pinton et al, 1995) |
| BD | 8 | ALA | 6 | 20 | PDT 700 | 570–750 | 150 | 180 | 50[3] | 12–24 | (Fritsch et al, 1998) |
| BD | 18 | ALA | 3 | 20 | Xenon Arc | 620–670 | 125–166 | 75–100 | 61 | 6 | (Wennberg et al, 1996) |
| BD | 3 | ALA | 3 | 20 | Slide Projector | 400–700 | 150 | 125 | >90 | 3 | (Stables et al, 1997) |
| BD | 20 | ALA | 4 | 20 | Xenon Arc | 600–660 | 70 | 125 | 75 | 2 | (Morton et al, 1996) |
| BD | 4 | ALA | 16 | 20 | LED | 590–670 | 40 | 240 | 100 | 20 | (Wong et al, 2001) |
| BD | 18 | ALA | 4 | 20 | Xenon Arc | 620–670 | 125, 166 | 75, 100 | 43, 100 | 6 | (Wennberg et al, 1996) |
| BD | 50 | ALA | 4 | 20 | PDT 1200 | 640 | 105–168 | 105 | 69 | 12 | (Warma et al, 2001) |
| BD | 40 | ALA | 4 | 20 | Xenon | 615–645 | 20–86 | 125 | 78 | 12–60 | (Morton et al, 2000) |
| BD | 45 | ALA | 4 | 20 | Xenon | 615–645 | 20–86 | 125 | 89 | 12–60 | (Morton et al, 2001) |

[1] Complete response rate is generally based on the results after one treatment. [2] Treatment was given either by surface irradiation or interstitially. [3] CR was dependent on the size of lesion and was improved by repetition of PDT (maximum 3 sessions): BD 75%

**Table 26D.** Clinical Studies on PDT Efficacy in Squamous Cell Carcinomas (SCC)

| Treated Lesion | n | Photosensitizer Type | Time [h] | Dose [mg/kg] | Light Source Type | λ [nm] | Intensity [mW/cm²] | Fluence [J/cm²] | CR[1] [%] | Follow up [mo] | Reference |
|---|---|---|---|---|---|---|---|---|---|---|---|
| | | **Intravenous** | | | | | | | | | |
| SCC | 32 | HpD | 72 | 5 | n.d. | 630 | n.d. | 30 | <50 | 6 | (Pennington et al, 1988) |
| SCC | 5 | Photofrin | 48–144 | 2 | Argon-PDL | 630 | 11–110 | 40–144[2] | 40 | 6 | (McCaughan et al, 1989) |
| SCC | 2 | NPe6 | 4–8 | 1 | Argon-PDL | 664 | 50–400 | 50–100 | 100 | n.d. | (Allen et al, 1992) |
| SCC | 7 | Photosan 3 | 48 | 2 | Argon-PDL | 630 | 100 | 100 | 86 | 54 | (Feyh et al, 1993) |
| SCC/BCC | 97 | mTHPC | 96 | 0.1–0.15 | Argon-PDL | 652 | 100 | 5–20 | 92.7 | 15 | (Kübler et al, 1999) |
| | | **Topical** | | [%] | | | | | | | |
| SCC | 8 | ALA | 3–6 | 20 | Slide-Projector | >600 | 150–300 | 54–540 | 80 | 2–3 | (Kennedy et al, 1990) |
| SCC nodular | 2 | ALA | 3 | 20 | Slide-Projector | red light | 19–44 | 100 | 0 | 17 | (Lui, Anderson, 1995) |
| SCC nodular | 6 | ALA | 6–8 | 20 | Argon-PDL | 630 | 100 | 60–80 | 67 | 29 | (Calzavara-Pinton et al, 1995) |
| SCC nodular | 4 | ALA | 6 | 20 | PDT 1200 | 570–750 | 150 | 180 | 0[3] | 12–24 | (Fritsch et al, 1998) |
| SCC superficial | 6 | ALA | 4–8 | 20 | Slide-Projector | >570 | 50–100 | 90 | 83 | 3–12 | (Wolf et al, 1993) |
| SCC superficial | 3 | ALA | 3 | 20 | Slide-Projector | red light | 19–44 | 100 | 67 | 17 | (Lui, Anderson, 1995) |
| SCC superficial | 12 | ALA | 6–8 | 20 | Argon-PDL | 630 | 100 | 60–80 | 92 | 29 | (Calzavara-Pinton et al, 1995) |
| SCC superficial | 10 | ALA | 6 | 20 | PDT 700 | 570–750 | 150 | 180 | 60[3] | 12–24 | (Fritsch et al, 1998) |
| SCC | 5 | ALA | 12 | 20 | Versa® | 585–720 | 150 | 50 | 80 | 8–12 | (Harth et al, 1998) |
| SCC | 35 | ALA | 4 | 20 | Slide-Projector | >600 | 50–100 | 5–180 | 8 | 36 | (Fink-Purches et al, 1998) |

[1] Complete response rate is generally based on the results after one treatment. [2] Treatment was given either by surface irradiation or interstitially. [6] CR was dependent on the size of lesion and was improved by repetition of PDT (maximum 3 sessions): BD 75%

**Table 26E.** Clinical Studies on PDT Efficacy in Solar Keratoses (SK)

| Treated Lesion | n | Photosensitizer Type **Topical** | Time [h] | Dose [%] | Light Source Type | λ [nm] | Intensity [mW/cm²] | Fluence [J/cm²] | CR[1] [%] | Follow up [mo] | Reference |
|---|---|---|---|---|---|---|---|---|---|---|---|
| SK | 10 | ALA | 3–6 | 20 | Slide Projector | >600 | 150–300 | 54–540 | 90 | 2–3 | (Kennedy et al, 1990) |
| SK | 9 | ALA | 4–8 | 20 | Slide Projector | >570 | 50–100 | 100 | 100 | 3–12 | (Wolf et al, 1993) |
| SK | 43 | ALA+Desferal | 20 | 20 | PTL-Penta | 570–680 | 150–250 | <300 | 81 | 20 | (Fijan et al, 1995) |
| SK | 50 | ALA | 6–8 | 20 | Argon | 630 | 100 | 60–80 | 100 | 29 | (Calzavara-Pinton et al, 1995) |
| SK | 52 | ALA | 6 | 10 | PDT 700 | 570–750 | 120 | 144 | 86–95[2] | 12–24 | (Fritsch et al, 1998) |
| SK | 36 | ALA | 6 | 10 | PDT 1200 | 580–740 | 160 | 150 | 0–71[3] | 1 | (Szeimies et al, 1996) |
| SK (face, scalp) | 218 | ALA | 3 | 10, 20, 30 | Argon PDL | 630 | 150 | 10–150 | 61, 78, 91 | 2 | (Jeffes et al, 1997) |
| SK (trunk,extrem.) | 218 | ALA | 3 | 10, 20, 30 | Argon PDL | 630 | 150 | 10–150 | 30, 38, 45 | 2 | (Jeffes et al, 1997) |
| SK | 6 | ALA | 4 | 10 | PDT | 543–548 | 20 | 30 | 83 | 15 | (Fritsch et al, 1997) |
| SK | 6 | ALA | 4 | 10 | PDT 1200 | 570–750 | 20 | 30 | 83[4] | 15 | (Fritsch et al, 1997) |
| SK | 6 | ALA | 4 | 10 | PDT 1200 | 570–750 | 120 | 144 | 86–95 | 12–24 | (Fritsch et al, 1998) |
| SK | 6 | ALA | 4 | 10 | PDT 1200 | 570–750 | 80 | 96 | 96 | 12–24 | (Fritsch et al, 1998) |
| SK (face, scalp) | 109 | ALA | 4 | 20 | Slide Projector | Visible | 50–100 | 70 | 93 | 52 | (Fink-Puches et al, 1997) |
| SK (face, scalp) | 45 | ALA | 4 | 20 | Slide Projector | >600 | 50–100 | 36 | 96 | 52 | (Fink-Puches et al, 1997) |
| SK (face, scalp) | 35 | ALA | 4 | 20 | Slide Projector | UVA | 50–100 | 27 | 100 | 52 | (Fink-Puches et al, 1997) |
| SK (face, scalp) | 29 | ALA | 3–6 | 20 | Xenon Lamp | n. d. | n. d. | 30–60 | 100[5] | 26–48 | (Stefanidou et al, 2000) |
| SK (extremities) | 29 | ALA | 3–6 | 20 | Xenon Lamp | n. d. | n. d. | 30–60 | 100[5] | 26–48 | (Stefanidou et al, 2000) |
| SK (face) | 10 | ALA | 4 | 20 | Dye Laser | 630 | 100 | 50–200 | 82[6] | 12 | (Itoh et al, 2000) |
| SK (extremities) | 53 | ALA | 4 | 20 | Dye Laser | 630 | 100 | 50–200 | 56 | 12 | (Itoh et al, 2000) |
| SK (face, scalp) | 36 | ALA | 14–18 | 20 | BLU-U | 417 | 3, 5, 10 | 2, 5, 10 | 66 vs. 171 | 2–4 | (Omrod, Jarvis, 2000) |
| SK (face, scalp) | 64 | ALA | 14–18 | 20 | BLU-U | 417 | 3, 5, 10 | 2, 5, 10 | 80 | 2–4 | (Omrod, Jarvis, 2000) |
| SK (face, scalp) | 241 | ALA vs. Placebo | 14–18 | 20 | BLU-U | 417 | 10 | 10 | 83 vs. 14 | 2–3 | (Omrod, Jarvis, 2000) |
| SK (face, scalp) | 855 | ALA-ME | 20 | 3 | CureLight | 570–670 | 70–200 | 75 | 91 vs. 68[7] | 3 | (Foley et al, 2001) |
| SK (hand, forearm) | 14 | ALA vs. FU | 20 | 4 | PDT 1200 | 570–750 | 80 | 150 | 73 vs. 70[8] | 6 | (Kurwa et al, 1999) |
| SK | 127 | ALA | 4 | 20 | PDT 1200 | 640 | 105–168 | 105 | 72 | 12 | (Warma et al, 2001) |

[1] Complete response rate is generally based on the results after one treatment. [2] CR was dependent on the body site location and the size of lesion (lesions on trunk responsed better than those on the extremities). [3] CR was dependent on the size of lesion. [4] In 6 patients with SK ALA-PDT was performed with green and red light for one front side. [5] 3 to 4 PDT sessions were performed. [6] 2–6 sessions were performed. [7] PDT vs. cryosurgery; cosmetic result was also better for Metvix-PDT than with cryosurgery (83% vs. 51% graded as excellent). [8] 3-week course of topical 5-FU (fluorouracil) applied twice per day.

**Table 26F.** Clinical Studies on PDT Efficacy in Metastatic and Other Skin Tumors

| Treated Lesion | n | Photosensitizer Type | Time [h] | Dose [mg/kg] | Light Source Type | λ [nm] | Intensity [mW/cm²] | Fluence [J/cm²] | CR[1] [%] | Follow up [mo] | Reference |
|---|---|---|---|---|---|---|---|---|---|---|---|
| **Intravenous** | | | | | | | | | | | |
| Kaposi's Sarcoma | 1 | Photofrin | 72 | 2.5 | Xenon | 600–700 | 100 | 120 | 100 | 24 | (Dougherty et al, 1981) |
| Kaposi's Sarcoma | 5 | Photofrin | 48–72 | 2 | Argon-PDL | 630 | 50–130 | 50–200[2] | 60 | 3 | (Schweitzer et al, 1990) |
| Kaposi | 289 | Photofrin | 48 | 1 mg/kg | | 630 | | 100–400 | 32,5 | 4 | (Bernstein et al, 1999) |
| Malignant Melanoma | 1 | Photofrin | 96 | 3.8 | Argon-PDL | 635 | n.d. | 60–140 | 70–80 | 5 | (Dougherty et al, 1981) |
| Malignant Melanoma | 27 | Photofrin | 48–144 | 2 | Argon-PDL | 630 | 11–110 | 40–144[2] | 7 | 6 | (McCaughan et al, 1989) |
| Recurrent Tu (Met.) | 34 | Photofrin | 48–72 | 1–2 | Argon-PDL | 630 | 40–172 | 25–100 | 47 | 3–5 | (Gilson et al, 1988) |
| Breast Ca | 174 | Photofrin | 48–144 | 2 | Argon-PDL | 630 | 11–110 | 40–144[2] | 4 | 6 | (McCaughan et al, 1989) |
| Breast Ca (Met.) | 37 | Photofrin | 48–72 | 1–2.5 | Argon-PDL | 630 | 120–200 | 104–244 | 13.5 | 1 | (Khan et al, 1993) |
| Breast Ca | 120 | Photofrin | 48 | 0.8 mg/kg | KTP:YAG-laser | 630 | | 135–170 | 89 | 6 | (Allison et al, 2001) |
| Papillary Ca (Met.) | 8 | NPe6 | 4–8 | 0.5/1 | Argon-PDL | 664 | 50–400 | 50–200 | 75 | n.d. | (Allen et al, 1992) |
| Papillary Ca | 6 | NPe6 | 4–8 | 1 | Argon-PDL | 664 | 50–400 | 50 | 0 | n.d. | (Allen et al, 1992) |
| Paget's Disease | 1 | Photofrin | 24–48 | | Argon-PDL | 630 | 150 | 200–250 | 100 | 6–12 | (Petrelli et al, 1992) |
| Verrucous Ca | 1 | NPe6 | 4–8 | 0.5 | Argon-PDL | 664 | 50–400 | 100 | 100 | n.d. | (Allen et al, 1992) |
| Adeno-Ca (Met.) | 50 | Photofrin | 72 | 1.5–2 | Cop. Vap-PDL | 630 | 5–1500 | 52–81[4] | 52 | n.d. | (Lowdell et al, 1993) |
| SCC (Met.) | 20 | Photofrin | 72 | 1.5–2 | Cop. Vap-PDL | 630 | 5–1500 | 150 | 25–74 | n.d. | (Lowdell et al, 1993) |
| **Topical** | | | | % | | | | | | | |
| Adeno-Ca (Met.) | 6 | ALA | 3–5 | 50 mg/cm² | Cop. Vap-PDL | 630 | <150 | 125–250 | 83 | 17 | (Cairnduff et al, 1994) |
| Breast Ca | 4 | ALA | 3–6 | 20 | Slide Projector | >630 | 150–300 | 54–540 | 0 | 2–3 | (Kennedy et al, 1990) |
| Breast Ca (Met.) | 9 | TPPS4 | n.d. | 0.15–0.3 | Argon-PDL | 630 | 312–680 | 150 | 30 | n.d. | (Lapes et al, 1996) |
| MM (Met.) | 8 | ALA | 4–8 | 20 | Slide Projector | >570 | 50–100 | 90 | 0 | 3–12 | (Wolf et al, 1993) |
| SCC (Met.) | 6 | ALA | 3–5 | 50 | Cop. Vap-PDL | 630 | <150 | 125–250 | 0 | 17 | (Cairnduff et al, 1994) |
| Paget's Disease | 1 | ALA | 4 | 20 | Visible light | >600 | 200 | 500 | 100 | n.d. | (Henta et al, 1999) |
| T-Cell-Lymphoma | n.d. | ALA | 4–6 | 2–10 | n.d. | 630 | n.d. | 75–200 | 100 | n.d. | (Shanler et al, 1993) |
| T-Cell-Lymphoma | 4 | ALA | 4–6 | 20 | Nd:YAG-PDL | 630 | 100 | 150 | 50 | 6–14 | (Svanberg et al, 1994) |
| Mycosis Fungoides | 2 | ALA | 4–6 | 20 | Slide Projector | >570 | 44 | 40 | 100 | 3–6 | (Wolf et al, 1994) |
| Keratoacanthoma | 4 | ALA | 6–8 | 20 | Argon-PDL | 630 | 100 | 60–80 | 29 | | (Calzavara-Pinton et al,1995) |

[1] Complete response rate is generally based on the results after one treatment. [2] Treatment was given either by surface irradiation or interstitially. [3] Oral lesions of AIDS-related Kaposi's sarcoma. [4] Light irradiation was performed interstitially. n.d. = no data available.

to achieve the highest penetration depth of the photons. However, compared to the commonly used ALA-PDT with red light, UVA-ALA-PDT was 40 times more potent in killing cultured human fibroblasts and 10 times more potent than ALA-PDT with green light (Buchczyk et al, 2000). Concerning these results on the influence of the wavelength on the cell death, further studies should focus on the use of UV / blue light in ALA-PDT. ALA-PDT in BCC (even of the nodular type) is justified due to the low metastatic risk, however, clinical follow up is mandatory. In contrast, SCC should be carefully selected for ALA-PDT due to its propensity for metastases. Nevertheless, in the case PDT is not applicable for tumors localized in difficult anatomical areas, FDAP should be performed to guide the surgical procedure.

Results of early clinical studies on PDT in epithelial skin tumors (Tables 26A–26F) should be evaluated critically due to methodological shortcomings of many studies. Histological examination demonstrated tumor tissue in a large proportion of tumors despite clinical regression after a single PDT cycle, and tumor recurrence was common after long term follow-up (Fritsch et al, 1998). In conclusion, the follow-up periods in most of these studies were too short.

In general, we strongly recommend to perform histopathological examination prior to any PDT session to confirm the clinical diagnosis and to prevent nonoptimum therapy due to failure in diagnosis (e.g., pigmented BCC vs. malignant melanoma, BCC vs. psoriatic lesions, etc.). In summary, ALA-PDT is highly efficient in the treatment of epithelial skin tumors with excellent cosmetic results superior to cryosurgery or surgery. In dermatology, the systemic use of ALA is rarely performed. In order to achieve a homogeneous porphyrin accumulation in deeper tumor tissues after oral ALA administration (Peng et al, 1995) as compared to topical ALA application, further clinical studies should focus on the efficacy of systemic ALA-PDT.

The use of ALA-PDT in **psoriasis lesions** is of great interest. However, various problems are limiting its practicability, such as light treatment of disseminated lesions, an expected high degree of burning pain using light doses higher than 30 J/cm$^2$, and the provocation of Koebner phenomenon (Fig. 220) (Stender et al, 1996). The most important question is if ALA-PDT will prove superior to established schedules in psoriasis treatment such as the use of topical psoralen-containing cream combined with UVA irradiation (cream-PUVA) or topical calcipotriol combined with narrow band UVB (311 nm) irradiation. Open questions are the total number of treatments necessary to achieve a CR and the duration of the disease-free interval after a successful PDT. At present, the treatment of psoriasis with PDT remains an experimental modality.

Concerning **verrucae vulgares** or **plantares**, it is premature to draw final conclusions. The published results are contradictory. In our experience, the treatment is accompanied by extreme pain and exhibits low efficacy. Pretreatment with salicylic acid containing tapes and mechanical removal of most of the wart is essential to achieve a remission with PDT. Viral warts are a common unsolved problem in dermatological clinics and we are skeptical that ALA-PDT will contribute to its solution. Modified route of administration of the photosensitizer, e.g., intralesional injection, or the combination with virustatic or immunomodulatory drugs may increase the response of warts to ALA-PDT.

**Condylomata acuminata** are amendable to treatment by topical imiquimod (5% cream) if the lesions are flat. In large papillomas electrocaustic surgery is very fast and effective, so that ALA-PDT seems to be of minor relevance in this disease. However, FDAP can be performed to optimize the detection of all lesions and to guide the treatment.

**Acne** is another dermatological disease of present interest in ALA-PDT research. Although many therapeutic strategies are available for acne treatment, the efficacy of ALA-PDT should be investigated, since the selective destruction of the propionibacteria, which play an important role in the pathogenesis of acne, can be achieved by ALA-PDT. Due to the proven antimicrobial effect of ALA-PDT (Zeina et al, 2001), skin diseases such as folliculitis might represent further indications for PDT.

The treatment of **hypertrichosis** by ALA-PDT is limited by the fact that many patients exhibit at least skin type III. Thus, PDT applied with the needed energy could frequently induce severe hyperpigmentation. Studies, which showed reduced hair regrowth in areas irradiated with 200 J/cm$^2$ should be critically evaluated because a thermal effect cannot be excluded.

**Atopic eczema** may also respond to ALA-PDT in analogy to the effect of high dose UVA1 treatment. The mechanism of UVA action in the treatment of atopic eczema is still not fully understood.

Successful phototherapy of atopic dermatitis was found to result from UVA radiation-induced apoptosis in skin-infiltrating T helper cells, leading to T cell depletion from eczematous skin (Morita et al, 1997). It is postulated that a selective accumulation of endogenous porphyrins in the lesions might be partly responsible for the efficacy of high dose UVA1 in atopic eczema. However, we could not verify this hypothesis by biochemical analyses (data not shown).

## J.3 Safety and Tolerability of ALA-PDT

*Contraindications for ALA-PDT*: Patients with cutaneous photosensitivity, porphyrias, or with other concomitant disorders, which are provoked or aggravated by UV-light, should be evaluated cautiously for PDT. In addition, allergies to porphyrins (which were not yet described), ALA or to any of the components of the formulation used are contraindications for PDT.

*Topical application of ALA* followed by light irradiation is a well tolerated procedure and adverse events are generally mild to moderate, localized and transient. Because systemic absorption of ALA after topical application is negligible (Figs. 20–23) (Fritsch et al, 1996), adverse effects are generally confined to the area of skin (lesion) treated.

*After topical ALA-treatment*: Following the topical application of ALA, the treated site will become photosensitive. Patients should be advised to avoid exposure of the treatment sites to sunlight or bright indoor light (e.g., examination lamps, theater lamps, tanning beds). Exposure may result in a stinging and burning sensation and may cause erythema and/or edema of the lesions. For patients, who only undergo fluorescence diagnosis, light exposed lesions have to be covered for 24 h after FDAP, (Fig. 72) to avoid any phototoxic reaction (Fritsch et al, 2000). Long-lasting generalized cutaneous photosensitivity is experienced in ALA-PDT even if ALA is applied systemically for FDAP or PDT. However, local cutaneous photosensitivity after topical PDT should not be underestimated. The potential of phototoxic reactions is usually of short duration and does not require any protective measures. Sunscreens will not effectively protect against photosensitivity reactions caused by visible light. Allergic contact dermatitis after exposure to a gel formulation and a dye laser (635 nm) was reported (Gniazdowska et al, 1998).

*During irradiation*: In contrast to many conventional therapeutic modalities directed against cancer, PDT has comparatively few and transient side effects. During light exposure, the patients may experience burning pain, stinging, or itching restricted to the illuminated area (Fritsch et al, 1998; Fritsch et al, 1997, Fritsch et al, 1996). The discomfort peaks within the first minutes of irradiation and may occasionally continue for several hours with decreasing intensity. Temperature monitoring studies have shown that skin tumors reach temperatures of between 39.5 and 42.5°C during ALA-PDT (Orenstein et al, 1995). The temperature in non-ALA-treated irradiated skin on the forehead was even 2 to 4°C higher. However, pain was associated only with the tumors, suggesting that stinging and/or burning during ALA-PDT is the result of the photochemical process, rather than hyperthermia. There is evidence that the severity of these effects of heat and pain is related to the wavelength of applied light and that shorter wavelengths (green instead of red light) cause less pain (Fig. 231–236) (Tables 23 and 24) (Fritsch et al, 1997). The discomfort is similar to that reported in patients suffering from erythropoietic protoporphyria exposed to sunlight and the reason for what is only partially understood. Most likely explanations refer to nerve stimulation and/or tissue damage by reactive oxygen species (Fig. 230). Local anesthesia or intensive cooling help to control the pain, especially when disseminated or large, ulcerative, or inflamed areas are treated. Generally, topical ALA-PDT of skin lesions such as disseminated SK, superficial BCC or SCC does not require analgesics. Erythema and mild edema of the treated area are common adverse effects occurring subsequent to illumination and may be treated by mild corticosteroid creams.

*After PDT*: All patients (100%) treated by ALA-PDT reported some degree of stinging and/or burning during and within 24 hours after PDT, compared to about 50% of vehicle-treated patients (Omrod and Jarvis, 2000). The complaints reached a plateau about 6 minutes after initiation of light treatment and subsided between 1 minute and 24 hours after end of irradiation. The normal course of clinical response to PDT usually comprises crusting, scaling, pruritus and healing within 1 to 4 weeks, depending on the extent and histopathologic features of the lesion (Fritsch et al, 1997). Urea (3%)-containing creams can be applied to remove dry crusts and accelerate re-epithelization. Pustules, dysesthesia, and excoriation may also occur. The cosmetic results of PDT are very good and often superior to cryosurgery, surgery or topical chemotherapy. Generally, scar formation is minimal or absent. A cosmetic disadvantage (10 to 30% of cases) is residual hyperpigmentation or hypopigmentation of the treated area.

The side effects associated with the *systemic administration of ALA* are more serious as compared to topical application of the substance and may include transient liver function abnormalities (Fig. 15), nausea and vomiting (Regula et al, 1995; Hermann et al, 1998). In a study on the treatment of Barrett's metaplasia additional side effects included malaise, headache, photosensitivity and alopecia occured. Fewer side effects and less hepatic toxicity were seen with 30 mg/kg b.w. (Ackroyed et al, 2000) or 10 to 20 mg/kg b.w. (Stummer et al, 1998) than with 50 mg/kg b.w. ALA. The mentioned symptoms are dependent on the total ALA amount administered and might be caused by increased ALA levels in serum and in liver tissue which are partly long-standing (Fritsch et al, 1997).

Among the photosensitizing (pro)drugs, ALA is the compound most widely applied. ALA esters, in particular ALA methylester, exhibit a high efficacy in PDT with a higher selectivity than free ALA. Systemically used porphyrin products, such as Photofrin or Photosan stimulated less interest in dermatological research during the last years. The major reason might be the easy use of ALA-PDT causing less cutaneous photosensitivity. However, it should be stated that for certain skin disorders, e.g., nodular BCC, the systemic administration of porphyrin products should prove more efficient than the topical application. Thus, although dermatologists generally prefer topical treatment, systemic ALA administration should be increasingly focused at in future investigations. Side effects such as nausea, circulatory disturbances and a transient rise of liver enzymes are closely correlated with the total amount of ALA administered. According to our experience the use of systemic ALA in doses up to 20 mg/kg b.w. is generally not linked to serious hemodynamic or other systemic effects.

Although ALA caused dose-dependent genotoxicity in cell culture, DNA damage was not detected in biopsies from patients receiving the clinically relevant systemic dose of 20 mg/kg.

An increase in the expression of the (proto)oncogenes c-myc and bcl-2 was measured following the exposure of transformed human fibroblasts to ALA and light (Verwanger et al, 1998). However, the over-expression was transient and not considered to represent a mutagenic risk.

## J.4 Regulatory Affairs Concernig Aminolevulinic Acid

The FDA announced the approval for the new drug application of ALA in December 1999. ALA hydrochloride is marketed by DUSA Pharmaceuticals (Inc. of Valhalla, NY) under the trade name Levulan® Kerastick™ (20% ALA hydrochloride for topical solution). The indication for Levulan® is the treatment of SK on the scalp and face. Levulan® is marketed in combination with blue light irradiation (Marcus et al, 1996). The German company Schering AG (Berlin) is presently trying to obtain the international rights to distribute this product. Levulan® Kerastick™ was planed to be available on the international market in 2002. There were also attempts to register the use of the product in combination with other light sources than blue light (such as red or green light) with proven efficacy in PDT procedures.

The German company medac GmbH (Wedel) is offering an ALA product for the diagnosis of bladder cancer and cerebral cancer. Developments are in progress to introduce this product also for the detection of cutaneous neoplasms and for the therapy of skin cancers, other skin diseases or psoriasis arthritis.

## J.5 Regulatory Affairs Concerning Aminolevulinic Acid Methylester

Photocure ASA (Oslo, Norway) is the company which has performed most preclinical and clinical studies in the field of dermatology concerning topical PDT in the last 4 years. The company's product Metvix® includes an oil in water formulation of ALA methylester. Photocure has applied for marketing authorisation of Metvix® in Scandinavian countries such as Sweden and Norway. Golderma (Freiburg, Germany) is responsible for the distribution of Metvix® in the rest of Europe. Phase III clinical studies of Metvix® for SK have been finalized in Europe, USA and Australia and are ongoing for high-risk BCC and primary BCC.

# K  Conclusion

The delineation of tumor borders, particularly in anatomically difficult sites such as the face, is a frequent problem in clinical routine. Multiple surgical procedures may be necessary for complete tumor removal. FDAP is a very effective method to detect neoplastic tissue in pretreated and sunlight-damaged skin and to demarcate clinically ill-defined tumor tissue. Therefore, FDAP can be recommended as a useful and easy technique to visualize and detect the size and extension of a certain tumor preoperatively. Similarly to urology, where FDAP is already used in various urological clinics as a routine technique for the detection of bladder cancers, this useful tool is now introduced into dermatology. FDAP should not be seen as an equivalent to histological examination that defines the malignancy or classification of skin tumors. The main advantage of FDAP is the identification of the borders between tumor and normal skin, thus improving the planning of further therapeutic strategies. Depending on the results of FDAP it can be decided whether a certain lesion should be treated by surgical excision, cryosurgery, $CO_2$-laser therapy, PDT or radiotherapy. Beyond this, FDAP can be used to detect post-operatively (or after any other tumor therapy) if any tumor tissue is remaining or regressing. The guidance of surgery, cryosurgery or PDT by FDAP represents an improvement in tumor therapy and follow up.

ALA-PDT is very effective to cure SK, small superficial BCC and SCC. Topical ALA-PDT is noninvasive and exhibits excellent cosmetic results. Most SK can be effectively treated by a single or two PDT sessions, performed after a healing phase of 1 to 4 weeks. The response of SK to PDT leads to cure rates similar to those achieved by the use of liquid nitrogen and chemical peels. PDT is less efficient in more deeply localized tumor parts due to the limited photophysical properties of PDT, the limited permeability for ALA due to overlying normal skin, and encapsulated tumor cell islands impermeable to ALA. Thus, re-treatment within 1–2 weeks is useful before normal skin will cover possible tumor remnants in deep tissue layers. Debulking of the superficial exophytic tumor parts prior to ALA application is mandatory to optimize FDAP / PDT efficacy especially in nodular tumors.

Future progress will be achieved with the development of more effective light sources and the development of new compounds such as esterified ALA derivatives. Dermatologists should not hesitate to perform research into the systemic administration of ALA, which may further enhance the efficacy of FDAP and PDT.

## L  Summary

The therapeutic concept of photodynamic therapy (PDT) with topically applied δ-aminolevulinic acid (ALA) relates to endogenously formed porphyrins which are acting as photosensitizers. Topical application of ALA induces porphyrin biosynthesis preferentially in tumors. Irradiation of porphyrin-enriched tumor tissue induces necrosis by formation of reactive oxygen species. Intratumoral accumulated porphyrins can be visualized by exciting their fluorescence under Wood's light irradiation (= UVA + visible light), which is used for fluorescence diagnosis with ALA-induced porphyrins (FDAP). In the present studies ALA-induced porphyrin synthesis was measured in cells, in organ culture systems and *in vivo*. The efficacy of FDAP and PDT was evaluated for several cutaneous diseases.

Cells incubated with 1 mM ALA synthesized high amounts of porphyrins (cell lines derived from malignant tissue more than those from normal skin). The major porphyrin metabolite was protoporphyrin IX. *Ex vivo*-incubation of human tumor tissues with 1 mM ALA resulted in an increased porphyrin formation in tumors as compared to surrounding normal tissue.

Biochemical analysis of human skin cancers, psoriasis lesions and normal skin revealed optimum ratios of porphyrin levels lesion/skin in basal cell carcinomas (BCC) and squamous cell carcinomas (SCC) 2–4 h after and in psoriasis lesions 6 h after topical application of 20% ALA ointment. ALA methylester led to a more selective porphyrin accumulation in solar keratoses (SK) as compared to free ALA.

Topically applied ALA did not induce any systemic side effects or increases of ALA or porphyrin levels in blood or urine. In contrast, orally administered ALA led to an early peak (4–6 hours) of ALA and porphyrin levels in plasma and red blood cells and, in addition, a delayed increase of porphyrins in urine (24–48 hours). Animal experiments proved that intravenously injected ALA caused long-lasting accumulation of porphyrins in liver tissue.

FDAP (topical application of 20% ALA ointment, application time of 4–6 hours and irradiation with Wood's light) was performed in several benign and malignant skin diseases. High fluorescence yields were measured in BCC, SCC, Bowen's disease (BD), SK and also in psoriasis lesions. In addition, plaques of mycosis fungoides, lesions of lupus erythematosus and extramammary Paget's disease did show a bright fluorescence in FDAP.

Performing FDAP preoperatively in BCC, SCC and BD improved the precise detection and delineation of tumor margins. Histopathological studies underlined that the macroscopically visible fluorescence area in FDAP corresponds with the extension of the tumor. FDAP was effectively used in guiding any type of tumor therapy and controlling the success of surgery, cryosurgery, $CO_2$-laser therapy or PDT.

PDT was shown to be highly effective for the treatment of cutaneous precanceroses and cancers. Up to 100% of SK and superficial BCC responded to topical ALA-PDT (maximum 3 sessions). BD and nodular BCC also showed high complete response rates (80–95%; 3 sessions). It was found that a pretreatment of nodular lesions by curettage of the exophytic tumor mass was necessary to achieve satisfactory results. The BCC of the sclerodermiform type showed a limited response to PDT (75%; maximum 3 sessions). Interestingly, also psoriasis lesions were cured with topical ALA-PDT (maximum 10 sessions).

The optimum concentrations of the prodrug ALA in FDAP or PDT were 20% for BCC, SCC and BD, 10% for SK and 1% for psoriasis lesions. Efficacy and side effects (burning pain during irradiation) in PDT were dependent on the amount of ALA applied and the type of light used. Pain was significantly lower using green instead of red light for irradiation. Optimum PDT efficacy was achieved with green light (SK, SCC, and superficial BCC) and red light (in part nodular BCC and BD).

The presented data clearly show that topical ALA-PDT is not longer an eperimental technique in the treatment of cutaneous diseases. In contrast, FDAP and ALA-PDT are presently included as a routine techniques in dermatological clinics.

# Acknowledgements

For their assistance with this project we would like to thank Dr. Kerstin Lang and Dr. Zuzana Horska for guidance, enthusiasm and support, and Prof. Dr. Helmut Sies for giving the opportunity to work in his laboratory. We also thank Prof. Wilhelm Stahl for his expertise and for many fruitful discussions. Many thanks to the research and technical staff of both the Department of Dermatology and the Institute for Physiological Chemistry I, namely Klaus Bolsen, PD Dr. Günter Michel, Dr. Klaus Werner Schulte, Prof. Dr. Percy Lehmann, PD Dr. Lars Oliver Klotz, Dr. Christine Gärtner, PD Dr. Karlies Briviba and Peter Graf for their generous information and time. We thank Mr. Wilfried Neuse, Diplom Fotodesigner, for his help preparing the high-quality color photographs. Clemens Fritsch would like to cordialy acknowledge Kerstin, Patrick, and his mother, father and brothers supporting every single step of this work.

# Bibliography

Abels C, Heil P, Dellian M, Kuhnle GEH, Baumgartner R, Goetz AE (1994): In vivo kinetic and spectra of 5-aminolevulinic acid induced fluorescence in an amelanotic melanoma of the hamster. Br J Cancer 70: 826–833

Ackroyd R, Brown NJ, Davis MF Stephenson TJ, Marcus SL, Stoddard CJ, Johnson AG, Reed MW (2000): Photodynamic therapy for dysplastic Barrett's oesophagus: A prospective, double blind, randomised, placebo controlled trial. Gut 47: 612–617

Agarwal R, Athar M, Elmets C, Bickers DR, Mukthar H (1992): Photodynamic therapy of chemically- and ultraviolet B radiation-induced murine skin papillomas by chloroaluminium phthalocyanine tetrasulfonate. Photochem Photobiol 56: 43–50

Allen RP, Kessel D, tharratt RS, Volz W (1992): Photodynamic therapy of superficial malignancies with Npe6 in man. Elsevier Science Publishers: Photodynamic therapy and biomedical lasers 441–445

Allison R, Mang T, Hewson G, Snider W, Dougherty D (2001): Photodynamic therapy for chest wall progression from breast carcinoma is an underutilized treatment modality. Cancer 91: 1–8

Ammann R, Hunziker T, Braathen LR (1995): Topical photodynamic therapy in verrucae. A pilot study. Dermatology 191: 346–347

Ammann R, Hunziker T (1995): Photodynamic therapy for mycosis fungoides after topical photosensitization with 5-aminolevulinic acid. J Am Acad Dermatol 33: 541

Anderson CY, Freye Kötubesing KA, Li Y-S, Kenney ME, Mukthar H, Elmets CA (1998): A comparative analysis of silicon phthalocyanine photosensitizers for in vivo photodynamic therapy of RIF-1 tumor in C3H mice. Photochem Photobiol 67: 332–336

Balasubramanian S, Elangovan V, Govindasamy S (1995): Fluorescence spectroscopic identification of 7,12-dimethylbenz[a]anthracene-induced hamster buccal pouch carcinogenesis. Carcinogenesis 16: 2461–2465

Basset-Seguin N, Bachmann I, Pavel S et al (2000) : A dose-finding study of photodynamic therapy (PDT) with Metvix® in patients with basal cell carcinoma (BCC). European Academy of Dermatology and venerology/EADV 14 (Suppl 1), 39

Baumgartner R, Fuchs N, Jocham D, Stepp H, Unsöld E (1992): Pharmacokinetics of fluorescent polyporphyrin Photofrin II in normal rat tissue and rat bladder tumor. Photochem Photobiol 55: 569–74

Baumgartner R, Huber RM, Schulz H, Stepp H, Rick K, Gamarra F, Leberig A, Roth C (1996): Inhalation of 5-aminolevulinic acid: A new technique for fluorescence detection of early stage lung cancer. J Photochem Photobiol B 36: 169–174

Becker-Wegerich PM, Fritsch C, Schulte KW, Neuse W, Lehmann P, Ruzicka T, Goerz G (1998): Carbon dioxide laser treatment of extramammary Paget's disease guided by photodynamic diagnosis. Br J Dermatol 138: 169–172

Ben-Hur E, Rosenthal I (1985): The phthalocyanines: A new class of mammalian photosensitizers with potential for cancer phototherapy. Int J Radiat Biol 47: 145–147

Bernstein ZP, Wilson BD, Oseroff AR, Jones CM, Dozier SE, Brooks JS, Cheney R, Foulke L, Mang TS, Bellnier DA, Dougherty TJ (1999): Photofrin photodynamic therapy for treatment of AIDS-related cutaneous Kaposi's sarcoma. AIDS 13: 1697–1704

Beutner KR, Geisse JK, Helman D, Fox TL, Ginkel A, Owens ML (1999): Therapeutic response of basal cell carcinoma to the immune response modifier imiquimod 5 % cream. J Am Acad Dermatol 41: 1002–1007

Bickers DR, Keogh L, Rifkind AB, Harber LC, Kappas A (1977): Studies in porphyria. VI. Biosynthesis of porphyrins in mammalian skin and in the skin of porphyric patients. J Invest Dermatol 68: 5–9

Bissonnette R, Lui H (1997): Current status of photodynamic therapy in dermatology. Dermatol Clin 15: 507–519

Bjerring P, Funk J, Roed-Petersen J, Söderberg U (June 2001): A randomized double blind study comparing photodynamic therapy (PDT) with Metvix® to PDT with placebo cream in actinic keratosis. Presented at the Nordic dermatology meeting, Gothenburg

Bloomer JR, Brenner DA, Mahoney MJ (1997): Study of factors causing excess protoporphyrin accumulation in cultured skin fibroblasts from patients with protoporphyria. J Clin Invest 60: 1354–1361

Boehncke WH, Elshorst-Schmidt T, Kaufmann R (2000): Systemic photodynamic therapy is a safe and effective treatment for psoriasis. Arch Dermatol 136: 271–2

Boehncke WH, Sterry W, Kaufmann R (1994): Treatment of psoriasis by topical photodynamic therapy with polychromatic light. Lancet 343: 801

Bolsen K, Lang K, Verwohlt B, Fritsch C, Goerz G (1996): In vitro induction of porphyrin biosynthesis in various human cells after incubation with d-aminolevulinic acid. Arch Dermatol Res 288: 320A

Braathen L, Paredes B, Fröhlich K et al (2000): A dose-finding study of photodynamic therapy (PDT) with Metvix® in actinic keratoses (AK). European Academy of Dermatology and Venerology/EADV 14 (Suppl 1), 38

Braichotte D, Savary JF, Glanzmann T, Westermann P, Folli S, Wagnieres G, Monnier P, Van den Bergh H (1995): Clinical pharmacokinetic studies of tetra(meta-hydroxyphenyl)chlorin in squamous cell carcinoma by fluorescence spectroscopy at 2 wavelengths. Int J Cancer 63: 198–204

# Bibliography

Braun-Falco O, Plewig G, Wolff HH, Burgdorf W (2000): Dermatology. Springer

Bruls WA, Slaper H, Van der Leun JC, Berrens L (1984): Transmission of human epidermis and stratum corneum as a function of thickness in the ultraviolet and visible wavelengths. Photochem Photobiol 40: 485–494

Buchanan RB, Carruth JAS, McKenzie AL, Williams SR (1989): Photodynamic therapy in the treatment of malignant tumours of the skin and head and neck. Eur J Surg Oncol 15: 400–406

Buchczyk DP, Klotz LO, Lang K, Fritsch C, Sies S (2001): High efficiency of 5-aminolevulinate-photodynamic treatment using UVA-irradiation. Carcinogenesis 22: 879–883

Cairnduff F, Stringer MR, Hudson EJ, Ash DV, Brown SB (1994): Superficial photodynamic therapy with topical 5-aminolevulinic acid for superficial primary and secondary skin cancer. Br J Cancer 69: 605–608

Calzavara-Pinton PG (1995): Repetitive photodynamic therapy with topical d-aminolaevulinic acid as an appropriate approach to the routine treatment of superficial non-melanoma skin tumours. J Photochem Photobiol B: Biol 29: 53–57

Canti G, Franco P, Marelli O, Cubeddu R, Taroni P, Ramponi R (1990): Comparative study of the therapeutic effect of photoactivated hematoporphyrin derivative and aluminium disulfonated phthalocyanines on tumor bearing mice. Cancer Lett 53: 123–127

Dalton JT, Meyer MC, Golub AL (1999): Pharmacokinetics of aminolevulinic acid after oral and intravenous administration in dogs. Drug Metab Dispos 27: 432–435

Dellian M, Abels C, Kuhnle GE, Goetz AE (1995): Effects of photodynamic therapy on leucocyte-endothelium interaction: Differences between normal and tumour tissue. Br J Cancer 72: 1125–1130

Dietel W, Bolsen K, Dickson E, Fritsch C, Pottier R, Wendenburg R (1996): Formation of water-soluble porphyrins and protoporphyrin IX in 5-aminolevulinic-acid-incubated carcinoma cells. J Photochem Photobiol B 33: 225–231

Diwu Z, Lown W (1994): Phototherapeutic potential of alternative photosensitizers to porphyrins. Pharmacol Ther 63: 1–35

Doiron DR, Keller GS (1986): Porphyrin photodynamic therapy: Principles and clinical applications. Curr Probl Dermatol 15: 85–93

Doiron DR, Profio E, Vincent RG, Dougerthy TJ (1979): Fluorescence bronchoscopy for detection of lung cancer. Chest 76: 27–32

Dougherty TJ, Gomer CJ, Henderson BW, Jori G, Kessel D, Korbelik M, Moan J, Peng G (1998): Photodynamic therapy. J Natl Cancer Inst 90: 889–905

Dougherty TJ (1981): Photoradiation therapy for cutaneous and subcutaneous malignancies. J Invest Dermatol 77: 122–124

Driver I, Lowdell CP, Ash DV (1991): In vivo measurement of the optical interaction coefficients of human tumours at 630 nm. Phys Med Biol 36: 805–813

Endlicher E, Knuchel R, Furst A, Scholmerich J, Messmann H (2001): Endoscopic fluorescence diagnosis of esophageal carcinoma after sensitization with 5-aminolevulinic acid. Med Klin 96: 157–160

Evensen JF (1985): Distribution of tetraphenylporphine sulphonate in mice bearing Lewis lung carcinoma. In: JORI G, PERRIA C (editors). Photodynamic therapy of tumors and other diseases. Padova: Libreria Progetto: 215–218

Evensen JF (1995): The use of porphyrins and non-ionizing radiation for treatment of cancer. Acta Oncol 8: 1103–1110

Fehr MK, Chapman CF, Krasieva T, Tromberg BJ, Mccullough JL, Berns MW, Tadir Y (1996): Selective photosensitizer distribution in vulvar condyloma acuminatum after topical application of 5-aminolevulinic acid. Am J Obstet Gynecol 174: 951–957

Fehr MK, Hornung R, Sschwarz VA, Simeon R, Haller U, Wyss P (2001): Photodynamic therapy of vulvar intraepithelial neoplasia III using topically applied 5-aminolevulinic acid. Gynecol Oncol 80: 62–66

Feyh J, Gutmann R, Leunig A (1993): Die photodynamische Lasertherapie im Bereich der Hals-, Nasen-, Ohrenheilkunde. Laryngorhinootologie 72: 273–278

Figge FHJ, Weiland GS, Manganiello LOJ (1948): Cancer detection and therapy: Affinity of neoplastic, embryotic, and traumatized tissues for porphyrins and metalloporphyrins. Proc Soc Exp Biol Med 68: 640–641

Fijan S, Hönigsmann H, Ortel B (1995): Photodynamic therapy of epithelial skin tumours using delta-aminolaevulinic acid and desferrioxamine. Br J Dermatol 133: 282–288

Fink-Puches R, Soyer HP, Hofer A, Kerl H, Wolf P (1998): Long-term follow-up and histological changes of superficial nonmelanoma skin cancers treated with topical delta-aminolevulinic acid photodynamic therapy. Arch Dermatol 134: 821–826

Fink-Puches R, Wolf P, Kerl H (1997): Photodynamic therapy of superficial basal cell carcinoma by instillation of aminolevulinic acid and irradiation with visible light. Arch Dermatol 133: 1494–1495

Foley P, Freeman M, Vinclullo C, Spelman L, Murell D, Weightman D, Anderson C, Raid C, Watson A, Fergin P (May 2001): A comparison of photodynamic therapy using Metvix® with cryotherapy in actinic keratosis. Presented at the Australasian annual scientific meeting in Adelaide

Frank RG, Bos JD (1996): Photodynamic therapy for condylomata acuminata with local application of 5-aminolevulinic acid. Genitourin Med 72: 70–71

Fraizer CC (1996): Photodynamic therapy in dermatolgy. Int J Dermatol 35: 312–316

Fritsch C, Abels C, Goetz AE, Stahl W, Bolsen K, Ruzicka T, Goerz G, Sies H (1997): Porphyrins preferentially accumulate in a melanoma following intravenous injection of 5-aminolevulinic acid. Biol Chem 378: 51–57

Fritsch C, Batz J, Bolsen K, Schulte KW, Zumdick M, Ruzicka T, Goerz G (1997): Ex vivo application of ALA induces high and specific porphyrin levels in human skin tumors. Possible basis for selective photodynamic therapy. Photochem Photobiol 66: 114–118

Fritsch C, Becker-Wegerich PM, Menke H, Ruzicka T, Goerz G, Olbrisch RR (1997): Successful surgery of multiple recurrent basal cell carcinomas guided by photodynamic diagnosis. Aesthetic Plast Surg 21: 437–439

Fritsch C, Becker-Wegerich PM, Schulte KW, Lehmann P, Ruzicka T, Goerz G (1996): Treatment of a large superficial basal cell carcinoma of the breast. Combination of photodynamic therapy and surgery controlled by photodynamic diagnosis. Hautarzt 47: 438–442

Fritsch C, Bolsen K, Ruzicka T, Goerz G (1997): Congenital erythropoietic porphyria. J Am Acad Dermatol 36: 594–610

Fritsch C, Goerz G, Ruzicka T (1998): Photodynamic therapy in dermatology. Arch Dermatol 134: 207–214

Fritsch C, Homey B, Stahl W, Lehmann P, Ruzicka T, Sies H (1998): Preferential relative porphyrin enrichment in solar keratoses upon topical application of delta-aminolevulinic acid methylester. Photochem Photobiol 68: 218–221

Fritsch C, Lang K, Neuse W, Ruzicka T, Lehmann P (1998): Photodynamic diagnosis and therapy in dermatology. Skin Pharmacol Appl Skin Physiol 11: 358–373

Fritsch C, Lehmann P, Bolsen K, Ruzicka T, Goerz G (1994): Photodynamische Diagnostik und Photodynamische Therapie von aktinischen Keratosen. Zeitschr Hautkr H+G 69: 713–716

Fritsch C, Lehmann P, Stahl W, Schulte KW, Blohm E, Lang K, Sies H, Ruzicka T (1999): Optimum porphyrin accumulation in epithelial skin tumours and psoriatic lesions after topical application of delta-aminolaevulinic acid. Br J Cancer 79: 1603–1608

Fritsch C, Neumann NJ, Ruzicka T, Lehmann P (2000): Photodiagnostic test methods III. Fluorescence diagnosis with aminolevulinic acid induced porphyrins. Hautarzt 51: 528–545

Fritsch C, Stege H, Saalmann G, Goerz G, Ruzicka T, Krutmann J (1997): Green light is effective and less painful than red light in photodynamic therapy of facial solar keratoses. Photodermatol Photoimmunol Photomed 13: 181–185

Fritsch C, Verwohlt B, Bolsen K, Ruzicka T, Goerz G (1996): Influence of topical photodynamic therapy with 5-aminolevulinic acid on porphyrin metabolism. Arch Dermatol Res 288: 517–521

Furukawa K, Yamamoto H, Crean DH, Kato H, Mang TS (1996): Localization and treatment of transformed tissues using the photodynamic sensitizer 2--hexyloxyethyl]-2-devinyl pyropheophorbide-a. Lasers Surg Med 18: 157–166

Gahlen J, Pietschmann M, Prosst RL, Herfarth C (2001): Systemic vs local administration of delta-aminolevulinic acid for laparoscopic fluorescence diagnosis of malignant intra-abdominal tumors. Experimental study Surg Endosc 15: 196–199

Garbo GM (1996): Purpurins and benzochlorins as sensitizers for photodynamic therapy. J Photochem Photobiol B Biol 34: 109–116

Gaullier JM, Berg K, Peng Q, Anholt H, Selbo PK, Ma LW, Moan J (1997): Use of 5-aminolevulinic acid esters to improve photodynamic therapy on cells in culture. Cancer Res 57: 1481–1486

Gilson D, Ash D, Driver I, Feather JW, Brown S (1988): Therapeutic ratio of photodynamic therapy in the treatment of superficial tumours of skin and subcutaneous tissue in man. Br J Cancer 58: 665–667

Gniazdowska B, Rueff F, Hillemanns P, Przybilla B (1998): Allergic contact dermatitis from delta-aminolevulinic acid used for photodynamic therapy. Contact dermatitis 38: 348–349

Goerz G, Link-Mannhardt N, Bolsen K, Zumdick M, Fritsch C, Schürer NY (1995): Porphyrin concentrations in various human tissues. Exp Dermatol 4: 218–228

Gomer CJ (1991): Preclinical examination of first and second-generation photosensitizers used in photodynamic therapy. Photochem Photobiol 54: 1093–1107

Gossner L, May A, Sroka R, Stolte M, Hahn EG, Ell C (1999): Photodynamic destruction of high grade dysplasia and early carcinoma of the esophagus after the oral administration of 5-aminolevulinic acid. Cancer 86: 921–928

Grant WE, Hopper C, Macrobert AJ, Speight PM, Bown SG (1993): Photodynamic therapy of oral cancer: Photosensitization with systemic aminolevulinic acid. Lancet 342: 147–148

Gregorie HB, Horger EO, Ward JL, Green JF, Richards T, Robertson HC, Stevenson TB (1968): Hematoporphyrin-derivative fluorescence in malignant neoplasms. Ann Surg 167: 820–828

Grossman M, Wimberly J, Dwyer P, Flotte T, Anderson RR (1995): PDT of hirsutism. Lasers Surg Med 7: 44

Gupta G, Morton CA, Whitehurst C, Moore JV, MacKie RM (1999): Photodynamic therapy with meso-tetra (hydroxyphenyl) chlorin in the topical treatment of Bowen's disease and basal cell carcinoma. Br J Dermatol 141: 385–386

Haddad R, Cohen M, Kaplan O, Greenberg R, Kashtan H (2001): Photodynamic therapy of nasal basal cell carcinoma. Harefuah 140: 25–27

Haller JC, Cairnduff F, Slack G, Schofield J, Whitehurst C, Tunstall R, Brown SB, Roberts DJ (2000): Routine double treatments of superficial basal cell carcinomas using aminolaevulinic acid-based photodynamic therapy. Br J Dermatol 143: 1270–1275

Hanania J, Malik Z (1992): The effect of EDTA and serum on endogenous porphyrin accumulation and photodynamic sensitization of human K562 leukemic cells. Cancer Lett 65: 127–31

Harth Y, Hirshovitz B (1998): Topical photodynamic therapy in basal and squamous cell carcinoma and penile Bowen's disease with 20% aminolevulinic acid, and exposure to red light and infrared light. Harefuah 134: 602–605, 672, 671

Hayata Y, Kato H, Konaka C, Ono J, Matsushima Y, Yoneyama K, Nishimiya K (1982): Fiberoptic bronchoscopic laser photoradiation for tumor localization in lung cancer. Chest 82: 10–14

Hendrich C, Huttmann G, Vispo-Seara JL, Houserek S, Siebert WE (2000): Experimental photodynamic laser therapy for rheumatoid arthritis with a second generation photosensitizer. Knee Surg Sports Traumatol Arthrosc 8: 190–4

Henta T, Itoh Y, Kobayashi M, Ninomiya Y, Ishibashi A (1999): Photodynamic therapy for inoperable vulval Paget's disease using delta-aminolaevulinic acid: Successful management of a large skin lesion. Br J Dermatol 141: 347–349

Herman MA, Webber J, Fromm D, Kessel D (1998): Hemodynamic effects of 5-aminolevulinic acid in humans. J Photochem Photobiol B 43: 61–65

Hillemanns P, Untch M, Dannecker C, Baumgartner R, Stepp H, Diebold J, Weingandt H, Prove F, Korell M (2000): Photodynamic therapy of vulvar intraepithelial neoplasia using 5-aminolevulinic acid. Int J Cancer 85: 649–653

Hillemanns P, Weingandt H, Baumgartner R, Diebold J, Xiang W, Stepp H (2000): Photodetection of cervical intraepithelial neoplasia using 5-aminolevulinic acid-induced porphyrin fluorescence. Cancer 88: 2275–2282

Hongcharu W, Taylor CR, Chang Y, Aghassi D, Suthamjariya K, Anderson RR (2000): Topical ALA-photodynamic therapy for the treatment of acne vulgaris. J Invest Dermatol 115: 183–192

Hua Z, Gibson SL, Foster TH, Hilf R (1995): Effectiveness of delta-aminolevulinic acid-induced protoporphyrin as a photosensitizer for photodynamic therapy in vivo. Cancer Res 55: 1723–31

Hürlimann AF, Hanggi G, Panizzon RG (1998): Photodynamic therapy of superficial basal cell carcinomas using topical 5-aminolevulinic acid in a nanocolloid lotion. Dermatology 197: 248–254

Itoh Y, Henta T, Ninomiya Y, Tajima S, Ishibashi A (2000): Repeated 5-aminolevulinic acid-based photodynamic therapy following electro-curettage for pigmented basal cell carcinoma. J Dermatol 27: 10–15

Itoh Y, Ninomiya Y, Henta T, Tajima S, Ishibashi A (2000): Topical delta-aminolevulinic acid-based photodynamic therapy for Japanese actinic keratoses. J Dermatol 27: 513–518

Jakus S, Edmonds P, Dunton C, King SA (2000): Margin status and excision of cervical intraepithelial neoplasia: A review. Obstet Gynecol Surv 55: 520–527

Jeffes EW, Mccullough JL, Weinstein GD, Kaplan R, Glazer SD, Taylor JR (1997): Photodynamic therapy of actinic keratosis with topical 5-aminolevulinic acid. A pilot dose-ranging study. Arch Dermatol 133: 727–732

Jesionek A, Von Tappeiner H (1905): Zur Behandlung der Hautcarcinome mit fluorescierenden Stoffen. Arch Klin Med 82: 72–76

Jichlinski P, Forrer M, Mizeret J, Glanzmann T, Braichotte D, Wagnieres G, Zimmer G, Guillou L, Schmidlin F, Graber P, Van den Bergh H, Leisinger HJ (1997): Clinical evaluation of a method for detecting superficial surgical transitional cell carcinoma of the bladder by light-induced fluorescence of protoporphyrin IX following the topical application of 5-aminolevulinic acid: Preliminary results. Lasers Surg Med 20: 402–408

Jones BB, Jessop LD, Samowitz WS, Bjorkman DJ (1993): Computer-assisted fluorescence identification of colon cancer in rats. Am J Gastroenterol 88: 1724–1728

Jones CM, Mang T, Cooper M, Wilson BD, Stoll HL (1992): Photodynamic therapy in the treatment of Bowen's disease. J Am Acad Dermatol 27: 979–982

Kalka K, Fritsch C, Bolsen K, Verwohlt B, Goerz G (1997): Influence of indoles (melatonin, serotonin and tryptophan) on the porphyrin metabolism in vitro. Skin Pharmacol 10: 221–224

Kalka K, Fritsch C, Ruzicka T, Goerz G, Eckel J (1998): 5-Aminolevulinic acid accumulates intracellularly mainly by transport mechanism and not via passive diffusion. Acta Haematol Suppl 1: 101

Kappas A, Sassa S, Galbraith RA, Nordman Y (1989): The porphyrias. In: STANBURY JB, WYNGAARDEN JB, FREDRICKSON DS (eds.): The metabolic basis of inherited disease. New York: McGraw-Hill, 1305–1365

Karrer S, Abels C, Landthaler M, Szeimies RM (2000): Topical photodynamic therapy for localized scleroderma. Acta Derm Venerol 80: 26–27

Keller P, Sowinska M, Tassetti V, Heisel F, Hajri A, Evrad S, Miehe JA, Marescaux J, Aprahamian M (1996): Photodynamic imaging of a rat pancreatic cancer with pheophorbide a. Photochem Photobiol 63: 860–867

Kennedy JC, Pottier RH, Pross DC (1990): Photodynamic therapy with endogenous protoporphyrin IX: Basic principles and present clinical experience. J Photochem Photobiol B: Biol 6: 143–148

Kessel D, Smith KM, Pandey RK, Shiau F-Y, Henderson B (1993): Photosensitization with bacteriochlorins. Photochem Photobiol 58: 200–203

Kessel D, Thompson P, Saatio K, Nantwi KD (1987): Tumor localization and photosensitization by sulfonated derivatives of tetraphenylporphine. Photochem Photobiol 45: 787–790

Kessel D, Woodburn K, Henderson BW, Chang CK (1995): Sites of photodamage in vivo and in vitro by a cationic porphyrin. Photochem Photobiol 62: 875–881

Khan SA, Dougherty TJ, Mang TS (1993): An evaluation of photodynamic therapy in the management of cutaneous matastases of breast cancer. Eur J Cancer 29A: 1686–1690

Kick G, Messer G, Goetz A, Plewig G, Kind P (1995): Photodynamic therapy induces expression of interleukin 6 by activation of AP-1 but not NF-kappa B DNA binding. Cancer Res 55: 2373–2379

King EG, Doiron D, Man G, Profio AE, Huth G (1982): Hematoporphyrin derivative as a tumor marker in the detection and localization of pulmonary malignancy. Recent Results Cancer Res 82: 90–96

Kinsey JH, Cortese DA, Sanderson DR (1978): Detection of hematoporphyrin fluorescence during fiberoptic bronchoscopy to localize early bronchogenic carcinoma. Mayo Clin Proc 53: 594–600

Klotz LO, Fritsch C, Briviba K, Tsacmacidis N, Schliess F, Sies H (1998): Activation of JNK and p38 but not ERK MAP kinases in human skin cells by 5-aminolevulinate-photodynamic therapy. Cancer Res 58: 4297–4300

Koenig F, McGovern FJ (1997): Fluorescence detection of bladder carcinoma. Urology 50: 778–779

Kreimeier-Birnbaum M (1989): Modified porphyrins, chlorins, phthalocyanines and purpurins: Second-generation photosensitizers for photodynamic therapy. Semin Hematol 26: 157–173

Kriegmair M, Baumgartner R, Knuchel R, Ehsan A, Steinbach P, Lumper W, Hofstädter F, Hofstetter A (1994): Photodynamic diagnosis of urothelial neoplasms after intravesicular instillation of 5-aminolevulinic acid. Urologe A 33: 270–275

Kriegmair M, Baumgartner R, Knuchel R, Steinbach P, Ehsan A, Lumper W, Hofstadter F, Hofstetter A (1994): Fluorescence photodetection of neoplastic urothelial lesions following intravesical instillation of 5-aminolevulinic acid. Urology 44: 836–841

Kriegmair M, Stepp H, Steinbach P, Lumper W, Ehsan A, Stepp HG, Rick K, Knuchel R, Baumgartner R, Hofstetter A (1995): Fluorescence cystoscopy following intravesical instillation of 5-aminolevulinic acid: A new procedure with high sensitivity for detection of hardly visible urothelial neoplasias. Urol Int 55: 190–196

Kriegmair M, Zaak D, Knuechel R, Baumgartner R, Hofstetter A (1999): Photodynamic cystoscopy for detection of bladder tumors. Semin Laparosc Surg 6: 100–103

Kubler A, Haase T, Kremer P, Rheinwald M, Kunze S, Muhling J (1999): An argon-dye laser system for photodynamic therapy and diagnosis. Neurol Res 21: 103–107

Kubler A, Haase T, Rheinwald M, Barth T, Muhling J (1998): Treatment of oral leukoplakia by topical application of 5-aminolevulinic acid. Int J Oral maxillofac Surg 27: 466–469

Kubler AC, Haase T, Staff C, Kahle B, Rheinwald M, Muhling J (1999): Photodynamic therapy of primary non-melanomatous skin tumours of the head and neck. Lasers Surg Med 25: 60–68

Kurwa HA, Barlow RJ, Neill S (2000) : Single episode photodynamic therapy and vulval intraepithelial neoplasia type III resistant to conventional therapy. Br J Dermatol 143: 1040–1042

Kurwa HA, Yong-Gee SA, Seed PT, Markey AC, Barlow RJ (1999): A randomized paired comparison of photodynamic therapy and topical 5-fluorouracil in the treatment of actinic keratoses. J Am Acad Dermatol 41: 414–418

Kyriazis GA, Balin H, Lipson RL (1973): Hematoporphyrin-derivative-fluorescence test colposcopy and colpophotography in the diagnosis of atypical metaplasia, dysplasia, and carcinoma in situ of the cervix uteri. Am J Obstet Gynecol 117: 375–380

Ladner DP, Steiner RA, Allemann J, Haller U, Walt H (2001): Photodynamic diagnosis of breast tumours after oral application of aminolevulinic acid. Br J Cancer 84: 33–37

Lam S, Macaulay C, Palcic B (1993): Detection and localization of early lung cancer by imaging techniques. Chest 103: 12S–14S

Lambah A, Dixon J: Breast cancer (2000): Detection and management. Practitioner 244: 884–898

Lambert R (2000): Treatment of oesophageogastric tumors. Endoscopy 32: 322–330

Lang K, Lehmann P, Bolsen K, Ruzicka T, Fritsch C (2001): Aminolevulinic acid: Pharmacological profile and clinical indication. Expert Opin Investig Drugs 10: 1139–1156

Lange N, Jichlinski P, Zellweger M, Forrer M, Marti A, Guilou L, Kucera P, Wagnieres G, Van den Bergh H (1999): Photodetection of early human bladder cancer based on the fluorescence of 5-aminolaevulinic acid hexylester-induced protoporphyrin IX: A pilot study. Br J Cancer 80: 185–193

Langer S, Abels C, Botzlar A, Pahernik S, Rick K, Szeimies RM, Goetz AE (1999): Active and higher intracellular uptake of 5-aminolevulinic acid in tumors may be inhibited by glycine. J Invest Dermatol 112: 723–728

Lapes M, Petera J, Jirsa M (1996): Photodynamic therapy of cutaneous metastases of breast cancer after local application of meso-tetra-(para-sulphophenyl)-porphin (TPPS4). J Photochem Photobiol B 36: 205–207

Lehmann P, Scharffetter K, Kind P, Goerz G (1991): Erythropoietic protoporphyria: Synopsis of 20 patients. Hautarzt 42: 570–4

Leunig A, Betz CS, Baumgartner R, Grevers G, Issing WJ (2000): Initial experience in the treatment of oral leukoplakia with high-dose vitamin A and follow-up 5-aminolevulinic acid induced protoporphyrin IX fluorescence. Eur Arch Otorhinolaryngol 257: 327–331

Leunig A, Betz CS, Mehlmann M, Stepp H, Arbogast S, Grevers G, Baumgartner R (2000): Detection of squamous cell carcinoma of the oral cavity by imaging 5-aminolevulinic acid-induced protoporphyrin IX fluorescence. Laryngoscope 110: 78–83

Leunig A, Rick K, Stepp H, Goetz A, Baumgartner R, Feyh J (1996): Photodynamic diagnosis of neoplasms of the mouth cavity after local administration of 5-aminolevulinic acid. Laryngorhinootologie 75: 459–464

Leunig A, Rick K, Stepp H, Gutmann R, Alwin G, Baumgartner R, Feyh J (1996): Fluorescence imaging and spectroscopy of 5-aminolevulinic acid induced protoporphyrin IX for the detection of neoplastic lesions in the oral cavity. Am J Surg 172: 674–677

Lim HW, Behar S, He D (1994): Effect of porphyrin and irradiation on heme biosynthetic pathway in endothelial cells. Photodermatol Photoimmunol Photomed 10: 17–21

Lipson RL, Baldes EJ, Olsen AM (1961): The use of a derivative of hematoporphyrin in tumor detection. J Natl Cancer Inst 26: 1–4

Lowdell CP, Ash DV, Driver I, Brown SB (1993): Interstitial photodynamic therapy. Clinical experience with diffusing fibres in the treatment of cutaneous and subcutaneous tumors. Br J Cancer 67: 1398–1403

Lowry OH, Rosenbrough NJ, Farr AL, Randall RJ (1951): Protein measurement with the folin phenol reagent. J Biol Chem 193: 265–275

Lui H, Anderson RR (1993): Photodynamic therapy in dermatology: Recent developments. Dermatol Clin 11: 1–13

Lui H, Anderson RR (1992): Photodynamic therapy in dermatology: Shedding a different light on skin disease. Arch Dermatol 128: 1631–1636

Lui H, Salasche S, Kollias N, Wimberly J, Flotte T, Mclean D, Anderson RR (1995): Photodynamic therapy of nonmelanoma skin cancer with topical aminolevulinic acid: A clinical and histologic study. Arch Dermatol 131: 737–738

Luna MC, Wong S, Gomer CJ (1994): Photodynamic therapy mediated induction of early response genes. Cancer Res 54: 1374–1380

Magne ML, Rodriguez CO, Autry SA, Edwards BF, Theon AP, Madewell BR (1997): Photodynamic therapy of facial squamous cell carcinoma in cats using a new photosensitizer. Lasers Surg Med 20: 202–209

Malik E, Berg C, Meyhofer-Malik A, Buchweitz O, Moubayed P, Diedrich K (2000): Fluorescence diagnosis of endometriosis using 5-aminolevulinic acid. Surg Endosc 14: 452–455

Malik Z, Kostenich G, Roitman L, Ehrenberg B, Orenstein A (1995): Topical application of 5-aminolevulinic acid, DMSO and EDTA: Protoporphyrin IX in skin and tumours of mice. J Photochem Photobiol B Biol 28: 213–218

Malik Z, Lugaci H (1987): Destruction of erythroleukaemic cells by photoactivation of endogenous porphyrins. Br J Cancer 56: 589–595

Mang TS, Mcginnis C, Liebow C, Nseyo UO, Crean DH, Dougherty TJ (1993): Fluorescence detection of tumors. Early diagnosis of microscopic lesions in preclinical studies. Cancer 71: 269–276

Marcus SL, Sobel RS, Golub AL, Carroll RL, Lundahl S, Shulman DG (1996): Photodynamic therapy (PDT) and photodiagnosis (PD) using endogenous photosensitization induced by 5-aminolevulinic acid (ALA): Current clinical and development status. J Clin Laser Med Surg 14: 59–66

Martin A, Tope DW, Grevelink JM, Starr JC, Fewkes L, Flotte TJ, Deutsch TF, Anderson RR (1995): Lack of selectivity of protoporphyrin IX fluorescence for basal cell carcinoma after topical application of 5-aminolevulinic acid: Implications for photodynamic therapy. Arch Dermatol Res 287: 665–674

Mayinger B, Reh H, Hochberger J, Hahn EG (1999): Endoscopic photodynamic diagnosis: Oral aminolevulinic acid is a marker of GI cancer and dysplastic lesions. Gastrointest Endosc 50: 242–246

Mccaughan JS, Guy JT, Hicks W, Laufmann L, Nims TA, Walker J (1998): Photodynamic therapy for cutaneous malignant neoplasms. Arch Surg 124: 211–216

Mccullough JL, Weinstein GD, Lemus LL, Rampone W, Jenkins JJ (1983): Development of a topical hematoporphyrin derivative formulation: Characterization of photosensitizing effects in vivo. J Invest Dermatol 81: 528–532

Medeiros MH, Di mascio P, Grundel S, Soboll S, Sies H, Bechara EJ (1994): Catabolism of 5-aminolevulinic acid to $CO_2$ by rat liver mitochondria. Arch Biochem Biophys 310: 205–209

Meffert H, Gaunitz K, Gutewort T, Amlong UJ (1990): Therapy of acne with visible light. Decreased irradiation time by using a blue-light high-energy lamp. Dermatol Monatsschr 176: 597–603

Mehlmann M, Betz CS, Stepp H, Arbogast S, Baumgartner R, Grevers G, Leunig A (1999): Fluorescence staining of laryngeal neoplasms after topical application of 5-aminolevulinic acid: Preliminary results. Lasers Surg Med 25: 414–420

Menon IA, Persad SD, Habermann HF (1989): A comparison of the phototoxicity of protoporphyrin, coproporphyrin and uroporphyrin using a cellular system in vitro. Clin Biochem 22: 197–200

Messmann H, Knuchel R, Baumler W, Holstege A, Schlmerich J (1999): Endoscopic fluorescence detection of dysplasia in patients with Barrett's esophagus, ulcerative colitis, or adenomatous polyps after 5-aminolevulinic acid-induced protoporphyrin IX sensitization. Gastrointest Endosc 49: 97–101

Messmann H (2000): 5-Aminolevulinic acid-induced protoporphyrin IX for the detection of gastrointestinal dysplasia. Gastrointest Endosc Clin N Am 10: 497–512

Moan J (1990): Properties for optimal PDT sensitizers. J Photochem Photobiol 5: 521–524

Morgan AR, Garbo GM, Keck RW, Selman SH (1988): New photosensitizers for photodynamic therapy: Combined effect of metallo-purpurin derivatives and light on transplantable tumors. Cancer Res 48: 194–198

Morita A, Werfel T, Stege H, Ahrens C, Karmann K, Grewe M, Grether-Beck S, Ruzicka T, Kapp A, Klotz LO, Sies H, Krutmann J (1997): Evidence that singlet oxygen-induced human T helper cell apoptosis is the basic mechanism of ultraviolet-A radiation phototherapy. J Exp Med 186: 1763–1768

Morton CA, Mackie RM, Whitehurst C, Moore JV, Mccoll JH (1998): Photodynamic therapy for basal cell carcinoma: Effect of tumor thickness and duration of photosensitizer application on response. Arch Dermatol 134: 248–249

Morton CA, Whitehurst C, Mccoll JH, Moore JV, Mackie RM (2001): Photodynamic therapy for large or multiple patches of Bowen disease and basal cell carcinoma. Arch Dermatol 137: 319–324

Morton CA, Whitehurst C, Moore JV, Mackie RM (2000): Comparison of red and green light in the treatment of Bowen's disease by photodynamic therapy. Br J Dermatol 143: 767–772

Morton CA, Whtehurst C, Moseley H, Mccoll JH, Moore JV, Mackie RM (1996): Comparison of photodynamic therapy with cryotherapy in the treatment of Bowen's disease. Br J Dermatol 135: 766–771

Navone NM, Polo CF, Frisardi AL, Andrade NE, Battle AM (1990): Heme biosynthesis in human breast cancer-mimetic "in vitro" studies and some heme enzymic activity levels. Int J Biochem 22: 1407–11

Nelson JS, Roberts WG, Berns MW (1987): In vivo studies on the utilization of mono-L-aspartyl chlorin (Npe6) for photodynamic therapy. Cancer Res 47: 4681–4685

Nilsson H, Johansson J, Svanberg K, Svanberg S, Jori G, Reddi E, Segalla A, Gust D, Moore AL, Moore TA (1994): Laser-induced fluorescence in malignant and normal tissue in mice injected with two different carotenoporphyrins. Br J Cancer 70: 873–879

Ochsner M (1997): Photodynamic therapy: The clinical perspective. Arzneim Forsch Drug Res 47: 1185–1194

Oleinick NL, Antunez AR, Clay ME, Rihter BD, Kenney ME (1993): New phthalocyanine photosensitizers for photodynamic therapy. Photochem Photobiol 57: 242–247

Omrod D, Jarvis B (2000): Topical aminolevulinic acid HCL photodynamic therapy. Am J Clin Dermatol 1: 133–139

Onizawa K, Saginoya H, Furuya Y, Yoshida H (1996): Fluorescence photography as a diagnostic method for oral cancer. Cancer Lett 108: 61–66

Onuki J, Medeiros MH, Bechara EJ, Di Mascio P (1994): 5-Aminolevulinic acid induces single-strand breaks in plasmid pBR322 DNA in the presence of $Fe^{2+}$ ions. Biochim Biophys Acta 1225: 259–263

Orenstein A, Kostenich G, Tsur H, Kogan L, Malik Z (1995): Temperature monitoring during photodynamic therapy of skin tumors with topical 5-aminolevulinic acid application. Cancer Lett 93: 227–232

Ortel B, Tanew A, Honigsmann H (1993): Lethal photosensitization by endogenous porphyrins of PAM cells: Modification by desferrioxamine. J Photochem Photobiol B Biol17: 273–278

Pahernik SA, Botzlar A, Hillemanns P, Dellian M, Kirschstein M, Abels C, Korell M, Mueller-Hoecker J, Untch M, Goetz AE (1998): Pharmacokinetics and selectivity of aminolevulinic acid-induced porphyrin synthesis in patients with cervical intra-epithelial neoplasia. Int J Cancer 78: 310–314

Pass HI (1993): Photodynamic therapy in oncology: Mechanism and clinical use. J Natl Cancer Inst 85: 443–456

Peng Q, Moan J, Warloe T, Iani V, Stehen A (1996): Build-up of esterified aminolevulinic-acid-derivative-induced porphyrin fluorescence in normal mouse skin. J Photochem Photobiol B Biol 34: 95–96

Peng Q, Moan J, Warloe T, Nesland JM, Rimington C (1992): Distribution and photosensitizing efficiency of porphyrins induced by application of exogenous 5-aminolevulinic acid in mice bearing mammary carcinoma. Int J Cancer 52: 433–43

Peng Q, Warloe T, Berg K, Moan J, Kongshaug M, Giercksky KE, Nesland JM (1997): 5-Aminolevulinic acid-based photodynamic therapy: Clinical research and future challenges. Cancer 79: 2282–2308

Peng Q, Warloe T, Moan J, Heyerdahl H, Steen HB, Nesland JM, Giercksky KE (1995): Distribution of 5-aminolevulinic acid-induced porphyrins in noduloulcerative basal cell carcinoma. Photochem Photobiol 62: 906–913

Pennington DG, Waner M, Knox A (1988): Photodynamic therapy for multiple skin cancers. Plast Reconstr Surg 82: 1067–1071

Petrelli NJ, Cebollero JA, Rodriguez-Bigas M, Mang T (1992): Photodynamic therapy in the management of neoplasms of the perianal skin. Arch Surg 127: 1436–1438

Policard A (1924): Etude sur les aspects offerts par des tumeurs expérimentales examinées à la lumière de Wood. C R Soc Biol 91: 1423–1424

Pomer S, Grashev G, Sinn H, Kalble T, Staehler G (1995): Laser-induced fluorescence diagnosis and photodynamic therapy of human renal cell carcinoma. Urol Int 55: 97–201

Popken G, Wetterauer U, Schultze-Seemann W (1999): Kidney-preserving tumour resection in renal cell carcinoma with photodynamic detection by 5-aminolaevulinic acid: Preclinical and preliminary clinical results. BJU Int 83: 578–582

Potter B (1967): Extramammary Paget's disease. Acta Derm Venereol 47: 259–62

Pres H, Meffert H, Sonnichsen N (1989): Photodynamic therapy of psoriasis palmaris et plantaris using a topically applied hematoporphyrin derivative and visible light. Dermatol Monatsschr 175: 745–750

Raab O (1900): Über die Wirkung fluorescierender Stoffe auf Infusoriera. Z Biol 39: 524

Razum NJ, Snyder AB, Doiron DR (1996): SnET2: Clinical update. In: DOUGHERTY TJ (ed.). Optical methods for tumor treatment and detection: Mechanisms and techniques in photodynamic therapy V. Proc SPIE 2675: 43–46

Regula J, Macrobert AJ, Gorchein A, Buonaccorsi GA, Thorpe SM, Spencer GM, Hatfield AR, Bown SG (1995): Photosensitisation and photodynamic therapy of oesophageal, duodenal, and colorectal tumours using 5-aminolaevulinic acid induced protoporphyrin IX – a pilot study. Gut 36: 67–75

Renschler MF, Yuen A, Panella TJ, Wieman TJ, Julius C, Panjepour M (1997): Photodynamic therapy trials with lutetium texaphyrin PCI-0123 (Lu-Tex). Photochem Photobiol 65(Suppl): 475

Reynolds T (1997): Photodynamic therapy expands its horizons. J NatI Cancer Inst 89: 112–114

Richter AM, Waterfield E, Jain AK, Canaan AJ, Allison BA, Levy JG (1993): Liposomal delivery of a photosensitizer, benzoporphyrin derivative monoacid ring A (BPD), to tumor tissue in a mouse tumor model. Photochem Photobiol 57: 1000–1006

Riedl CR, Plas E, Pfluger H (1999): Fluorescence detection of bladder tumors with 5-amino-levulinic acid. J Endourol 13: 755–759

Robinson DJ, Collins P, Stringer MR, Vernon DI Stables GI, Brown SB, Sheehan-Dare RA (1999): Improved response of plaque psoriasis after multiple treatments with topical 5-aminolaevulinic acid photodynamic therapy. Acta Derm Venereol 79: 451–455

Robinson PJ, Carrith JAS, Fairris GM (1988): Photodynamic therapy: A better treatment for widespread Bowen's disease. Br J Dermatol 119: 59–61

Ross EV, Romero R, Kollias N, Crum C, Anderson RR (1997): Selectivity of protoporphyrin IX fluorescence for condylomata after topical application of 5-aminolaevulinic acid: Implications for photodynamic treatment. Br J Dermatol 137: 736–742

Rud E, Gederaas O, Hogset A, Berg K (2000): 5-aminolevulinic acid, but not 5-aminolevulinic acid esters, is transported into adenocarcinoma cells by system BETA transporters. Photochem Photobiol 71: 640–647

Santoro O, Bandieramonte G, Melloni E, Marchesini R, Zunino F, Lepera P, De Palo G (1990): Photodynamic therapy by topical meso-tetraphenylporphinesulfonate tetrasodium salt administration in superficial basal cell carcinomas. Cancer Res 50: 4501–4503

Savary JF, Monnier P, Fontolliet C, Mizeret J, Wagnieres G, Braichotte D, Van den Bergh (1997): Photodynamic therapy for early squamous cell carcinomas of the esophagus, bronchi, and mouth with m-tetra (hydroxyphenyl) chlorin. Arch Otolaryngol Head Neck Surg 123: 162–8

Schweitzer VG, Visscher D (1990): Photodynamic therapy for treatment of AIDS-related oral Kaposi's sarcoma. Otolaryngol Head Neck Surg 102: 639–649

Seubert A, Seubert S (1982): High performance liquid chromatographic analysis of porphyrins and their isomers with radial compression columns. Anal Biochem 124: 303–307

Shanler SD, Wan W, Whitaker JE, Mang TS, Jones C, Wilson BD, Stoll HL, Pincus S, Oseroff AR (1993): Topical d-aminolevulinic acid for photodynamic therapy of cutaneous carcinomas and cutaneous T-cell lymphoma. J Invest Dermatol 101: 406a

Smetana Z, Malik Z, Orenstein A, Mendelson E, Ben-Hur E (1997): Treatment of viral infections with 5-aminolevulinic acid and light. Lasers Surg Med 21: 351–8

Soler AM, Angell-Petersen E, Warloe T, Tausjo J, Steen HB, Moan J, Giercksky KE (2000): Photodynamic therapy of superficial basal cell carcinoma with 5-aminolevulinic acid with dimethylsulfoxide and ethylendiaminetetraacetic acid: A comparison of two light sources. Photochem Photobiol 71: 724–729

Soler AM, Warloe T, Berner A, Gierckscky KE (2001): A follow-up study of recurrence and cosmesis in completely responding superficial and nodular basal cell carcinomas treated with methyl 5-aminolaevulinate-based photodynamic therapy alone and with prior curettage. Br J Dermatol 145: 467–471

Soler AM, Warloe T, Tausjo J, Berner A (1999): photodynamic therapy by topical aminolevulinic acid, dimethylsulphoxide and curettage in nodular basal cell carcinoma: A one-year follow-up study. Acta Derm Venereol 79: 204–206

Soler AM, Warloe T, Tausjo J, Giercksky KE (2000): Photodynamic therapy of residual or recurrent basal cell carcinoma after radiotherapy using topical 5-aminolevulinic acid or methylester aminolevulinic acid. Acta Oncol 39: 605–609

Soret JL (1883): Recherches sur l'absorption des rayons ultra violets par diverses substances. Arch Sci Phys Nat 10: 430–485

Spikes JD (1990): Chlorins as photosensitizers in biology and medicine. J Photochem Photobiol B Biol 6: 259–274

Spikes JD (1986): Phthalocyanines as photosensitizers in biological systems and for the photodynamic therapy of tumors. Photochem Photobiol 43: 691–699

Sroka R, Beyer W, Gossner L, Sassy T, Stocker S, Baumgartner R (1996): Pharmacokinetics of 5-aminolevulinic-acid-induced porphyrin in tumour-bearing mice. J Photochem Photobiol B Biol 34: 13–19

Stables GI, Stringer MR, Ash DV (1995): The treatment of erythroplasia of Queyrat by topical aminolevulinic acid photodynamic therapy. Br J Dermatol 133 (Suppl 45): 30

Stables GI, Stringer MR, Robinson DJ, Ash DV (1997): Large patches of Bowen's disease treated by topical aminolevulinic acid photodynamic therapy. Br J Dermatol 136: 957–960

Stefanidou M, Tosca A, Themelis G, Vazgiouraki E, Balas C (2000): In vivo fluorescence kinetics and photodynamic therapy efficacy of delta-aminolevulinic acid-induced porphyrins in basal cell carcinomas and actinic keratoses; implications for optimization of photodynamic therapy. Eur J Dermatol 10: 351–6

Steinbach P, Kriegmair M, Baumgartner R, Hofstadter F, Knuchel R (1994): Intravesical instillation of 5-aminolevulinic acid: The fluorescent metabolite is limited to urothelial cells. Urology 44: 676–681

Steiner RA, Tromberg BJ, Wyss P, Krasieva T, Chandanani N, Mccullough J, Berns MW, Tadir Y (1995): Rat reproductive performance following photodynamic therapy with topically administered Photofrin Human Reprod 10: 227–233

Stender IM, Na R, Fogh H, Gluud C, Wulf HC (2000): Photodynamic therapy with 5-aminolaevulinic acid or placebo for recalcitrant foot and hand warts: Randomised double-blind trial. Lancet 355: 963–966

Stender IM, Wulf HC (1996): Kobner reaction induced by photodynamic therapy using delta-aminolevulinic acid. A case report. Acta Derm Venereol 76: 392–393

Stender IM, Wulf HC (1996): Photodynamic therapy with 5-aminolevulinic acid in the treatment of actinic cheilitis. Br J Dermatol 135: 454–456

Stringer MR, Collins P, Robinson DJ, Stables GI, Sheehan-Dare RA (1996): The accumulation of protoporphyrin IX in plaque psoriasis after topical application of 5-aminolevulinic acid indicates a potential for photodynamic therapy. J Invest Dermatol 107: 76–81

Stummer W, Novotny A, Stepp H, Goetz C, Bise K, Reulen HJ (2000): Fluorescence-guided resection of glioblastoma multiforme by using 5-aminolevulinic acid-induced porphyrins: A prospective study in 52 consecutive patients. J Neurosurg 93: 1003–1013

Stummer W, Stocker S, Wagner S, Stepp H, Fritsch C, Goetz C, Goetz AE, Kiefmann R, Reulen HJ (1998): Intraoperative detection of malignant gliomas by 5-aminolevulinic acid-induced porphyrin fluorescence. Neurosurgery 42: 518-525; Discussion 525–526

Svanberg K, Anderson T, Killander D, Wang I, Stenram U, Andersson-Engels S, Berg R, Johansson J, Svanberg S (1994): Photodynamic therapy of non-melanoma malignant tumours of the skin using topical d-amino levulinic acid sensitization and laser irradiation. Br J Dermatol 130: 743–751

Szeimies RM, Abels C, Fritsch C, Karrer S, Steinbach P, Bäumler W, Goerz G, Goetz AE, Landthaler M (1995): Wavelength dependency of photodynamic effects after sensitization with 5-aminolevulinic acid in vitro and in vivo. J Invest Dermatol 105: 672–677

Szeimies RM, Karrer S, Sauerwald A, Landthaler M (1996): Photodynamic therapy with topical application of 5-aminolevulinic acid in the treatment of actinic keratoses: An initial clinical study. Dermatology 192: 246–251

Szeimies RM, Sassay M, Landthaler M (1994): Penetration potency of topical applied delta aminolevulinic acid for photodynamic therapy of basal cell carcinoma. Photochem Photobiol 59: 73–76

Taber SW, Fingar VH, Coots CT, Wieman TJ (1998): Photodynamic therapy using mono-L-aspartyl chlorin e[6] (Npe6) for the treatment of cutaneous disease: A phase I clinical study. Clin Cancer Res 4: 2741–2746

Tan WC, Fulljames C, Stone N, Dix AJ, Shepherd N, Roberts DJ, Brown SB, Krasner N, Barr H (1999): Photodynamic therapy using 5-aminolaevulinic acid for oesophageal adenocarcinoma associated with Barrett's metaplasia. J Photochem Photobiol B 53: 75–80

Thissen MR, Schroeter CA, Neumann HA (2000): Photodynamic therapy with delta-aminolaevulinic acid for nodular basal cell carcinomas using a prior debulking technique. Br J Dermatol 142: 338–339

Tierney AC (2000): Laparoscopic radical and partial nephrectomy. World J Urol 18: 249–256

Tope WD, Ross EV, Kollias N, Martin A, Gillies R, Anderson RR (1998): Protoporphyrin IX fluorescence induced in basal cell carcinoma by oral delta-aminolevulinic acid. Photochem Photobiol 67: 249–255

Tschudy DP, Collins A (1957): Reduction of d-aminolevulinic acid dehydratase activity in the livers of tumor-bearing animals. Cancer Res 17: 976–980

Van den Boogert J, Van Hillegersberg R, De Rooij FW, De Rooij FWM, Edixhoven-Bosdijk A, Siersema PD, Van Hillegersberg R (1998): 5-Aminolaevulinic acid-induced protoporphyrin IX accumulation in tissues: Pharmacokinetics after oral or intravenous administration. J Photochem Photobiol B 44: 29–38

Varma S, Wilson H, Kurwa HA, Gambles B, Charman C, Pearse AD, Taylor D, Anstey AV (2001): Bowen's disease, solar keratoses and superficial basal cell carcinomas treated by photodynamic therapy using a large-field incoherent light source. Br J Dermatol 144: 567–574

Verwanger T, Schnitzhofer G, Krammer B (1998): Expression kinetics of the (proto) oncogenes c-myc and bcl-2 following photodynamic treatment of normal and transformed human fibroblasts with 5-aminolaevulinic acid-stimulated endogenous protoporphyrin IX. J Photochem Photobiol B 45: 131–135

Von rueden DG, Mcbrearty FX, Clements BM, Woratyla S (1993): Photo detection of carcinoma of the colon in a rat model: A pilot study. J Surg Oncol 53: 43–46

Von Tappeiner H, Jesionek A (1903): Therapeutische Versuche mit fluorescierenden Stoffen. Münch Med Wschr 50: 2042–2044

Von Tappeiner H, Jodlbauer A (1904): Über die Wirkung der photodynamischen (fluorescierenden) Stoffe auf Ptotozoen und Enzyme. Arch Klin Med 80: 427–487

Waidlich R, Stepp H, Baumgartner R, Weninger E, Hofstetter A, Kriegmair M (2001): Clinical experience with 5-aminolevulinic acid and photodynamic therapy for refractory superficial bladder cancer. J Urol 165: 1904–1907

Waldow SM, Rocco VL, Kohler IK, Wallk S, Fritts TF (1987): Photodynamic therapy for treatment of malignant cutaneous lesions. Laser Surg Med 7: 451–456

Wang I, Clemente LP, Pratas RM, Cardoso E, Clemente MP, Montan S, Svanberg S, Svanberg K (1999): Fluorescence diagnostics and kinetic studies in the head and neck region utilizing low-dose delta-aminolevulinic acid sensitization. Cancer Lett 135: 11–19

Wang X (1984): Preliminary study of the diagnosis of early-stage oral cancer by the hematoporphyrin derivative-fluorescence technic. Zhonghua Yi Xue Za Zhi 64: 594–597

Warloe T, Peng Q, Heyerdahl J, Moan J, Steen B, Giercksky KE (1995): Photodynamic therapy with 5-aminolevulinic acid induced porphyrins and DMSO/EDTA for basal cell carcinoma. Proc SPIE2371: 226–235

Warloe T, Peng Q, Moan J, Qvist HL, Giericksky KE (1992): Photochemotherapy of multiple basal cell carcinoma with endogenous porphyrins induced by topical application of 5-aminolevulinic acid. In: Photodynamic therapy and biochemical lasers. Spinelli P, Del Fante M, Marchesini R (eds.). Amsterdam, Elsevier, 449–453

Warloe T, Peng Q, Stehen HB, Giericksky KE (1992): Localization of porphyrins in human basal cell carcinoma and normal skin induced by topical application of 5-aminolevulinic acid. In: Photodynamic therapy and biochemical lasers. Spinelli P, Del Fante M, Marchesini R (eds.). Amsterdam, Elsevier, 454–458

Wennberg AM, Gudmundson F, Stenquist B, Ternesten A, Molne L, Rosen A, Larko O (1999): In vivo detection of basal cell carcinoma using imaging spectroscopy. Acta Derm Venereol 79: 54–61

Wennberg AM, Lindholm LE, Alpsten M, Larko O (1996): Treatment of superficial basal cell carcinomas using topically applied delta-aminolaevulinic acid and a filtered xenon lamp. Arch Dermatol Res 88: 561–564

Wennberg AM (2000): Basal cell carcinoma – new aspects of diagnosis and treatment. Acta Derm Venereol (Suppl 209): 5–25

Whitaker M (1994): Fluorescence imaging in living cells. In: Celis JE (ed.). Cell biology. A laboratory handbook, Vol. 2, San Diego New York Boston London Sidney Tokyo Toronto: Academic Press: 37–43

Wilson BC (1986): The physics of photodynamic therapy. Phys Med Biol 31: 327–360

Wilson BD, Mang T, Stoll H, Jones C, Cooper M, Dogherty TJ (1992): Photodynamic therapy for the treatment of basal cell carcinoma. Arch Dermatol 128: 1597–1601

Wilson BD, Mang T (1995): Photodynamic therapy for cutaneous malignancies. Clin Dermatol 13: 91–96

Winkelman JW, Collins GH (1987): Neurotoxicity of tetraphenylporphine sulfonate TPPS4 and its relation to photodynamic therapy. Photochem Photobiol 46: 801–807

Wolf P, Fink-Puches R, Cerroni L, Kerl H (1994): Photodynamic therapy for mycosis fungoides after topical photosensitization with 5-aminolevulinic acid. J Am Acad Dermatol 31: 678–680

Wolf P, Kerl H (1991): Photodynamic therapy on a patient with xeroderma pigmentosum. Lancet 337: 1613–1614

Wolf P, Rieger E, Kerl H (1993): Topical photodynamic therapy with endogenous porphyrins after application of 5-aminolevulinic acid: An alternative treatment modality for solar keratoses, superficial squamous cell carcinomas, and basal cell carcinomas? J Am Acad Dermatol 28: 17–21

Wolf P, Wulf HC, Warloe T, et al: A pivotal study of photodynamic therapy with Metvix cream 160 mg/g in patients with basal cell carcinoma unsuitable to conventional therapy. In press

Wong TW, Sheu HM, Lee JY, Fletcher RJ (2001): Photodynamic therapy for Bowen's disease (squamous cell carcinoma in situ) of the digit. Dermatol Surg 27: 452–456

Woodburn KW, Fan Q, Kessel D, Wright M, Mody TD, Hemmi G, Magda D, Sessler JL, Dow WC, Miller RA, Young SW (1996): Phototherapy of cancer and atheromatous plaque with texaphyrins. J Clin Laser Med Surg 14: 343–348

Young SW, Woodburn KW, Wright M, Mody TD, Fan Q, Sessler JL, Dow WC, Miller RA (1996): Lutetium texaphyrin (PCI-0123): A near-infrared, water-soluble photosensitizer. Photochem Photobiol 63: 892–897

Zaak D, Kriegmair M, Stepp H, Baumgartner R, Oberneder R, Schneede P, Corvin S, Frimberger D, Knuchel R, Hofstetter A (2001): Endoscopic detection of transitional cell carcinoma with 5-aminolevulinic acid: Results of 1012 fluorescence endoscopies. Urology 57: 690–694

Zaidi SIA, Oleinick NL, Zaim MT, Mukhtar H (1993): Apoptosis during photodynamic therapy-induced ablation of RIF-1 tumors in C3H mice: Electron microscopic, hisopathologic and biochemical evidence. Photochem Photobiol 58: 771–776

Zeina B, Greenman J, Purcell WM, Das B (2001): Killing of cutaneous microbial species by photodynamic therapy. Br J Dermatol 144: 274–278

Zenk W, Dietel W, Schleier P, Gunzel S (1999): Visualizing carcinomas of the mouth cavity by stimulating synthesis of fluorescent protoporphyrin IX. Mund Kiefer Gesichtschir 3: 205–209

# SpringerMedicine

## Michael Hertl (ed.)
## Autoimmune Diseases of the Skin

Pathogenesis, Diagnosis, Management

2001. XVII, 373 pages. Numerous figures, partly in colour.
Hardcover **EUR 49,–**
(Recommended retail price) Net-price subject to local VAT.
ISBN 3-211-83598-9

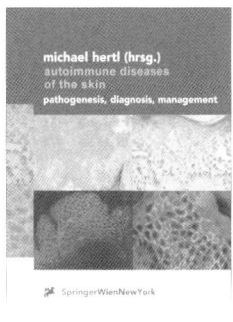

Cutaneous autoimmune diseases of the skin remain an enigma for many clinicians and scientists who are not familiar with these mostly severe and chronic diseases. The book presented provides an overview and the latest information on the broad spectrum of cutaneous autoimmune disorders for clinicians, scientists and practitioners in dermatology, medicine, rheumatology, ENT, pediatrics and ophthalmology.

The book is unique since it presents the state-of-the-art knowledge on pathophysiology, clinical diagnosis and management of these disorders provided by the world experts in the field. The primary intention is to broaden the understanding of the pathophysiology of cutaneous autoimmune disorders and to provide a practical guide to how to identify and handle these conditions.

The book is illustrated with many tables, illustrative figures and clinical color photographs.

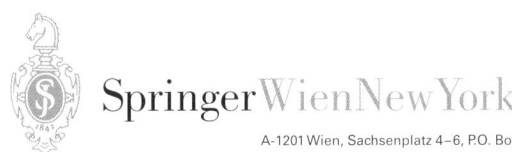

A-1201 Wien, Sachsenplatz 4–6, P.O. Box 89, Fax +43.1.330 24 26, e-mail: books@springer.at, Internet: **www.springer.at**
D-69126 Heidelberg, Haberstraße 7, Fax +49.6221.345-229, e-mail: orders@springer.de
USA, Secaucus, NJ 07096-2485, P.O. Box 2485, Fax +1.201.348-4505, e-mail: orders@springer-ny.com
Eastern Book Service, Japan, Tokyo 113, 3–13, Hongo 3-chome, Bunkyo-ku, Fax +81.3.38 18 08 64, e-mail: orders@svt-ebs.co.jp

**Springer** Medicine

M. R. Nowrousian (ed.)

# Recombinant Human Erythropoietin (rhEPO) in Clinical Oncology

Scientific and Clinical Aspects of Anemia in Cancer

2002. IX, 502 pages. 66 figures, partly in colour.
Hardcover **EUR 98,–**
(Recommended retail price).
Net-price subject to local VAT.
ISBN 3-211-83661-6

Anemia is a frequent complication of cancer and its treatment. A number of clinical studies shows that the impact of anemia is much greater than previously thought. Beyond clinical symptoms, anemia significantly impairs physical and metabolic functions as well as patients' activity, well-being and quality of life. Life expectancy is also affected.

In this book, written by a group of outstanding international experts, the current knowledge on anemia in cancer and its treatment with rhEPO is presented and future developments are discussed. Based on a broad spectrum of topics, the book describes the scientific and clinical aspects of anemia in various fields of oncology and gives diagnostic and therapeutic recommendations on when and how to use rhEPO.

The book will serve as an authentic and essential source of information for radiotherapists, oncologists, hematologists, internists, pediatricians, surgeons, specialists in transfusion or laboratory medicine and pharmacologists.

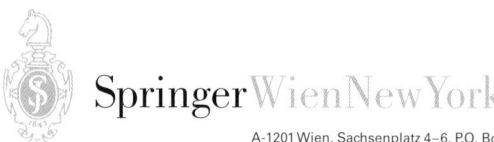

A-1201 Wien, Sachsenplatz 4–6, P.O. Box 89, Fax +43.1.330 24 26, e-mail: books@springer.at, Internet: **www.springer.at**
D-69126 Heidelberg, Haberstraße 7, Fax +49.6221.345-229, e-mail: orders@springer.de
USA, Secaucus, NJ 07096-2485, P.O. Box 2485, Fax +1.201.348-4505, e-mail: orders@springer-ny.com
Eastern Book Service, Japan, Tokyo 113, 3–13, Hongo 3-chome, Bunkyo-ku, Fax +81.3.38 18 08 64, e-mail: orders@svt-ebs.co.jp

# SpringerMedicine

## Nikolai N. Korpan (ed.)

### Atlas of Cryosurgery

2001. XIX, 524 pages.
Over 1200 figures, mostly in colour.
Hardcover **EUR 180,–**
(Recommended retail price)
Net-price subject to local VAT.
ISBN 3-211-83449-4

The "Atlas of Cryosurgery" is the first publication to document the modern era of this discipline. The use of low temperatures to destroy abnormal tissues, the basis of cryosurgery, is now being successfully applied in many branches of medicine, especially in the treatment of different malignancies. This atlas aims at presenting the fundamental aspects of modern cryosurgery and the advantages it offers to cancer patients compared to conventional surgical approaches.

The presentation includes definitions of the most frequently used terms, short descriptions of the historical and scientific background of cryosurgery as well as an outline of cryosurgical equipment and techniques. Given, too, is the whole spectrum of experimental and clinical cryosurgery and the results of cryosurgical treatment of tumors in, for example, the liver, lung, or skin and bone.

Over 1200, mostly coloured illustrations collected from a wide variety of international sources, serve to demonstrate the cryosurgical approach.

## Nikolai N. Korpan (ed.)

### Basics of Cryosurgery

2001. XXII, 325 pages.
Numerous figures and illustrations, mostly in colour.
Hardcover **EUR 130,–**
(Recommended retail price)
Net-price subject to local VAT.
ISBN 3-211-83701-9

"Basics of Cryosurgery" is the first publication specialising in the fundamentals of modern cryosurgery. It is dedicated to surgeons and all doctors throughout the world – especially those working in cryosurgery and cryotechnology, who are helping patients in their fight against malignant tumours.

This book presents what is currently known in modern cryosurgery and is the first on the subject to appear at the start of the third millennium. It aims to contribute to the further development of this branch of medicine, which is set to become indispensable in treating patients. "Basics of Cryosurgery" is a unique contribution – no previous work has compiled in one source all available scientific data on the theoretical, experimental, and clinical investigations that have been undertaken in this field.

The chapters were written by authorities in the field who have not only experienced the triumphs but have learnt from their own and others' failures, and how to avoid these.

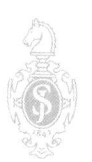

## SpringerWienNewYork

A-1201 Wien, Sachsenplatz 4–6, P.O. Box 89, Fax +43.1.330 24 26, e-mail: books@springer.at, Internet: **www.springer.at**
D-69126 Heidelberg, Haberstraße 7, Fax +49.6221.345-229, e-mail: orders@springer.de
USA, Secaucus, NJ 07096-2485, P.O. Box 2485, Fax +1.201.348-4505, e-mail: orders@springer-ny.com
Eastern Book Service, Japan, Tokyo 113, 3–13, Hongo 3-chome, Bunkyo-ku, Fax +81.3.38 18 08 64, e-mail: orders@svt-ebs.co.jp

## Springer-Verlag
## and the Environment

WE AT SPRINGER-VERLAG FIRMLY BELIEVE THAT AN international science publisher has a special obligation to the environment, and our corporate policies consistently reflect this conviction.

WE ALSO EXPECT OUR BUSINESS PARTNERS – PRINTERS, paper mills, packaging manufacturers, etc. – to commit themselves to using environmentally friendly materials and production processes.

THE PAPER IN THIS BOOK IS MADE FROM NO-CHLORINE pulp and is acid free, in conformance with international standards for paper permanency.